Praise

THE ALZHEIMER'S REVOLUTION

"In an era of continued improvements in healthcare, we have not yet made great gains against the burdens of dementia. *The Alzheimer's Revolution* represents the most current, thorough, and exhaustive review of the available research on this overwhelming topic. Our friends, families, and patients all need to understand how daily decisions can impact their future risk. Although we do not yet have all the answers, this book provides a single source to access what IS known. *The Alzheimer's Revolution* will help us all learn how to beat the odds."

—FARROKH FARROKHI, MD, neurosurgeon

"In *the Alzheimer's Revolution*, Joseph Keon once again demonstrates his ability to bring together a large amount of scientific data in an organized manner that is enticing and easy to understand. He not only lays out a clear picture of the wide range of known and emerging risk factors, he also provides a road map of actionable steps each of us can take to reduce the risk of developing this devastating disease. This book is a must read for anyone concerned about optimizing long-term quality of life for both themselves and their loved ones."

—ANDREW COOK, MD, surgeon and author
of *Stop Endometriosis and Pelvic Pain*

"In the Alzheimer's Revolution, Joseph Keon has taken an incredibly deep dive into understanding and explicating the deeply nuanced and devastating disease of Alzheimer's dementia. Keon has done his homework, and he manages to explain the complicated science behind Alzheimer's in an accessible way that empowers the reader to take back their health with simple and direct changes to their diet and lifestyle. Keon's careful explanations make this debilitating disease less scary and overwhelming and turn it into something we can manage, and potentially prevent. I believe this book will be an important resource for anyone who wants a healthier brain and healthier life."

—BROOKE GOLDNER, MD, author of *Goodbye Lupus* and *Goodbye Autoimmune Disease*

"Joseph Keon's exposition is wonderfully readable and empowering. All of us, from individuals to society, need to increase their understanding of Alzheimer's Disease (AD) and take bold steps to mitigate the contributors to this tragic, degenerative condition. The Alzheimer's Revolution gives us easy access to an enormous amount of scientific research, gentle insights, and steps we can all embrace. As you read through this impressive litany, and if you are as convinced as I am of Keon's insights, skip to Chapter 23 and put your own plan in place to decrease your risk or the risk of someone you love, from AD."

—JOHN W. PEABODY, MD, PhD, FACP, Founder, Qure Healthcare

THE ALZHEIMER'S REVOLUTION

AN EVIDENCE-BASED LIFESTYLE PROGRAM TO BUILD COGNITIVE RESILIENCE AND REDUCE YOUR RISK OF ALZHEIMER'S DISEASE

JOSEPH KEON

Hatherleigh Press is committed to preserving and protecting the natural resources of the earth. Environmentally responsible and sustainable practices are embraced within the company's mission statement.

Visit us at www.hatherleighpress.com and register online for free offers, discounts, special events, and more.

THE ALZHEIMER'S REVOLUTION

Library of Congress Cataloging-in-Publication Data is available.

ISBN: 978-1-57826-943-3

NOTE TO THE READER

Please do not make any adjustments to your diet, medications, or begin any type of exercise program without first consulting your personal physician. If you are experiencing memory problems, please let your healthcare provider know so that you can be properly assessed.

Maintaining order rather than correcting disorder is the ultimate principle of wisdom. To cure a disease after it has manifest is like digging a well when one feels thirsty or forging a weapon when the war has already begun.

—Yellow Emperor of China

All scientific work is incomplete . . . that does not confer upon us a freedom to ignore the knowledge we already have, or to postpone the action that it appears to demand at a given time.

—Sir Austin Bradford Hill

CONTENTS

PART III

EMERGING RISK FACTORS

PART IV

THE ALZHEIMER'S REVOLUTION LIFESTYLE PLAN

FOREWORD

O NE OF THE most exciting breakthroughs in medicine in recent decades is the understanding that we can reduce our risk of developing Alzheimer's disease. According to the best evidence we have, we can cut this risk easily and dramatically.

The findings came from carefully conducted research studies. Researchers tracked the diets of thousands of people over many years to see how foods, exercise, and other factors affect brain health. The Chicago Health and Aging Project, for example, took a close look at what people ate for breakfast, lunch, and dinner. They found that people who ate in certain healthful ways were much less likely to develop Alzheimer's disease. But certain not-so-healthful foods turned out to be strongly linked to the loss of mental function.

One of the culprits identified by the Chicago researchers was something I knew a lot about. As a child growing up in the Midwest, I often woke up in the morning to the smell of bacon emanating from the kitchen. Running downstairs, I found my mother pulling bacon strips out of the fry pan with a fork and setting them onto a paper towel to cool. When the bacon was out of the pan, she carefully poured the bacon grease into a jar to save it. That jar did not go in the refrigerator. My mother just kept it on the shelf. Because as bacon cools, it turns into a waxy solid that does not need to be refrigerated. The next day, she would spoon the grease back into the pan to fry eggs (hold onto your coronary arteries!).

The fact that bacon grease is solid at room temperature is a sign that it is loaded with what doctors call *saturated fat*—that is, "bad fat." It's called "bad" because it raises cholesterol levels. But the Chicago researchers also found a connection with Alzheimer's disease. It turned out that people who generally avoid saturated fat cut their Alzheimer's risk by more than half.

They made other findings. It also paid to avoid trans fats, which are sometimes used in snack foods. And vegetables, fruits, and foods rich in vitamin E, such as nuts and seeds, turned out to be protective.

Other research teams extended these findings. And they found that exercise can help, as well. As years went by, we have gained more and more knowledge on ways to prevent Alzheimer's disease and to maintain brain health lifelong.

As you read through the practical steps in this book, let me encourage you to share them with others. So many people have had a parent or grandparent who succumbed to Alzheimer's disease, and they fear that that fate awaits them as well. With the power you will gain from this book, you can help others to understand that there are steps they can take right now to gain a measure of protection for themselves and their families.

Neal D. Barnard, MD, FACC
Adjunct Faculty, George Washington University School of Medicine
President, Physicians Committee for Responsible Medicine
Washington, DC

INTRODUCTION

As a teen I spent a few summers earning pocket money by working in my grandparents' yard in Mattoon, Illinois. Using a putty knife, I would uproot the thick moss that grew between bricks in the footpath bordering my Grandmother Mollie's flower garden. It was often hot and remarkably humid, and except for the cicada bugs that serenaded me from the nearby white oak trees, quiet. It was mindless work that allowed me to sink deep into thought and, ultimately, earn enough money to buy my favorite NFL player's football jersey or a coveted pair of athletic shoes. Occasionally, Mollie would join me in the yard. Working from a stoop or on her knees, and stopping occasionally to sip hot coffee, she could spend hours deadheading roses, delphiniums, and oleander, reducing the height of heather, and replenishing other flowers from which she composed indoor bouquets. Sometimes I'd stop to admire her dedication to her garden. Despite the oppressive heat and humidity, she found pleasure in every opportunity to tend to her plants.

In addition to her passion for floriculture, the grandmother I had grown up with was a prolific reader and founding member of the local literary club, a Cub Scout leader, and she taught Sunday school and volunteered at the local library for years. She relished long walks with her two English Setters alongside the acres of corn that grew adjacent to her home. She was fond of baking confections and treated her Sunday school students to homemade fudge each week. A world traveler and family historian, she captivated the attention of her 13 grandchildren with stories of our family's past.

All that changed when she was 84 and stricken with Alzheimer's. Her once nimble mind that enabled her to recount the details of decades-past travel, a special relationship from her youth, or to faithfully recall the birthday of each of her grandchildren so she could send them a card in the mail, was now failing her on even the most momentous occasions. Just hours after attending the funeral of her beloved husband, Richard, she asked whether the ceremony had taken place yet. As the vibrant colors from her forgotten garden dissipated and the formerly generative soil contracted into desiccated beds of weeds, Mollie's interests narrowed to just a few things that took on a distorted significance.

One activity that provided Mollie reassurance was a visit to the bank. She told her caregivers and my uncle, who lived next door, that she felt better if she had some pocket money. What began as a distraction that allowed for a short excursion to town evolved into an obsession. Enlisted as an accomplice by my Uncle Dick, the bank manager had been told the reason behind her increasingly frequent visits to the bank, and always greeted Mollie with warmth and feigned surprise. These outings became essential to easing her anxiety and buoying her spirit, if only temporarily. Otherwise, her life had been reduced to hours of anxious contemplation, watching news broadcasts, and anticipating another trip to town.

Five years ago, I found it no easier to witness another neurological disease that struck my father. Because he was experiencing progressive physical and cognitive changes, we took him to the Memory and Aging Center at the University of California San Francisco. After completing a battery of tests, he received a diagnosis of Parkinson's disease with Lewy body dementia (LBD). Neither my siblings nor I could imagine just how rapidly he would deteriorate and how profound the consequences of his decline would be.

Within six months of his diagnosis, my father's spatial perception had diminished such that it was no longer safe for him to drive a car. Almost worse, his executive function was compromised to the point that his neurologist advised he no longer make financial decisions. Up until two years before his diagnosis my father had been a shrewd businessman who ran an international manufacturing firm, enjoyed speaking French, and was studying Mandarin. He was a world traveler, a real estate investor, and a trader in stocks from companies all over the world. He delighted in performing complex mathematical computations without pen and paper and retained an encyclopedic recall of movies and the names of the actors and actresses who performed in them. As his disease progressed, his recollection of his former life, including Ellie, his beloved partner of 20 years, rapidly dissolved. He could no longer read the time on a clock, make change for a dollar, or easily construct a thoughtful sentence. Rigidity settled into his legs, arms, face, and mind.

The man who once held court in our family, entertained with his relentless sense of humor, traveled the world to take in foreign cultures, and dazzled people with his prodigious mental capacity had become mentally and physically inept, while suffering bouts of paranoia. Save for occasional sparks of humor, he retained few of the personality traits of his former self.

Although Parkinson's is a movement disorder, people with LBD share many symptoms seen in AD including problems with memory and reasoning. Cognitively, he became very similar to someone who suffers from Alzheimer's.

As his condition worsened, my dad at age 82 needed to be bathed, diapered, dressed, fed, and constantly reassured. The independent and exciting life he had formerly lived had been reduced to residence in a memory care facility apartment, where he preferred to sit in front of a TV and indulge in movie-watching marathons, unaware of the outside world. After a team was assembled that consisted of a neurologist, psychologist, physical therapist, legal guardian, attorney, and caregivers, the task of unwinding his highly complex life began. Friends, family, and business associates needed to be informed of his state, complex business holdings needed to be sorted out and dismantled, and real estate and other property needed to be liquidated. We were faced with the looming costs of long-term care. Through a lengthy process of trial and error, we finally felt that we had found the right caregivers and then the right living environment.

While my siblings and I were still struggling to accept our father's prognosis, more impossible news came. One of my five sisters, a physician just 55 years old, called to tell me that she had received a diagnosis of Parkinson's disease. I recall thinking that this just couldn't happen. My father and now my sister? My initial reaction was to tell myself there must have been a mistake in the diagnosis and if my sister consulted the right doctor, she'd find that to be so. While all neurological disease is cruel, her diagnosis seemed particularly so. She wasn't retired and reflecting on a life well lived. She was at the height of her career as a radiologist. Ever since the beginning of her work in medicine, as an oncology nurse, she had devoted her life to caring for and helping to guard the health of others. Her three daughters were embarking on academic and professional careers of their own and her husband had recently found success with his own business. Now everything needed to be reassessed.

I began to reflect on all that had happened in so short a time. What was the cause of my father's condition? My sister's? Were they in any way related to what had triggered my grandmother's Alzheimer's? Was there a genetic component? Or had we all unknowingly been exposed to something at some point in our lives that placed us at risk? What did this portend for my mother, for my other four siblings, and for me? I wondered if our genetic heritage had determined our fate, and if there was anything we could do to reduce our chances of succumbing to a neurological disease.

I decided to take a cursory look at a few public health websites to learn more of the conventional wisdom about neurologic disease, but the information I came across was limited, vague, and generally unhopeful. I also noted the focus on drug research and genetics. The picture presented could be summed up in just a few sentences: 1) we don't know what causes most neurological disease; 2) genetics play a big role; 3) there's little anyone can do to reduce their risk.

As an investigative medical writer, I had researched and written about heart disease, hypertension, breast and prostate cancer, and osteoporosis. I had discovered that the conventional wisdom about these conditions was misconceived and greatly disempowering to individuals who wished to reduce their risk. There was so much more to know about these diseases than was shared on the websites of nonprofits and public health organizations or in pamphlets at doctors' offices. I found relevant material buried in scientific studies—some of it decades old—and yet absent from mainstream discussions. For example, there were numerous studies, including some from Harvard University, which showed a strong association between consumption of cow's milk and the risk of developing metastatic prostate cancer.[1] Why was this not common knowledge among men so that they could make informed choices? Based upon my past experiences of investigating disease, I couldn't help but wonder if I might find similar "hidden" information about neurological disease.

Were there factors that the medical community had not yet embraced? Was there anything that had been published in the scientific literature but had not received the attention it warranted in mainstream literature? Were there practical steps my family and I could take to lower our own risk and possibly improve or slow the progression of my father's and sister's conditions? These and other questions inspired me to begin looking beyond conventional wisdom at what the body of scientific research might reveal.

What I uncovered was intriguing! Scientific studies had indeed found lifestyle and other factors that could compromise cognition and heighten risk of dementia. As I became familiar with the lexicon of neurological disease, I found myself increasingly attuned to the cognitive health of others. When somebody failed to recall a name or date or repeated themselves in a casual conversation, I wondered if that might be a sign of mild cognitive impairment (MCI), a possible precursor to dementia. Then a day came when I was in conversation with another of my five sisters who was 54 at the time.

We were reminiscing with a group of friends about events from our childhood. She recounted something we had spoken about only ten minutes before, but as though it had just come to her mind. At that moment, although I didn't say anything, I became hypervigilant, listening acutely to what she said next. Over the next few weeks, I began to see a pattern in which she repeated herself. I also noted that although she seemed to initially recall my girlfriend's name after I introduced them, she referred to her as "your sweetheart" thereafter. A few months later, my sister became disoriented while driving with another sister. Rather than enter the freeway in the northbound direction to reach her house, she entered the roadway heading southbound, diverting her from a course she had followed for 18 years.

After discussing with her some of the things I had noticed, I encouraged her to make an appointment to be assessed, as a precaution, with a full neuropsychiatric evaluation and imaging studies at the nearby University of California San Francisco Memory and Aging Clinic. I reassured her that memory problems can sometimes be brought about by medications, such as sleeping aids or pain pills, or just bouts of insomnia, and that it was important to find out what was going on. She acknowledged that she was aware of some of her memory lapses and agreed to make an appointment. When the day came for the neurologist to share his findings, my sister invited me to be on the phone, thinking I could be helpful in asking questions she might not think to ask. At the designated time, my sister, her partner, my mother, and I all joined a conference call initiated by her neurologist.

He wasted no time getting to the point. "I wish that I had more encouraging news to share with you today," he began, "but the MRI we performed confirmed what the interview and other tests made us suspect. The region of your brain responsible for memory and emotion, the hippocampus, and the parietal lobe, show volume loss, and we don't see this in healthy women as young as you. Although we can perform other tests, such as a PET scan and a spinal tap to corroborate these findings, we believe that you are in the first stages of early-onset Alzheimer's disease."

For a moment, none of us spoke. I was frozen by my own shock and devastation hearing my sister was diagnosed with early-onset Alzheimer's. The neurologist pierced the silence to share a few perfunctory details about follow-up protocols and to ask if there were any questions he could answer about the diagnosis. There were questions about what my sister could expect in terms of a timeline, and what, if anything, one should do after such a diagnosis. Was there an action plan? A defensive protocol to follow to slow the advancement of the disease or reduce its symptoms? In short, the answer was no. The neurologist seemed to have nothing further to offer, save for the possibility of enrolling in a future drug trial and joining a support group.

After hanging up the phone, I sat at my desk feeling the weight of the news. The role of genes crept back into my mind. Two siblings, a parent, and a grandparent had now all been touched by neurological disease. I was frightened and couldn't help but wonder what would come next.

It took some days before I began to regain my emotional footing. I thought about genes and my family again. Whatever role they might be playing in our risk, we could do nothing to change them. We couldn't excise the ones we didn't want, but could we take actions that might influence how our genes are expressed? Were there things that my sisters could do to slow the rate at which their disease progressed? Hoping to learn more about our situation, I began looking at studies about the role of genetics, and in particular, studies of identical twins. If two people share the exact same genes and one developed a neurological disease, is it not a certainty the other will do so as well? The assumption is logical, but the science shows otherwise.

What I discovered is substantial evidence that Alzheimer's and other neurological diseases are *not* primarily genetic, that they have over-lapping risk factors, and that there are many practical steps—lifestyle strategies—anyone can adopt that studies show could lower our risk, and even slow progression when a diagnosis has already been made.

I went to sleep thinking about neurons and synapses and woke up reviewing daily actions I would take to thwart processes like oxidative stress, inflammation, and brain shrinkage. At the end of the day, I would ask myself if I had done everything I could in my waking hours to promote neurogenesis, the process whereby the brain produces new neurons, and build cognitive reserve in my own brain. That virtually nobody close to me had the slightest idea what these terms meant didn't bother me. I shared my findings with friends and family, whether they listened to me or not, while I also developed an entirely new awareness of choices that all of us were making. Mainly, it felt good to know I was beginning to exercise influence over my own cognitive health.

After a year of research, I became convinced that, as with other major chronic diseases, the portrayal of Alzheimer's reaching the public was incomplete and disempowering. The evidence indicating that we can take control of our Alzheimer's risk is so compelling, and the global threat of this disease so great, I knew I had to devote myself to making this information more broadly known.

In 1902 Thomas Edison was asked about the future of medicine and prophesized, "The doctor of the future will give no medicine but will interest his patient in the care of the human frame, in diet and in the cause and prevention of disease."[2] We are living at a time of increasingly rapid advances in healthcare technology. Our attention has been captured by such innovations as the artificial heart, prosthetics, synthetic blood, a growing array of vaccines, robotic surgery, greater precision in diagnostics, and blockbuster drugs. While these innovations have been lifesaving and life-changing, it's understandable that they may also cause us to forget that as individuals we have much greater influence over our health than we might believe. Preventive actions we can take to safeguard our health are relatively simple to perform. The day-to-day choices that each of us makes have a profound effect on whether we preserve our health or allow it to deteriorate.

While we're more than 100 years beyond Edison's prediction, and a gap exists between what he envisioned and our current reality, the research-backed findings and guidance in the pages that follow are consistent with Edison's belief. They affirm that we will be much better off if, rather than cede responsibility for our health to others, we take that responsibility into our own hands. In short, the conventional perception of Alzheimer's is dated, ill-informed, and consequently demoralizing. Understandably, in the absence of any useful information about prevention, it's no surprise that many people have lost hope and are terrified by this disease.

Since the quest that began in 1984 for a miracle drug that will eradicate Alzheimer's disease has been so far unsuccessful, I propose that we focus our resources on something better than the so-far elusive cure: prevention. Because prevention is always better than cure.

We have gained an understanding of many of the pathological changes that occur in Alzheimer's disease. We know they develop years before symptoms are apparent. We also know some of the causes of those changes. Therefore, it's plausible that if we stop these changes from happening in the first place, we may be able to disrupt the processes that lead to the disease.

The lifestyle plan that I propose is simple, practical, and, as I hope I will be able to convince you, logical.

Because they are based upon large, long-term studies showing very encouraging outcomes, I am convinced that the preventive measures outlined in this book will give you and your family the best chance of preventing Alzheimer's and other degenerative diseases. For example, while the focus of this book is on Alzheimer's, some risk factors for the condition are shared by Parkinson's disease (PD) and amyotrophic lateral sclerosis (ALS), commonly known as Lou Gehrig's disease.[3]

One need not be formally diagnosed with neurological disease to suffer from cognitive decline. So, while the steps that I outline in this book are aimed at preventing a diagnosis, they also reflect the best insight available today for keeping one's mind as sharp and nimble as possible, and possibly even arresting cognitive decline that has begun. Moreover, the same measures that address the risk for Alzheimer's will also reduce your risk for the number-one killer in the United States: heart disease. Conveniently, they will also give you the means to sharply decrease risk for stroke, hypertension, diabetes, obesity, osteoporosis, depression, and even some forms of cancer. Thus, what you hold in your hands is truly a wellness book.

Together, I hope we can revolutionize how we think about protecting cognitive health and working to prevent Alzheimer's. Please join me in embracing the Alzheimer's Revolution Lifestyle.

PART I

UNDERSTANDING ALZHEIMER'S DISEASE

1

INCURABLE BUT LARGELY PREVENTABLE

THE DISEASES THAT have touched my own family are becoming startlingly more common. A study found that between 1989 and 2010, the death rate from neurological diseases—including Alzheimer's disease (AD), Parkinson's disease (PD), and motor neuron disease (MND)—in men aged 55 to 74 increased 82 percent. In women of the same age, the rate jumped 48 percent.[4] Today in the USA and the UK, more elderly women are dying from neurological diseases than from cancer. In fact, the rates of death from neurological disease have risen all over the world, with the highest increases occurring in developed nations.[5]

Another tragic fact is that neurological diseases are occurring more frequently in younger victims.[6] Two decades ago, it was highly rare for people in their forties to be told they have dementia. Not anymore. The U.K., with the third-greatest increase worldwide, has seen so many younger people affected by dementia that a nonprofit charity, The Young Dementia Network, formed.[7]

Drawing upon data from the 48 million customers they insure, in 2020 the Blue Cross Blue Shield Association (BCBSA) reported that in the brief time between 2013 and 2017 diagnoses of early-onset dementia and Alzheimer's increased 143 percent among those aged 55 to 64 and 311 percent in those aged 45 to 54. Even more shocking, it increased 373 percent among patients aged 30 to 44.[8] "The increase in early-onset dementia and Alzheimer's diagnoses among a generation who typically wouldn't expect to encounter these conditions for several decades is concerning," noted Dr. Vincent Nelson, vice president of medical affairs at BCBSA.

Some of the rise in incidence overall can be attributed to the *Gompertzian* effect, which says that degenerative disease increases in populations as lifespan increases. But because of the relatively rapid rise, as well as the increasingly early age of diagnosis, it's clear that environmental factors are at play here. And while these findings are sufficiently disturbing, it's likely they fail to capture the entire picture. Because deaths from dementia tend to be underreported, the situation may be even worse.[9]

Families with a member stricken with neurological disease pay a great price emotionally and often financially. But the dramatic rise in diseases of the brain also brings great costs to society, because it threatens to overwhelm the stability of healthcare systems in the USA and other Western countries.

As far back as the 2009 International Conference on Alzheimer's disease in Vienna, Dr. William Thies, chief medical and scientific officer for the Alzheimer's Association, was already warning that the Alzheimer's epidemic would "devastate the world's economies and healthcare systems, and far too many families."[10] This was echoed by Dr. Richard J. Hodes, director of the National Institute on Aging, who said, "I don't know of any other disease predicting such a huge increase, it's going to swamp the system."[11]

According to the Alzheimer's Association, $355 billion is spent annually treating Alzheimer's in the USA alone. That's more money than is spent on heart disease and cancer combined, making it the most expensive disease we face.[12] Presently, one of every five Medicaid and Medicare dollars is devoted to Alzheimer's care. In another decade it's expected to be one of every three dollars.[13] Yet this does not even account for the 11 million hours of unpaid care provided to patients by family members. The Alzheimer's Association values that contribution at an additional $257 billion.[14] Medicaid will cover an average of just $8,700 per year for low-income patients 65 and older; Medicare covers an even smaller portion.[15] Currently, the lifetime cost for providing care to a person with Alzheimer's is estimated at $357,000.

Public health officials who monitor disease predict that within the next 30 years, Alzheimer's will strike nearly one in two Americans aged 85 and older. By then, there will be one million new cases annually, and health-care costs for the disease will have doubled, making the financial burden to the nation simply unmanageable.[16] By 2050 Alzheimer's is expected to be a trillion-dollar disease that may drive Medicare into bankruptcy.[17]

It's not just the financial challenges we face. The medical system is simply not prepared to contend with the inevitable surge in new cases. In a 2020 report, half of primary physicians surveyed said they expect a rise in cases of dementia and feel the medical system is not prepared to contend with the increased demand the disease will bring. More than half said that there are already not enough dementia specialists in their area to handle patient demand. Nearly one-third reported they are "never" or only "sometimes" comfortable answering their patients' questions about dementia. Twenty-two percent said they had no residency training in dementia diagnostics and care. The 78 percent who did have such training said that it was "very little."[18] This is tragic, because in large part diagnosing and caring for patients with dementia is currently managed by primary care physicians.

Japan is offering a preview of what's to come as it already struggles with what some have called a "dementia crisis." Japan's health ministry projects that by 2025 the disease will strike one in five Japanese citizens aged 65 and older.[19] The cases are already overwhelming both the medical system and, due to a shortage of professional caregivers, families as well. The *Japan Times* reported that 100,000 people are quitting their jobs each year in order to provide care to a dementia-stricken family member. Yet in 2019 a record 17,479 Japanese with dementia went missing after wandering from their homes, presumably because they were not receiving adequate care.

Presently, it takes 14 years and between $800 million and $1 billion to develop a new drug. If an effective drug treatment were to make it to market, an estimated $10 billion in annual sales would be generated for the pharmaceutical company that created the drug. But the lure has not worked. Since 2000, the pharmaceutical industry has tested 245 Alzheimer's drugs, which have resulted in a 99 percent failure rate.[20]

The five drugs that received approval prior to 2021 do no more than mildly alleviate symptoms for several months, while doing nothing to treat the underlying cause of the disease.[21] "What's available now," says Dr. Reisa Sperling, a leading Alzheimer's researcher at Harvard Medical School, "are symptomatic treatments that simply give a patient maybe six to twelve months of doing just a little bit better."

In early 2018, the world's third-largest pharmaceutical company, Pfizer, announced it was dropping Alzheimer's drug research altogether. After 99 trials of 24 Alzheimer's drugs brought only failure, Pfizer threw in the towel. Dr. Mikael Dolsten, president of Pfizer Worldwide Research, said, "We're simply not making the progress necessary to translate into truly transformational therapies for patients." [22] In 2021, Biogen's controversial drug, Aducanumab, marketed as Aduhelm, was green-lighted by the FDA even after 10 of 11 members of an FDA advisory board voted against its approval. This was the first new drug for Alzheimer's patients in 18 years. So, when news broke that the drug would soon be in the distribution pipeline, Alzheimer's patient advocacy groups were thrilled. This drug is not a cure. The drug maker, Biogen, suggested Aduhelm could slow cognitive decline in some patients for about four months over 18 months of treatment, a benefit that may be tough to justify when the drug's side effects are considered. It's been reported that 40 percent of those who have taken the drug have experienced swelling or bleeding in the brain.[23] The drug is administered by a monthly infusion at what was originally a cost of $56,000 per year. After weak sales and a storm of criticism directed toward the FDA for its approval of the drug, and some scientists petitioning the FDA to remove it from the market, Biogen slashed the price to $28,200.[24]

ABSENT A CURE, THERE EXISTS ONE COMPELLING PATH TO FOLLOW: PREVENTION.

Our approach to illness has historically been preferentially focused on treatment over prevention. The tendency is to permit disease to take up residence in the body and then try to manage it with drugs and surgery, interventions that carry with them the risk of serious side effects. This is a wildly expensive way to treat our health problems and assures that the USA will continue to have the costliest healthcare in the world with some of the poorest outcomes for that care.[25] Moreover, when it comes to Alzheimer's disease, this approach is useless.

Dr. Bruce Miller, director of the Memory and Aging Center at the University of California San Francisco, shifts the focus away from treatment, saying, "We know now that prevention of this disease is feasible and something our field will conquer."[26] There are several leaders in the field whose research is illuminating just what may be possible when one is willing to adopt powerful lifestyle changes.

Kristine Yaffe, M.D., and Deborah E. Barnes, Ph.D., also at the University of California San Francisco, estimate that up to 50 percent of the Alzheimer's cases worldwide can be accounted for by just seven risk factors: diabetes, hypertension, obesity, smoking, depression, cognitive inactivity, and physical inactivity.[27] Doctors Yaffe and Barnes estimate that even a small reduction in these risk factors could cut the incidence of Alzheimer's in the U.S. by up to 492,000 cases, and worldwide by up to 10 million cases.[28] Such estimates tempt one to imagine what could be achieved were we to address these risk factors much more aggressively.

Dr. Klodian Dhana and colleagues at the Rush University Medical Center in Chicago reported findings from a ten-year study tracking the lifestyle habits of 2,765 participants, including physical activity, diet, smoking, alcohol consumption, and cognitive activities. The researchers found a dose-response relationship between how many healthful habits were adopted and the level of AD risk a participant faced. The adoption of two or three healthy lifestyle choices was good for a 39 percent reduction in risk of developing AD compared to subjects who embraced one or none of the healthy strategies. Four or five healthy choices reduced risk by 60 percent. Regardless of how many protective lifestyle changes individuals adopted, each additional change lowered the risk of developing Alzheimer's another 22 percent. These results were consistent regardless of the race or gender of participants.[29]

A study led by neurologist Dr. Richard Isaacson from New York-Presbyterian/Weil Cornell Medical Center affirms that lifestyle changes can have a potent effect in not only arresting cognitive decline but boosting memory and brain function as well.[30] All subjects in the study had a history of Alzheimer's in their families and all showed signs of cognitive deterioration. Each was given a list of 20 lifestyle changes to make, the most important of which were to address their diet and increase the amount of exercise they were getting. Upon reevaluation 18 months later, those who adopted the greatest number of changes not only halted their cognitive decline but saw significant improvement in thinking skills and memory. This study affirms again that there is no silver bullet—addressing multiple factors together yields the best outcomes.

Dr. Miia Kivipelto, a professor, senior geriatrician, and director of research, development, education and innovation at the Karolinska University Hospital in Stockholm, is another trailblazer in research on protecting cognitive health through lifestyle. Her landmark FINGER (Finnish Geriatric Intervention Study to Prevent Cognitive Impairment and Disability) study is having a worldwide impact.

FINGER was the first large-scale, long-term randomized controlled study to determine if changes in multiple lifestyle factors could prevent cognitive decline and disability in elderly subjects at increased risk for dementia. Initially, 1,260 individuals aged 60 to 77 were recruited to participate, with half assigned to receive lifestyle interventions related to diet, exercise, cognitive and social stimulation, and management of vascular and metabolic risk factors, while the other served as a control group and were given general health advice. Based upon initial test scores, all participants were considered at risk for developing dementia. After two years, cognitive test scores for the intervention group were 25 percent higher overall, with complex memory tasks improved by 40 percent and executive function and processing speed up 83 percent and 150 percent respectively. Don't worry about the terminology—what's important is that brain function improved significantly in those who adopted the lifestyle changes. Meanwhile the control group that did not make changes were 30 percent more likely to experience cognitive *decline* in that same period.

The outcomes of this study were so encouraging they spawned the Worldwide FINGER Network, a series of ongoing trials in various countries modeled after the original study.[31] It's expected that the study will be replicated in 25 countries including the USA, China, Spain, Germany, and Japan. Dr. Kivipelto believes that up to 50 percent of Alzheimer's cases are driven by risk factors we can influence.[32]

In Washington, D.C., Harvard-trained neurologist Majid Fatuhi, M.D., is having remarkable success addressing early stages of cognitive decline. Participants are enrolled in a lifestyle modification program that includes exercise, dietary intervention, stress reduction, and strategies to ensure quality sleep. Eighty-four percent of those enrolled saw significant improvements in three areas of cognitive function, and 17 of the participants experienced growth (as shown by MRI) in their hippocampus equivalent to a one- to two-year reversal in cognitive decline.

As this book was going to press yet another encouraging study was published. Drawing on data from the Chinese Longitudinal Healthy Longevity Survey, which included over 6,000 adults aged 80 and older, a research team from Duke Kunshan University in China found once again that certain lifestyle choices provide significant protection. The greater the number of healthful choices individuals adopted the greater their protection. Those who follow a moderately healthy lifestyle were 28 percent less likely to develop dementia. Those who adopted the greatest number of healthful choices were 55 percent less likely to develop dementia.[33]

These findings are so encouraging, and yet I am convinced that we have reason to be even more optimistic about how much we may be able to reduce risk for Alzheimer's by adopting an even wider spectrum of lifestyle changes that will provide powerful protection. No study has yet addressed all the risk factors addressed in the Alzheimer's Revolution, while all have employed only moderate dietary improvements. But before I get to my recommendations for protecting our brains, let's look at how the brain works.

2

UNDERSTANDING ALZHEIMER'S BY UNDERSTANDING THE BRAIN

I N 1906, GERMAN psychiatrist and neuroanatomist Alois Alzheimer made an unsettling discovery. Under Dr. Alzheimer's care was Auguste Deter, a 51-year-old woman who was suffering from memory disturbances, confusion, insomnia, paranoia, crying, and aggressiveness.[34] After five years of these travails, she died and became the first known case of a disease later named after her doctor. At the 37th Meeting of South-West German Psychiatrists in Tubingen, Alzheimer gave a presentation about Deter's case, describing it as "a peculiar severe disease process of the cerebral cortex."[35]

"Peculiar" suggests that what the doctor found in Ms. Deter's brain, including amyloid plaques and neurofibrillary tangles—about which more later—was previously unknown to him. In contrast, today a person is diagnosed with this disease roughly every minute.

We have learned a lot about the brain since Dr. Alzheimer performed an autopsy on Ms. Deter. In just the past 20 years, 100,000 or so scientific papers on Alzheimer's disease have been published. This research has yielded remarkable discoveries about the brain's resiliency and its vulnerabilities, how it grows and adapts in response to its environment, and how it ultimately may succumb to pathological changes. We have gained new insights about what we can do to best support brain health and protect cognitive function throughout our lives.

Not too long ago, the brain was believed to be fixed in its size and structure. We now see the brain through the lens of *plasticity*, which describes the brain's lifelong ability to change its structure and its functions as a result of learning, life experiences, environmental factors, and injury.[36] It does this through the reorganization of existing pathways, the formation of new pathways, and adding and subtracting synapses (the junctions between brain cells). If one part of the brain is injured, the brain can remap or rewire itself, forming new connections that work around an injured zone and reassign tasks to another part of the brain. In other words, our brains are always changing and adapting. This is a wonderful characteristic because it gives us the opportunity to affect the brain's very structure and functionality by the choices we make.

In 1963 scientists first proposed that the brain, specifically the hippo-campus region, was able to produce new neurons in adulthood, a process called *adult hippocampal neurogenesis*. Many in the scientific community rejected the notion. At the time, it was firmly believed the brain stopped making new neurons after childhood. Still, the possibility remained enticing since the hippocampus is severely compromised in Alzheimer's disease.[37] This region of the brain, named for the Greek word that means seahorse because of a vague resemblance, is critical to the formation, organization, and storage of new memories, and it's highly susceptible to damage in Alzheimer's disease. If we could somehow promote the birth of new neurons in this region, what would that mean to our effort to protect memory function?

Adult hippocampal neurogenesis has been conclusively demonstrated in many mammalian species including non-human primates,[38] and some scientists have asserted that, depending on our lifestyle, humans may produce as many as 700 new hippocampal neurons a day.[39] Yet postmortem studies on the human brain have been fraught with tech-nological and methodological challenges that have contributed to the controversy. Some show evidence for neurogenesis, while others have not. So, the topic has been hotly debated for decades and numerous studies have been published that claim to either prove or refute the phenomena,[40] including one in support of it that was published as this book went to press.[41] No doubt, due to the intense interest in the topic, more studies will be forthcoming, and hopefully we will soon have the imaging technology that enables us to confirm neurogenesis in living adults. Until then, as we will later see, the strategies believed to promote neurogenesis in humans also happen to lower the risk of AD.

The brain is an energy hog, using more energy (20 percent of oxygen and blood) than any other organ in your body. Its 100 billion neurons, each about one-hundredth the size of the period at the end of this sentence, together have a memory capacity equivalent to one million gigabytes.[42] A personal computer with that much memory could store 200 million songs or 500 million eBooks. What's fascinating, and very different from how computers function, is how neurons work together.

Neurons need to communicate with one another. This communication begins with an electrical signal sent down the axon (nerve fiber) of the neuron. Think of the axon as a hand outstretched to reach other hands. The hand is super charged to find other hands; that is, the axon produces a signal carried by a chemical messenger called a neurotransmitter across the synapse (the junction between brain cells). That signal contacts the neighboring neuron and attaches itself to a receiver. Axon meets axon, all but ad infinitum. A single neuron may be connected to thousands of other neurons by many thousands of synapses. The brain has 100 trillion of these synapses, connections that enable neurons to form networks that work together.[43] These networks produce and hold our thoughts, feelings, and memories. They enable learning and remembering, processing and expression of emotions, planning, and the ordering of movement. In short, these connections—the synapses—are essential to our networks of neurons working correctly.

The relative strength of synapse connections determines the volume of the conversation between two neurons. They may, as it were, talk in a whisper or a shout. A synapse can change in shape and strength in response to our experiences and stimulation.

As with other parts of our brains and our bodies, the synapse connections are vulnerable to a lack of stimulation as well as a variety of assaults, including poor nutrition, alcohol, pesticides, heavy metals, stress, and physical trauma.

When the brain gets assaulted, synapses can deteriorate and be lost. In the initial stages of Alzheimer's disease, the loss of synapses precedes the loss of neurons.[44] As synapses are lost, they no longer wire together the networks of neurons, which then become disintegrated. When neurons that worked together efficiently no longer do so, brain function suffers. That means our memory, our basic cognitive ability, and even our personality suffers.

When it comes to synapse health, the adage "use it or lose it" applies. Aside from minimizing assaults, to retain synapse health we must stimulate our brains. Specifically, the more the brain is stimulated through learning and new experiences, the stronger the signal between neurons via synapses becomes. And with greater repetition comes better signal transmission.

On the "lose it" end of the spectrum, synaptic connections can be lost with reduced stimulation. This loss factor leads to increasingly impaired cognitive function and changes in mood. This is why a person you have known your whole life may come to seem like a stranger when they are afflicted with Alzheimer's.

But "losing it" goes beyond just synaptic connections being lost. An unconnected neuron's ability to metabolize energy, communicate, and perform self-repair is also disrupted, and eventually it will die. Subsequently, as with muscle and bone, the brain will lose actual volume and will atrophy, or shrink, over time.[45]

These changes, including what Dr. Alzheimer described, are now known under the umbrella term of *dementia*. Dementia describes a syndrome, a broad range of symptoms that include a decline in memory, reasoning, judgment, spatial perception, and language that eventually interferes with a person's ability to perform simple daily tasks, known as Activities of Daily Living (ADL). ADL includes things we all take for granted: eating, bathing, walking, dressing, toileting, and continence.

For a diagnosis of dementia, two or more of these functions must be significantly impaired. By itself, a decline in memory isn't necessarily a sign of dementia and can be brought about by many factors, including common medications, stress, depression, alcohol use, nutritional deficiencies, and sleep deprivation. Anyone over 40 knows what it's like to experience sporadic lapses of memory or to feel organizationally challenged at times, yet these episodes are not necessarily a sign of impending dementia.

FOUR CAUSES OF REVERSIBLE DEMENTIA

In 2016, singer Kris Kristofferson revealed that after years of believing doctors who told him he had Alzheimer's disease, he sought another opinion from a curious doctor who decided to test the singer for Lyme disease. To his great relief, Kristofferson learned that he had been misdiagnosed and did not have Alzheimer's. He was suffering from cognitive impairment brought about by Lyme disease, a condition caused by spirochete bacteria that are transmitted by a bite from an infected deer tick.[46] With a proper diagnosis, he was successfully treated, and his impairment was resolved.

In up to four percent of long-term Lyme cases, the bacteria enter the nervous system and result in a dementia-like syndrome known as Lyme neuroborreliosis (LNB). The condition is treated with intravenous antibiotics, such as ceftriaxone, that cross the blood–brain barrier and eradicate the bacteria.

Pseudodementia, which is also frequently reversible, is the name given to cognitive impairments that develop as a result of one's psychiatric health status and not because of neurodegenerative events in the central nervous system. This type of impairment is most frequently associated with protracted bouts of depression. It manifests like authentic dementia in that an individual loses executive function and memory; however, in pseudodementia, individuals typically have trouble recalling both recent events and events from the past, whereas in authentic dementia, at least in the early stages, memory loss is chiefly relegated to recent memories. Pseudodementia is treated with both antidepressant medications and talk therapy.

Vitamin B12 deficiency is another cause of reversible cognitive impairment. Conditions such as gastritis, Crohn's disease, and Celiac disease can significantly impede absorption of vitamin B12. Surveys suggest about 16 percent of 20 to 59-year-olds and 20 percent of those aged 60 or older are deficient. As we will see later, vitamin B12 sufficiency is critical to cognitive health and a supplement is strongly advised.

The use of corticosteroids, such as prednisone, which are prescribed for a wide number of ailments, including allergies, arthritis, immune disorders, and skin diseases, can cause some individuals to suffer memory loss. While most cases are resolved within a couple of months after the medications are stopped, for some, the memory impairment persists.[47] Elderly users of steroids seem to be more susceptible. In Chapter 19 we will explore other common prescription medications that may heighten the risk for not just temporary impaired memory, but Alzheimer's disease as well.

DEMENTIA IS A PROGRESSIVE DISEASE

People used to think dementia could show up in someone suddenly, as if a switch were flipped. We now have evidence that dementia is progressive. Gradual cognitive decline is the result of damage to neurons and the loss of connections between them (synapse loss).[48] In fact, development of dementia may take place over a couple of decades, until the pathological changes occurring in the brain finally reach a point critical enough that symptoms become apparent. When we first diagnose Alzheimer's, it is usually relatively late in the disease process.

The very first symptoms are referred to as mild cognitive impairment (MCI). MCI is a condition in which you or your family and friends become aware that your memory is consistently compromised. You might have a creeping sense that your forgetfulness is worsening, but the problem hasn't progressed to the point where you need intervention. MCI is believed to be an intermediary stage that indicates brain changes are occurring—changes that often, but not always, progress to Alzheimer's disease. MCI frequently remains stable for years. However, almost 40 percent of those with MCI will go on to develop Alzheimer's within five years.[49]

Over time, a host of other symptoms may become apparent including disorientation; mood and behavior changes; confusion about events, times, and places; suspicions about family, friends, and professional caregivers; and difficulty speaking, swallowing, and walking. When these symptoms arise, one begins grappling with Activities of Daily Living and a marked decline in the quality of life.

WHAT CHANGES IN THE BRAIN

The brain of an Alzheimer's patient contains four primary physical pathological features, all with dire-sounding names: amyloid plaques, tau tangles, neuronal death, and brain shrinkage.

Amyloid Plaques

Most researchers subscribe to the amyloid hypothesis, which posits that the main culprit in Alzheimer's is a protein called beta amyloid. In the brain, a healthy neuron does its job of connecting to other neurons through the tiny space of a synapse. Keeping those synapses healthy are small amounts of amyloid precursor proteins. These proteins regularly get cut up and reassembled in a recycling process, but in Alzheimer's cases, they get reassembled wrong, like deformed origami.[50] This is referred to as protein misfolding. The amyloid also becomes sticky, clustering together into plaques, thus the "amyloid plaques" of Alzheimer's.

Normally, amyloid is routinely cleared from the brain by special cells called microglia. In Alzheimer's disease it may be that the brain starts overproducing amyloid or that the microglia are unable to sufficiently clear it away—or both. So, the levels of amyloid in a person with Alzheimer's disease are between 100 and 1,000 times higher than levels in healthy people.[51]

How do amyloid plaques cause problems? Plaques form on the outsides of neurons as well as in the synapses, disrupting these neurons' ability to communicate with other neurons. Also, as amyloid builds up, the microglia go into overdrive in an effort to get control of the deposits. In doing so, they trigger inflammation of the neurons, and this may even result in the loss of some synapses.

Using relatively new specialized PET scans, doctors can inject a patient with a contrast dye that attaches to a brain's amyloid protein. This dye allows a doctor to visually confirm the presence of plaques decades before symptoms become apparent.[52]

What remains a mystery is why plaques may be found in about 30 percent of those aged 65 and older who demonstrate no symptoms of Alzheimer's, as well as in people much younger, even in their 20s.[53] It may be that plaques themselves are not enough to cause Alzheimer's and that a co-conspirator, tau protein, is required.

Tau Tangles

Inside a neuron is a protein called tau. In a healthy brain, tau forms a stabilizing structure, somewhat like scaffolding, to help transport nutrients from one location to another.[54] In diseased brains, however, tau forms *neurofibrillary tangles*, twisted thread-like filaments. These filaments, which are 10,000 times thinner than human hair, can become tangled up with one another and damage the ability of neurons to send signals. In Alzheimer's disease, the tau "scaffolding" inside neurons collapses and can no longer do its job. The neurons themselves then become dysfunctional and perish. Some research has suggested that inflammation may be a factor in what triggers tau to change into its dysfunctional form.[55]

While it's been known for some time that Alzheimer's has a gender bias, only very recently have scientists begun to understand why two-thirds of cases occur in women. One reason may be that tau accumulates in the brains of women much more rapidly than it does in men. In one study, tau accumulated in female subjects 75 percent faster than in male subjects. [56]

Neuronal Death and Brain Shrinkage

As Alzheimer's progresses, there's a loss of neurons, synapses, (the junctions between neurons) and white matter, the deep tissue composed of nerve fibers that connects different regions of the brain. This results in a loss of connectivity, coupled with growing inflammation. As a result of this death of neurons, synapses, and white matter, the brain begins to lose volume and shrinks at an accelerated rate, especially in the hippocampus, a part of the brain that is critical to memory and emotion. Some scientists believe that the loss of synapses may be in large part driven by microglia, which we will learn more about in the next chapter. As we'll see later, one need not be diagnosed with dementia to experience brain shrinkage, and there's much we can do to thwart a loss of brain volume. A brain that is deprived of adequate blood, oxygen, fuel, and sufficient levels of social engagement, physical exercise, and cognitive stimulation is prone to excessive shrinkage.

THE INTRIGUING IDEA OF COGNITIVE RESERVE

Just as some people smoke and do not develop lung cancer, some people develop the pathology of Alzheimer's—amyloid plaques and tau tangles—yet do not manifest the symptoms of the disease. In other words, their brains undergo the physical changes of the disease, but they remain cognitively healthy.

Autopsies of these brains reveal them to be heavier than average and to contain more neurons and synapses. Scientists believe that these individuals may have had more brain matter (neurons and synapses) to spare and were therefore better able to compensate for AD's debilitating changes.[57] In other words, these people had *cognitive reserve*. The presence of more neurons and synapses fosters greater resilience and flexibility, allowing the brain to "work around" the plaques and tangles.

The theory of cognitive reserve came from a study of 137 residents of a nursing home who had been cognitively assessed for some years before they died. Upon autopsy, researchers found physical evidence of Alzheimer's disease (plaques and tangles) in those who died with dementia as well as those who remained cognitively normal.[58] The outliers (those with plaques and tangles who nevertheless remained cognitively normal) scored as well as or better on cognitive function checklists than age-matched control residents who were free of Alzheimer's pathology. The researchers noted that the subjects who had Alzheimer's pathology but remained dementia-free had heavier brains, a greater number of neurons, and more synapses, presumably as a result of overall brain stimulation. What also caught their attention was that while the outliers' brains did have plaques and tangles, they did not show significant loss of neurons and total brain volume. Factors such as total years of education, other forms of mental stimulation, social engagement, level of physical activity, and job status are thought to contribute to building cognitive reserve and the resilience it affords.

In other studies researchers have found that some individuals, particularly those who pursue higher education and skill development, have up to 17 percent more synapses for each neuron compared to those with less education and training. This greater number of synaptic connections seems to create a more robust and impervious network of connectivity between neurons. In addition, the brain's ability to rewire itself in response to a changing environment—via the aforementioned brain plasticity—may enable these more robust neuronal networks to recruit other neurons and synapses that would not normally be utilized in a healthy brain to compensate for areas that have been lost.

Because our cognitive reserve may permit us to delay cognitive decline and the onset of Alzheimer's symptoms, later I will discuss several key strategies you can adopt to build your own reserve.

In brief, that's some of what can go wrong in a brain. Promoting this havoc are two conditions that deserve our attention next.

3

RUST AND FIRE, BY OTHER NAMES

TWO CONDITIONS—OXIDATIVE STRESS and inflammation—are dangerous for our brains but potentially manageable if we maintain healthy habits. Unfortunately, each can promote the other and both are major drivers of the Alzheimer's disease process. I'll be referencing oxidative stress and inflammation throughout this book, so let's start with a solid understanding of what they are and what actions you can take to keep them in check.

OXIDATIVE STRESS

All chemical reactions in the body that are required to sustain life result in *oxidation*. A familiar example of oxidation is when iron-containing tools are left outside and exposed to oxygen and moisture. The oxidation manifests as rust. If you cut an apple open, its flesh quickly turns brown. That's oxidation as well.

Oxidation in the body produces elements called *free radicals*, and here we must go briefly back to chemistry class. A free radical is a molecule that has lost one or more electrons, making it unstable and highly reactive. A free radical has a need to bond with or steal an electron from another molecule. When it takes an electron from another molecule, it turns *that* molecule into a free radical, which in turn destabilizes another molecule by absconding with one of *its* electrons. This chain reaction of molecules becoming destabilized can cause damage to cell membranes, make fat more prone to stick to blood vessel walls, and even damage DNA.

The process of oxidation and free-radical production is intrinsic, meaning it is naturally occurring. Basic metabolism produces small amounts of free radicals as a matter of course. To avoid oxidative stress, the body has a defense system. Our internal *antioxidants* neutralize free radicals. That's where the trendy word comes from: antioxidants promote anti-oxidation.

Some antioxidants, like superoxide dismutase, catalase, and glutathione peroxidase, are obscure, while others like beta-carotene and vitamins C and E are well known to most of us. The job of all of them is simple: disarm free radicals before they can wreak havoc.

The body works to control damage caused by free radicals both *preventatively*, by suppressing free-radical production, as well as *reactively*, by scavenging for free radicals and eliminating them. However, as we age, the free radical defense system becomes less robust.

Oxidative stress occurs when the number of free radicals exceeds the capacity of the body's antioxidant defense system.[59] Simply put, it's an imbalance between free radicals and antioxidants.

Our brains are especially vulnerable. Partly because of its high rate of metabolism, the brain is easily susceptible to free radical assaults.[60] Free radicals can damage neurons, prevent their growth and development, and ultimately kill them. This is why oxidative stress has been implicated as a driving force in Alzheimer's and other neurological diseases.[61]

Scientists who have tested people with mild cognitive impairment have found lower levels of antioxidants in both their brains and their blood.[62] As Alzheimer's advances, certain indicators that confirm oxidative damage is occurring become elevated in the brain, blood, and cerebrospinal fluid of patients.[63] Some researchers believe that oxidative stress may be one of the first important changes in the cascade that leads to AD.[64]

In addition to the direct damage it causes, oxidative stress boosts the production and depositing of amyloid protein, which forms the plaques seen in AD. The accumulation of these plaques in turn causes more oxidative stress.[65]

We can fortify our body's defense against oxidative stress by consuming a diet rich in antioxidants. This means creating meals with fruits, vegetables, nuts, legumes, herbs, and spices.[66] Remember the apple that turns brown shortly after exposure to oxygen? A squeeze of fresh lemon juice prevents the browning. Because the lemon contains citric acid, an antioxidant, it protects the apple from oxidation. Other ways to help our bodies defend against runaway free radicals are regular exercise, stress management, and even the quality of our sleep.[67]

INFLAMMATION

Inflammation is a normal, healthy process within the body that helps protect us from infection, pathogens, and pollutants, and accelerates healing. The inflammatory response involves immune cells and blood vessels that work along with special molecules to eliminate damaged tissue and support the production of healthy new tissue. Think of the inflammation you've had around a wound or cut. The affected area becomes red, swollen, and painful, and the surrounding area may become stiff. After the critical work of inflammation is done, other special molecules are released to shut it down and return the body to its normal healthy state.

We encounter problems with inflammation when it is low-grade and chronic, meaning it persists beyond the need to heal an acute injury or to fight a pathogen. In this case, instead of being restorative, inflammation is injurious and can encourage various diseases.[68] For years experts have highlighted the role of chronic inflammation in advancing heart disease, cancer, arthritis, and other conditions. With aging, greater inflammation in both the brain and other parts of the body is seen. This has been dubbed *inflammaging*. Biomarkers found in blood that are the signature of such inflammation are accurate predictors of impending health problems, not the least of which includes dementia. At least ten large studies have shown an association between chronic inflammation and the risk of developing Alzheimer's.[69]

Let's take a closer look at how inflammation works in the brain. Here, inflammation is activated by cells called microglia, part of the brain's own immune system. You can think of microglia as the janitor cells of the brain. Their job is to sweep up and dispose of viruses, toxins, and cellular debris. Microglia can be activated by a virus or an allergen. But they can also be triggered by head trauma from an accident, fall, or sports injury.

What we now know is that pro-inflammatory molecules triggered outside the brain can also lead to inflammation inside the brain.[70] After crossing the blood-brain barrier, they activate microglia, and thus trigger inflammation there as well, and increasingly so with age.[71]

Inflammation is believed to play a role in the very early stages of AD, even before any symptoms are evident.[72] And once Alzheimer's has developed, chronic inflammation of neurons remains a central feature and primary driver of the condition.[73] "Plaques and tangles may set the stage," says Rudi Tanzi, Director of the Alzheimer's Genome Project. "But at the end of the day, it's neuroinflammation that kills enough neurons to get to dementia."

A research team at Johns Hopkins University School of Medicine tested 1,633 participants with an average age of 53 for blood levels of five different markers for inflammation. The participants were then monitored for an average of 24 years, at which point they were given memory tests and brain scans. Compared to those with no increased levels of markers for inflammation, the participants with three or more elevated markers had significantly less brain volume, especially in the hippocampus region. They also performed more poorly on memory tests. The researchers concluded that midlife inflammation in the body may be an indicator for inflammation in the brain and a harbinger for neuron loss and other changes that lead to dementia years later.[74]

Other researchers have corroborated the Johns Hopkins team's finding that as the level of inflammation increases, so does the severity of cognitive impairment.[75] For example, those with mild cognitive impairment (MCI) already have heightened levels of inflammation. And over time their inflammatory markers will rise to increasingly higher levels if their conditions advance to AD. Higher inflammation levels may lead to a faster rate of mental decline. Both the progression and the severity of Alzheimer's disease correlate with how much inflammation is present.[76]

One of the blood markers for inflammation is called C-reactive protein (CRP). Studies have shown that those who are overweight have significantly elevated CRP levels. However, as they lose weight, CRP levels drop by as much as 48 percent.[77]

A troubling thing is that we may not even know we have chronic body and brain inflammation. If it *is* happening, it can stimulate a cascade of deleterious effects in the brain. It reduces blood flow to certain regions of the brain, deprives brain cells of oxygen and nutrients, promotes oxidative stress, and ultimately damages and kills neurons.[78] All this while we remain oblivious to the harm going on inside our own heads.

The good news—and yes, there is *plenty* of good news—is that many of the major promoters of inflammation are things we can control. We can all take practical steps to significantly reduce inflammation, and therefore our risk for Alzheimer's, starting today.

Significantly, *lifestyle choices* we make as we age can determine our propensity for inflammation.[79] Diet is a major player, as are cardiovascular disease, obesity, high blood pressure, diabetes, alcohol consumption, and insomnia. And because of the tight relationship between the nervous system and the immune system, inflammation also can be brought about by chronic or traumatic psychological stress.[80] In Chapter 42, we'll look at several strategies to help keep the stress response under control.

The foods we eat can either promote or cool the flames of systemic inflammation. For example, foods rich in dietary fiber suppress inflammation whereas sugary foods and those made from refined white flours turn the flames up.[81] Meat, processed meat, fast foods, fried foods, and processed and sweetened snack foods promote inflammation, whereas almonds, walnuts, leafy greens, and berries cool the flames.

PROMOTERS OF INFLAMMATION	
High-fat Diet	High Blood Pressure
Refined Sugars	Diabetes
High Fructose Corn Syrup	Inactivity
Trans fats	Insomnia
Fried foods	Overweight/Obesity
Refined Sweeteners	Psychological stress
Meat /Processed Meat	Pesticides
Soft drinks	Air Pollutants
Dairy Products	Cigarette Smoke
Heavy Metals	Alcoholic beverages
Margarine, Shortening, Lard	Artificial colors & flavors

What we eat *really* matters. Multiple studies have confirmed that people who follow the typical Western diet have significantly elevated levels of inflammation.[82] Foods that are the centerpiece of the Western diet, as well as smoking and drinking alcohol, stoke the flames of inflammation.[83] Even short-term consumption (seven days) of a diet high in saturated fat and sugar can drive up inflammation.[84] Conversely, the dietary plan in the Revolution Lifestyle outlined in Chapter 24 can slash levels of inflammation by 30 percent in just two weeks.[85]

Another big help with lowering inflammation is regular aerobic exercise.[86] In fact, after just 20 minutes of moderate intensity exercise inflammation levels are lowered markedly.[87] We'll look more closely at this topic in Chapter 32.

The next topic we will address is genetics. Too many people have been led to believe that their genes are their destiny. Such thinking is not only disempowering, you're going to learn that it's simply wrong.

PART II

PRIMARY CONTROLLABLE RISK FACTORS FOR ALZHEIMER'S DISEASE

4
WHAT ABOUT GENETICS?

ARE NEUROLOGICAL DISEASES, including Alzheimer's, caused by particular gene mutations? Yes and no. Many people are drawn to the growing business of internet-based genetic-testing services, but when it comes to AD, these tests are not a reliable predictor of risk. While there are genetic risk factors for neurological disease, they most certainly do not act alone.

Until recently, the message implied by discussions of genetics and the risk of Alzheimer's has been one of little hope: if you carry a particular gene, you're essentially doomed. Fortunately, this could not be farther from the truth. There are basically two types of Alzheimer's disease: (1) early onset and (2) late onset. Early onset AD, which is linked to genetics, has historically occurred between the early forties and mid-fifties and results from a mutation in three genes: amyloid precursor protein (APP), presenilin 1(PS1) and presenilin 2(PS2). Only four to six percent of all AD cases can be attributed to the early-onset, genetically-driven form of AD.[88]

Now stay with me on this genetics discussion because I'm certain you're going to be encouraged by what you read.

The other kind of Alzheimer's disease—late onset—involves a gene called apolipoprotein E (APOE). There are three variations of the APOE gene: E_2 E_3, and E_4. Each of us caries two copies of the gene in various combinations. Your gene combination specifies your APOE genotype.[89] APOE2, the rarest of them, may reduce risk of Alzheimer's disease by 40 percent.[90] APOE3, the most common of them, doesn't increase risk. APOE4, which is present in 10 to 15 percent of people, increases risk and reduces the age of onset for Alzheimer's.[91] If you carry one copy of

APOE4 your risk of developing Alzheimer's is three times higher than that of people without the gene.[92] However, if you carry two copies of APOE4 your risk may be 8 to 12 times higher.[93]

If you have two copies of APOE4 is there no hope, then? Fortunately, genes are not always destiny. It's true that APP, PS1, and PS2 are *deterministic* genes—genes that directly cause a disease. However, APOE4 is a *risk* gene that simply increases the likelihood but offers no certainty. You are not necessarily condemned to get the disease. We know that people in certain parts of the world with distinctly different lifestyles than those of people in the USA rarely develop Alzheimer's despite having APOE genotypes that increase risk.

The black population in Nigeria has one of the highest frequencies of the APOE4 gene in the world,[94] yet Nigeria has a relatively low rate of Alzheimer's disease.[95] One of the biggest differences between Nigeria and the USA is diet.

The rapidly growing field of *epigenetics* challenges the belief that we have no influence over our genetic heritage. The prefix *epi* refers to something that is on top of or in addition to genetics. We are learning that our environment and lifestyle can change what's called *gene expression*. Our genome, which can be thought of as our genetic blueprint, is dynamic and responsive to its environment. The choices we make related to nutrition, exercise, response to stress, and exposure to toxins may turn our genes on or off, thereby changing how our cells function and interact, and ultimately influence our risk. For example, a person may have the APOE4 genotype, but by making certain dietary choices their genetic status may not be as significant when it comes to the risk of developing Alzheimer's. What may matter more is nutrition.[96]

A growing body of evidence is emerging that indicates lifestyle and environment play a much greater role in the development of neurological impairment than previously imagined. A landmark study of 20,000 pairs of identical twins demonstrated that genetics are not the sole determinant of risk.[97] The study found that if Alzheimer's developed in one identical male twin, the other twin developed the disease only 45 percent of the time; for female identical twins, the result was 60 percent. Moreover, there may be as much as a 16-year difference in the age at which the disease is diagnosed as well as differences in the severity of the disease.[98] Identical twins, of course, have identical genes so some other factor must account for the discrepancies.

In another twin study, from the Sun Health Research Institute, researchers described a pair of identical twins in which one was occupationally exposed to pesticides and diagnosed with Alzheimer's disease at age 60, struggling with the disease for 16 years before he died. His twin, cognitively intact, died from cancer at age 79. An autopsy found the first brother's brain riddled with plaques and tangles, the hallmark pathological features of Alzheimer's disease.[99] Yet the lead researcher, Paul Coleman, reported that in the unaffected brother, "We had to hunt through the brain sections in order to find even one neurofibrillary tangle."[100] Yet these men shared the same genetic heritage.

Even in general populations we can see discrepancies in neurological disease rates based on where people come from and where they move to. Japanese natives who move to Hawaii and adopt the lifestyle of their new homeland have a dramatically increased risk of Alzheimer's disease.[101] A similar tendency is seen in African Americans who live in the USA compared to Black residents of Nigeria.[102] An individual can be cognitively healthy in one society and more likely to be cognitively diseased in another. The risk of AD may be five times lower for a person who stays in Nigeria rather than moving to the USA. Their genes don't change but their environment and lifestyle do.

A further indication that genetic issues are not the only factors in the development of neurological disease is the incidence of concussion and correspondingly high risk of dementia in professional football players. Retired players between the ages of 50 and 59 have been shown to have a risk of becoming cognitively impaired that is five times greater than that of the general population.[103]

Lifestyle factors we can influence significantly determine our susceptibility to Alzheimer's.[104] This is illustrated in a 21-year Swedish study. The research revealed that if a person carrying one copy of the APOE4 gene that increases the risk of developing AD by 2.83 times also avoids exercise, drinks alcohol, smokes, and eats a typical high-fat American diet, their risk for AD increases more than ten times.[105] The interplay between genetics and lifestyle illustrates the adage "genetics loads the gun, but lifestyle pulls the trigger."

In the next chapter we're going to look at cardiovascular disease, one of several key risk factors we'll examine that are controllable (preventable) by making healthful lifestyle choices. Since this disease kills more Americans than all forms of cancer combined and is a major risk factor for dementia, you'll want to be sure to stay tuned.

5

CARDIOVASCULAR DISEASE

RIGHT AROUND HIS 100th birthday, California heart surgeon, Dr. Ellsworth Wareham, was interviewed by CNN's Sanjay Gupta, MD. The medical journalist wanted to know the secret to Dr. Wareham's longevity. The surgeon credited his careful attention to cholesterol, explaining that if your cholesterol level is under 150 mg/dl, "your chances of having a heart attack are pretty small." Determined to keep his cholesterol levels low, the doctor ate a plant-based diet. The result? Dr. Wareham had a total cholesterol level of 117 mg/dl at the time of the interview. The average American has a level of 189 mg/dl, 100 million American adults are at 200 mg/dl, and 28 million have cholesterol levels higher than 240mg/dl.[106]

Your cardiovascular system includes your heart and all your blood vessels. Cardiovascular disease (CVD)* is the number-one killer of Americans, and it can have a serious negative impact on the brain long before it strikes a fatal blow. Because it's very likely that the pathological changes that occur with CVD have already been seeded in your own body, I want you to pay close attention to the pages that follow. Don't worry, CVD is a disease that doesn't have to advance and that is also reversible. But you must understand it first.

When cardiovascular disease sets in, so does atherosclerosis, a buildup of plaque composed of cholesterol, fat, and cellular debris. That plaque is deposited on blood vessel walls and eventually narrows the blood

---

*Cardiovascular disease includes heart valve problems, arrhythmia, and heart failure which will not be included in this discussion.

vessels and makes them less flexible, thereby restricting the free flow of blood to both the heart and to the brain.

With often fatal results, a piece of this plaque can break away and block an artery feeding the heart. What happens next is, literally, a heart attack, killing off part of the heart muscle (if not the person as well). Likewise, when an artery feeding the brain becomes completely blocked, the result is a stroke, and brain tissue will die. Stroke is a major cause of memory loss. Yet CVD can take a serious toll on the brain and advance cognitive decline even without a heart attack or stroke.

As new insight has revealed, what's good or bad for the heart and blood vessels is also good or bad for the brain. Put simply, if an artery feeding one's heart is compromised, chances are very good that an artery feeding one's brain is compromised as well.

In his interview, Dr. Wareham shared that not only was he still assisting with complicated surgeries at age 95, but he also boasted that if given new information to memorize, he could commit it to memory as quickly as he did when he was 20. The same lifestyle strategies he used to protect his heart and blood vessels appeared to have benefited his cognitive health as well.

The Alzheimer's Association reports that 80 percent of those who die with Alzheimer's also have cardiovascular disease. The presence of what is called *atherosclerotic* plaque in arteries was noted back in 1907 by Dr. Alzheimer himself, when he performed an autopsy on the brain of his patient, Auguste Deter.[107] However, not until the 1970s was it suggested that clogged blood vessels played a role in dementia, rather than being coincidentally present.

Brain damage can be insidious, occurring well before a heart attack or a stroke. Imperceptible and slowly growing plaques that develop inside arteries over decades can choke the heart and the brain in slow motion. The damage done by risk factors such as an unhealthy diet, inactivity, smoking, being overweight, diabetes, and high blood pressure may not be evident until it has significantly progressed.

With the buildup of plaque in blood vessels, the amount of blood and oxygen reaching the brain is incrementally reduced. By age 65, many of us will already have a 20 percent reduction in blood flow to our brain.[108] Studies have indicated that, depending on lifestyle factors, between ages 30 and 89 cerebral blood flow may decline between 25 and 40 percent.[109] This reduction in blood flow is a significant contributor to cognitive decline. The brain cells require an unimpeded supply of blood to function properly, so a reduction in blood flow may set off a chain of events sufficient to damage or kill neurons.[110]

New research from the University of Southern California has shown a link between a reduction in blood flow to the brain and the development of tau tangles. Researchers followed a group of men and women for four years and used magnetic resonance imaging (MRI) and positron emission tomography (PET) scans to image their brains. As blood flow to the brain was reduced, tau tangles flourished.[111] Scientists at Vanderbilt University's Memory and Alzheimer's Center showed that people with the poorest blood flow to the brain had much greater cognitive impairment, and their brains appeared to be 20 years older than their chronological age when examined at autopsy.[112] Twenty years! There is no question: to protect against Alzheimer's, the heart must be strong and healthy and the blood vessels clear and flexible, so blood pressure remains low and sufficient levels of blood and oxygen are consistently transported to the brain.

CLOGGED BRAIN BLOOD VESSELS

In those who die from Alzheimer's, there is frequently atherosclerosis in the brain blood vessels.[113] As parts of the brain get deprived of blood flow and oxygen, imperceptible mini strokes may occur that progressively kill off brain tissue and are an important contributor to memory loss and dementia.[114] Only recently have experts realized how widespread these events may be, occurring in as many as 50 percent of those aged 60 and older, and up to 70 percent of those with severe dementia.[115]

Dr. Joel Kramer, professor of neuropsychology at the UCSF Memory and Aging Center, led a study on the influence of atherosclerosis on mental decline. Using ultrasound imaging, his colleagues studied elderly subjects by first measuring the amount of atherosclerotic plaque in the walls of their carotid arteries, the major blood vessels in the neck that feed blood to the brain. Over four years following the initial imaging, the people with the most plaque in their blood vessels experienced the greatest decline in cognitive function.[116]

The evidence is clear: people with the most severe levels of plaque in their blood vessels move from mild cognitive impairment to dementia and decline more rapidly than those with the least amount of arterial plaque.[117]

There is also an association between reduced blood flow to the brain and the accumulation of amyloid plaques. When blood flow is restricted, the brain boosts an enzyme, BACE1, which in the short term offers some degree of protection, but over the long term encourages the production of amyloid plaques. Reduced blood flow, and thus reduced oxygen, to the brain also increases oxidative stress and inflammation.[118]

In one study, researchers measured the levels of atherosclerosis in blood vessels and then imaged subjects' brains to check for the presence of amyloid plaques. With each unit of increase in atherosclerosis, they found a two- to four-fold increase in the likelihood of finding amyloid plaques and brain tissue damage.[119]

WHAT CAUSES ATHEROSCLEROSIS?

The development of atherosclerosis is a protracted process that begins early in life. If you follow the typical Western diet, the first damage to your arteries can begin as early as age ten when pre-plaques, called fatty streaks, develop on the arterial walls.[120]

Full-blown cardiovascular disease has many contributing factors, including obesity, diabetes, high blood pressure, an unhealthy stress response, inactivity, and smoking. But by far the largest contributor to risk are the foods we eat and how they affect the cholesterol circulating in our blood. The problems begin when cholesterol levels become too high, a condition that 100 million Americans struggle with today.

A waxy, fat-like substance, cholesterol is not all bad. It's essential to the integrity of every cell in our body, (including brain cells) required for hormone production and our ability to make vitamin D. Fortunately our body manufactures all the cholesterol it needs for these purposes and the brain manufactures its own personal supply. Unfortunately, the diet that many people follow is packed with unnecessary dietary cholesterol, as well as a type of fat that causes the body to make more cholesterol. Consequently, many Americans have unhealthy high cholesterol levels. According to the Centers for Disease Control and Prevention, one in five American teens already has dangerously high cholesterol levels because of what they eat.

Let's investigate the terms "good cholesterol" and "bad cholesterol." Cholesterol won't dissolve in blood so it must be packaged for transport by *lipoproteins*, including low-density lipoprotein (LDL) and high-density lipoprotein (HDL). In a normal, healthy process, cells in our bodies regularly die off. After a cell dies, it no longer needs its cholesterol. So the cholesterol "garbage truck," HDL, picks up the cholesterol and returns it to the liver, where it is either excreted from the body or used to make hormones. Higher levels of HDL are considered desirable because HDL sweeps up LDL and lowers the chance it will become deposited on blood vessel walls. High levels of LDL spell trouble and portend more deposits on artery walls.

When your blood cholesterol levels are checked, you'll get a number representing your total cholesterol level along with the two of the numbers that make up that total: your HDL and LDL levels. You will also see your level of triglycerides, which are fat particles in your blood and also linked to cardiovascular disease. The total figure is very important, because high total cholesterol is predictive of cardiovascular disease and the likelihood of a heart attack or stroke.

But the *ratio* of HDL to LDL in the total cholesterol is also important because it reflects how well your body is sweeping up the bad cholesterol. A high LDL level in relation to HDL indicates a greater risk of arterial plaque buildup. Higher levels of LDL cholesterol specifically have also been linked to Alzheimer's pathology and the risk of earlier onset of the disease.[121] In one study, participants with elevated LDL cholesterol (155 mg/dl or higher) were eight times more likely to have Alzheimer's pathology in their brain when they died than those with LDL levels lower than 106 mg/dl.

Plaques form when there is inflammation of the delicate lining (endothelium) of arteries. What inflames it? Eating food rich in cholesterol, saturated fat, or trans fat; smoking; having high blood pressure; being inactive; having insulin resistance; and diabetes. Once the lining is inflamed, LDL cholesterol, calcium, fat, and other material in the bloodstream begins to accumulate on the injured wall. Then white blood cells move in to try to break down the plaque. This causes further inflammation and more deposits. Over time, the artery becomes increasingly narrowed by the deposits.

IS THERE A CHOLESTEROL/ALZHEIMER'S CONNECTION?

Although not clear why, high blood cholesterol levels contribute not only to plaques in blood vessels but are associated with higher levels of amyloid protein and the development of amyloid plaques in the brain.[122] The higher one's blood cholesterol level, the greater the number of plaques in the brain.

Researchers measured blood cholesterol levels in 2,587 individuals at midlife, and again 10 to 15 years before their deaths.[123] They found that those who had cholesterol levels over 224 mg/dl were up to seven times more likely to have beta amyloid plaques in their brains at the time of death compared with those who kept their blood cholesterol levels below 173 mg/dl.[124]

A Kaiser Permanente study of over 9,000 individuals showed that, compared to individuals who maintain a cholesterol level under 200 mg/dl, a blood cholesterol level of 220 mg/dl at midlife increased risk of Alzheimer's later in life by about 25 percent.[125] A cholesterol level of 250 mg/dl increased risk by 50 percent. Even moderately elevated levels of blood cholesterol at midlife have been shown to increase the likelihood of dementia later in life.[126]

Once Alzheimer's has developed, it also seems to advance more rapidly in those who have high blood cholesterol levels.[127]

WHAT RAISES BLOOD CHOLESTEROL LEVELS?

While dietary cholesterol can contribute to a rise in blood cholesterol levels, dietary saturated fat is the big player as it stimulates the liver to make more cholesterol and raises LDL (bad) cholesterol levels. There's another co-conspirator, trans fats, which we will examine in Chapter 10. Saturated fat is concentrated in foods derived from animals, including beef, chicken, fish, milk, cheese, and butter, as well as a few plant-derived tropical oils (coconut, palm, and palm kernel). The popular notion that eating chicken in place of beef will somehow protect your heart and blood vessels has been proven false. Regardless of whether one consumes beef or chicken, the adverse effect on cholesterol levels has been found to be identical.[128]

Plant-based meals can be a potent weapon against rising cholesterol levels—including LDL cholesterol. Such a diet has been shown to reduce LDL levels by up to 30 percent. This is comparable to the effect of popular statin drugs.[129] When other lifestyle changes are added to the mix, the outcome can be even more impressive. In many people, a plant-based diet combined with aerobic exercise and stress reduction strategies can bring total cholesterol levels to around 150 mg/dl. When I adopted a plant-based diet in combination with a robust exercise program, my total cholesterol plummeted from 178 mg/dl to 116 mg/dl.

CULTURES THAT POINT TO SOLUTIONS

Although few populations in the developed world have resisted adopting the Western diet, several holdouts show us what our cardiovascular health could be like. As mentioned, even with the highest concentration of the APOE4 gene, Nigeria is not a hot bed of Alzheimer's Disease.[130] The Nigerians' diet is likely affecting the expression of their genes. Nigerians as a rule do not fry food. Corn, sorghum, millet, okra, plantains, rice, tomatoes, and sweet potatoes—all cholesterol-free and low in saturated fat—are at the heart of the average Nigerian's diet. As a result, they maintain low cholesterol levels and are not burdened with cardiovascular disease like we are in the West.

Sardinia, Italy; Okinawa, Japan; the Nicoya Peninsula in Costa Rica; Icaria, Greece; and the Seventh Day Adventist area of Loma Linda, California, are places where people have very low rates of chronic disease and tend to live longer than in any other areas. Sometimes referred to as the Blue Zones, because when researcher Dan Buettner and colleagues first identified these regions they drew blue circles around them on a map, these regions are home to the greatest number of nonagenarians (people who live over 90 years) and centenarians (people who live over 100 years).[131] The inhabitants of these regions tend to follow diets that are 90 percent or more plant derived. Their superior vascular health and relative lack of degenerative disease reflect that. Dr. Wareham was a Seventh Day Adventist, vegan, and died at the age of 104—cognitively intact.

The people believed to have the cleanest arteries of any population in the world belong to a subsistence agriculture community in lowland Bolivia known as the Tsimane (pronounced *chee-mon-ee*). Randall Thompson MD, who led a study of the Tsimane, reported that compared to the average sedentary urban dweller, the arteries of the Tsimane appear 25 to 30 years younger.[132] Their diet is composed primarily of plant foods, including plantains, rice, nuts, fruits, and vegetables with little wild game. They are physically active for hours each day and have low blood sugar, low blood pressure, low cholesterol, and rarely develop diabetes or heart disease.[133] The Tsimane also have the lowest rate of dementia in the world; just 1 percent of their population is afflicted.[134]

The great news is that a landmark study has shown that by adopting a plant-based diet and other healthful lifestyle changes, 90 percent of patients studied were able to open up their clogged arteries and restore vital blood flow.[135] In addition to the recommended dietary changes, later we will learn about other strategies that support a strong heart and healthy blood vessels.

6

HIGH BLOOD PRESSURE

MOST OF US have sat in a chair at the doctor's office and had our blood pressure measured. An inflatable cuff wrapped around the upper arm constricts as it is pumped full of air, then is slowly deflated, and a reading is taken. More recently, this task is performed by an electronic system that self-inflates the cuff.

A blood pressure reading is an indication of how hard blood is pushing against the walls of your arteries. The systolic (top) number represents the pressure when the heart beats. The diastolic (bottom) number represents the pressure when the heart is at rest.

There is blood pressure . . . and then there is high blood pressure. Everyone has heard someone in a movie or in their own lives talk about something being "bad for my blood pressure." Sometimes it's even joked about. As the culprit behind 50 percent of all heart attacks and up to 70 percent of strokes, high blood pressure is not only potentially deadly; it's associated with structural brain changes, cognitive decline, and it's a potent risk factor for Alzheimer's disease.[136]

Based on current American Heart Association guidelines for healthy blood pressure (see box), half of American adults now have high blood pressure, also known as hypertension.[137] By 2025 the disease will affect 1.5 billion people worldwide, including a growing number of children.[138] This is an astonishing number, nearly one-fifth of the earth's entire population.

Blood Pressure Categories

American Heart Association.

BLOOD PRESSURE CATEGORY	SYSTOLIC mm Hg (upper number)		DIASTOLIC mm Hg (lower number)
NORMAL	LESS THAN 120	and	LESS THAN 80
ELEVATED	120-129	and	LESS THAN 80
HIGH BLOOD PRESSURE (HYPERTENSION) STAGE 1	130-139	or	80-89
HIGH BLOOD PRESSURE (HYPERTENSION) STAGE 2	140 OR HIGHER	or	90 OR HIGHER
HYPERTENSIVE CRISIS (consult your doctor immediately)	HIGHER THAN 180	and/or	HIGHER THAN 120

In the USA alone, consumers spend $30 billion a year on prescription drugs to control the condition[139] when they might instead be able to keep their blood pressure in check through lifestyle changes.

Elevated blood pressure is associated with the brain changes characteristic of MCI and Alzheimer's disease: plaques, tau tangles, and shrinkage of the brain.[140] Left unchecked, high blood pressure stiffens the carotid arteries that bring blood to the brain and damages the small blood vessels in the brain, restricting blood flow and the delivery of glucose and oxygen.[141] It boosts inflammation, causes oxidative stress, and increases brain damage.[142]

This damage occurs because when you have high blood pressure, your blood vessels, including the tiny fragile ones inside your brain, become inflamed and stiff. That stiffness can lead to imperceptible micro-bleeding or lesions in brain tissue, which kill brain cells and contribute to cognitive impairment.[143] As these lesions increase, more tau tangles tend to develop.[144]

Examined at autopsy, the areas with micro-bleeding or lesions appear as little holes in the brain.[145] An estimated 25 percent of people 65 and older are victims of micro-bleeds but don't know it.[146] When researchers from Rush University looked at the brains of deceased people who had maintained varying rates of blood pressure, one thing became clear. The higher a subject's blood pressure was before death, the more brain lesions could be found at autopsy.

HIGH BLOOD PRESSURE AND STROKE

High blood pressure dramatically increases the risk of suffering a stroke. There are two types of stroke: *ischemic*, which involves a blockage or clot that deprives part of the brain of oxygen, and *hemorrhagic*, which involves bleeding in or around the brain. Hemorrhagic stroke occurs when a blood vessel that has been weakened ruptures, usually from an aneurysm which is a part of the vessel that has ballooned from pressure. In either case, serious brain injury may result and one in four stroke survivors will go on to develop dementia.

In another compelling study, researchers tracked a group of 5,646 subjects to better understand the link between high blood pressure at midlife and the risk of future dementia. Women in the study with an average age of 44 who had elevated blood pressure had a 70 percent greater risk of dementia later in life when compared to same-aged women who maintained healthy blood pressure.[147]

LOWERING HIGH BLOOD PRESSURE WITH DRUGS

Looking specifically at the formation of plaques in the brain, Dr. Karen Rodrigue, assistant professor at the University of Texas Dallas Center for Vital Longevity, conducted a study of individuals aged 30 to 89.[148] The subjects were required to undergo cognitive testing and MRI and PET scans using a compound that when injected travels to the brain and binds with amyloid proteins, allowing the scientists to visualize the amount of amyloid plaque present. Blood pressure was also measured at each visit.

Some participants in the study had high blood pressure but were not getting treated and others were taking high blood pressure medication. Even participants who had a genetic propensity for Alzheimer's (i.e., they carried the APOE4 gene) showed less brain plaque formation if their high blood pressure was being treated with medication—about the equivalent of subjects who didn't have elevated blood pressure or a genetic risk for Alzheimer's.

Several studies in the U.S. and in Europe have shown a 50 to 70 percent reduction in the risk of developing AD in those who undergo long-term treatment with antihypertensive medications, when compared to those whose hypertension is left untreated.[149]

Antihypertensive medication improves blood flow to the brain.[150] In one recent study those who took the blood pressure drug Nilvadipine for six months saw a 20 percent increase in blood flow to the hippocampus.[151] Even in people who are already experiencing MCI, getting high blood pressure under control may reduce the risk that their condition will advance to Alzheimer's disease by 80 percent.[152]

The studies show very clearly that keeping your blood pressure in the "normal" range reduces the risk of Alzheimer's even if you have a genetic propensity for the disease. And this is something you may be able to do without medication.

LOWERING HIGH BLOOD PRESSURE WITHOUT DRUGS

Prescription medications often present their own risks. For example, high blood pressure medication may cause dizziness, weight gain, headaches, constipation, insomnia, fatigue, sun sensitivity, electrolyte imbalance, damage to the kidneys, and an elevated risk of stroke.[153] Some, such as beta-blockers, are associated with an increased risk of memory impairment thought to result because they block two key neurotransmitters, norepinephrine and epinephrine.[154] So, it's worthwhile first taking control of elevated blood pressure with a few lifestyle adjustments.

High blood pressure can be caused by several factors including smoking, stress, excess body weight, lack of exercise, alcohol intake, and, for many, a high intake of sodium. These are all things over which we have control. The fact is, before antihypertensive medications were available, lifestyle intervention was the main treatment—and was generally successful.[155] Let's look at how it can work.

It was 1920 when the association between being overweight or obese and high blood pressure was first noted.[156] In 1995 the Harvard Nurses Health Study reported between a twofold and sixfold greater prevalence of high blood pressure in subjects depending on how severely overweight they were.[157] Depending on the individual and the amount of weight reduced, shedding excess pounds can cut blood pressure by four to ten points.

Decades of research has repeatedly affirmed that adopting a diet centered on plant foods can cause blood pressure to drop precipitously. Conversely, a diet rich in saturated fat causes the blood to become viscous so the heart must work harder to push it through blood vessels, leading to elevated pressure.[158] Imagine the difference between sucking water or a very thick milkshake through a straw and you get the idea. A diet high in saturated fat, trans fat, and cholesterol leads to inflammation, promotes stiffening of arteries, contributes to plaque formation on the artery walls, and ultimately means greater force is required to move blood through the vessels. Do you sometimes think of rewarding yourself with a fatty meal? Even a single high-fat meal can temporarily impair the endothelium, the inner lining of blood vessels, preventing it from expanding to permit greater blood flow.[159]

Removing meat and dairy products from one's diet can significantly lower blood pressure in as little as a week.[160] The Adventist Health Study found that, compared to omnivores, those who follow an entirely plant-based diet (vegans) have significantly lower blood pressure.[161] In a review of 32 studies, when compared to omnivores vegetarians also had blood pressure that was lower on average, even lower than those who were still eating fish and dairy. When fish and dairy are avoided, blood pressure drops even more.[162] The reason is basic: plant-based foods are low in total fat and saturated fat, low in sodium, and rich in potassium (a nutrient that helps reduce arterial inflammation), all of which help to reduce blood pressure.

By contrast, meat-centered diets can raise blood pressure, in part by increasing cortisol levels. Cortisol is a stress hormone that elevates blood pressure by causing blood vessels to constrict.[163] We will look at cortisol more closely in later chapters.

In the European Prospective Investigation into Cancer and Nutrition—an Oxford study of 11,000 British men and women aged 20 to 78, subjects were grouped according to dietary preferences. There was a meat-eating group, a fish-eating group, a vegetarian group, and a group following a dairy-free plant-based (vegan) diet. The highest blood pressure counts were among the meat-eaters. The lowest were seen in the vegans.[164]

In another study that included analysis of the food intake of 188,000 subjects, meat, processed meat, poultry, and fish were all associated with elevated blood pressure, whereas whole grains, fruits, and vegetables were not.[165]

The Coronary Artery Risk Development in Young Adults (CARDIA) study, which looked at 4,304 subjects aged 18 to 30, showed that the potent role of diet in influencing high blood pressure applies to younger as well as older people. In this study researchers found a dose-dependent relationship between plant foods and improved blood pressure. The greater the proportion of plants in the diet, the lower blood pressure could be expected to be.

Some plants contain elements that can lead to significant reductions in blood pressure within hours of their consumption. For example, a reduction of 4-10 mm/Hg has been seen within three to six hours after beet or beet juice consumption. Beets contain nitrates which are converted by our body into nitric oxide, a compound that relaxes and dilates our blood vessels causing pressure to fall. Other elements found in plants collaboratively help one to lower and maintain healthful blood pressure levels.

In a study of subjects who had been taking antihypertensive medications for an average of eight years, the adoption of a completely plant-based diet allowed nearly all of them to stop taking these medications altogether.[166]

YES, SODIUM DOES PLAY A ROLE

Five thousand years ago, the Chinese had already figured out that excess dietary salt could cause high blood pressure. They cautioned in the *Huangdi Neijing*, or *The Yellow Emperor's Classic of Internal Medicine*, "Hence if too much salt is used for food, the pulse hardens."[167]

Throughout history salt has been a prized substance, and due to its initial scarcity, it was very valuable. In ancient Rome soldiers were sometimes paid in salt, hence the expression "worth one's salt." With today's abundant salt mines and modern salt evaporation ponds that harvest salt from the oceans, there is no shortage of the substance. Today we consume more salt than ever before, and we pay a serious price for doing so.

One of the simplest shifts we can make is to reduce our often-heavy salt intake. More than 100 studies have confirmed the potent role that sodium added to foods can play in boosting blood pressure. And even though you have probably heard about the relationship between salt and blood pressure, you may not know how dangerous the connection is.

As salt intake increases, the ability of the kidneys to remove water from the blood is reduced. The extra fluid causes greater blood volume, which in turn increases blood pressure and causes changes in heart function.[168]

Public health messaging has advised keeping sodium intake to less than 2,300 mg—about one teaspoon of table salt—per day. Ninety percent of Americans take in seven times that amount.[169] Yet the Institute of Medicine, a branch of the National Academy of Sciences, suggests a goal of 1,500 mg or less. A lot of the excess sodium we consume is from prepared foods—especially fast food and processed meats, including bacon, beef jerky, canned meat, cold cuts, corned beef, ham, hot dogs, pepperoni, salami, and sausage.

But plenty also comes from the saltshaker on the table. Here's a modern motivator to get you to cut back on salting your dinner: Because much of it is derived from sea water, 90 percent of table salt now contains microplastics too small to be seen with the naked eye. Yes, plastic in your salt. As a result of the vast plastic contamination in the world's oceans, the average American now consumes about 20,000 pieces of microplastics a year just in the salt they sprinkle over their food.[170] When one adds the microplastics from bottled water and fish and shellfish, the average American today consumes the weight of a credit card in plastic each week.[171]

A single high salt meal can boost blood pressure and stiffen arteries for hours afterward. Yet cutting the added salt out of one's diet can cause blood pressure to drop in a mere two days. In populations where no salt is added to food and a low-fat plant-centered diet prevails, hypertension is rare and blood pressure does not rise with age. This includes the Tsimane of the Bolivian Amazon, the highlanders of New Guinea, residents of the Kotyang community in Nepal, the Polynesian islanders, and the Yanomamo of Brazil.[172]

Decoding Sodium-Related Terms on Food Labels

- Sodium-free – Less than 5 mg of sodium per serving and contains no sodium chloride

- Very low sodium – 35 mg or less per serving

- Low sodium – 140 mg or less per serving

- Reduced (or less) sodium – At least 25 percent less sodium per serving than the usual sodium level

- Light (for sodium-reduced products) – If the food is "low calorie" and "low fat" and sodium is reduced by at least 50 percent per serving from the usual sodium level

- Light in sodium – If sodium is reduced by at least 50 percent per serving from the usual sodium level

Even better than trying to decode product marketing is to check the nutrition information for the amount of sodium per serving—while making careul note of the serving size, of course

The Dietary Approach to Stop Hypertension (DASH), prescribed by nutritionists for modifying blood pressure, can result in a drop of systolic pressure by 8 to 14 points in as little as two weeks.[173] The diet emphasizes fruits, vegetables, whole grains, and nuts, and restricts sodium to 2,300 mg per day. It allows dairy, fish, and poultry, which limit the improvements the change in diet can offer. And it presents other problems specific to AD risk. Therefore, while the DASH diet modifications are an effective move in a healthful direction, for maximum risk reduction of Alzheimer's my recommendation is to move even further into the plant kingdom and away from problematic foods.

Although seldom mentioned, sugary foods and drinks also contribute to high blood pressure. A high sugar intake inhibits the production of an important substance called nitric oxide (NO), which works as a vasodilator, relaxing blood vessels and keeping pressure down.[174] A high intake of sugar also causes the body to absorb more sodium from the diet, which in turn boosts blood volume and in so doing raises blood pressure.[175] Cutting back on all sources of added refined sugars, including sodas, so-called sports drinks, and other common culprits can be helpful to lowering blood pressure.

WHAT ELSE TO DO?

The basics have not changed. Among the most obvious is to stop smoking. Smoking raises blood pressure immediately and over time damages the lining of the blood vessels, making them stiffer and making elevated blood pressure harder to fight. There's no soft-pedaling it: if you are serious about protecting your brain, stop smoking! Also, avoid using popular high caffeine "energy drinks" such as Red Bull and Rockstar because they raise blood pressure significantly within 90 minutes of consumption, and for as long as 24 hours.[176] They also raise markers of inflammation and reduce artery function.

Another basic strategy: move. A regular exercise program that involves at least 30 minutes of aerobic conditioning most days of the week can lower systolic pressure by four to nine points, which is similar to what blood pressure medications can achieve.[177] Also, strength training exercises performed five times per week have shown impressive reductions of 10 points systolic pressure and nine points diastolic pressure in as little as five weeks.[178] With regular exercise your heart becomes stronger, which enables it to pump more blood with less effort. Exercise also reduces blood vessel stiffness, allowing blood to flow with less resistance.

Lastly, prioritize stress reduction strategies. People who have a negative response to unavoidable life stressors may have elevated levels of the stress hormone cortisol, which can cause elevated blood pressure.[179] Chronic stress, therefore, may contribute to sustained elevated blood pressure.[180] We'll look at stress and many ideas for reducing it in the Alzheimer's Revolution Lifestyle Plan later in the book.

7

OBESE OR OVERWEIGHT

WHETHER CALLED FAT acceptance, body positivity, or body neutrality, today there are new attitudes emerging around body weight and image. I commend those leading the movement to lessen the emotional and psychological burden that may be fueled by advertising imagery that all too frequently presents impractical, if not unhealthy, standards for how both women and men should look. At the same time, I've included this section because there are very real risks to cognitive health from being overweight that should not be ignored. More than 1,000 studies have explored the relationship between being overweight and brain function, finding that excess body weight is predictive of poor cognitive function and increased risk of Alzheimer's later in life.[181] This is particularly so when fat has accumulated in the belly region.

In 2020 the Centers for Disease Control and Prevention reported that more than 40 percent of the US population is obese.[182] This includes 20 percent or more of residents in every US state. Worldwide, more than two billion people are overweight, and another one billion people are obese.[183]

You may be aware that being overweight or obese increases the risk for 13 different cancers and shortens one's lifespan.[184] But obesity is also strongly linked to cognitive impairment and is associated with an increased risk of AD by about twofold.[185] However, researchers with Kaiser Permanente tracked medical records for 6,583 members who were assessed for obesity centered around the abdominal area in the 1960s and 1970s. The researchers found that, accounting for the comorbidities of diabetes, heart disease, hypertension, stoke, marital status, race, and sex, those who carried the most excess weight in the abdominal region had nearly a threefold increased risk that they would be diagnosed with dementia 36 years later.[186]

Why has the world's population become so overweight? There are several contributing factors including what we eat and how much we eat, as well as how many calories we expend. A worldwide negative change in nutrition quality, dramatic globalization of food markets, and economic growth have led to unprecedented access to the very foods most effective at promoting weight gain. The proliferation of high-fat, highly sweetened, calorie-dense foods, including beverages, has made it easier than ever to consume too many calories in a day.[187]

Shopping malls are teeming with snack shops emanating the aromas of freshly baked, calorie-swamped enticements from which only the most self-restrained can turn away. Gas station convenience stores now offer little automotive related merchandise. Instead, they sell a miscellany of hit-and-run, calorie-dense and nutritionally bankrupt snacks and beverages. Even coffee has become a major source of unwanted calories and sugar. Why have a five-calorie, 16-ounce cup of coffee when you can have a Mocha Frappuccino that socks you with 500 calories and 79 grams of sugar? Lest you think you are doing yourself a favor by ordering the healthful-sounding Green Tea Frappuccino at Starbucks, think again. It clocks in at 550 calories—about the same as a McDonald's Big Mac.

Add to this the fact that people are simply moving less and burning fewer calories as they adopt passive activities in their leisure time, harness technology in the home and office, and avoid exercise.[188] Today, less than 22 percent of Americans get the minimum level of daily physical activity recommended by the Centers for Disease Control and Prevention—an all-time low. The national lockdown triggered by the COVID-19 pandemic made things even worse. Quarantine brought stress-induced eating, sedentarism, and thus a further increase in unhealthful weight gain. In an online survey almost half of women and one-quarter of men said they had gained weight during the first months of the lockdown. Other surveys found that candy consumption more than doubled and alcohol consumption (which adds calories) was up 55 percent during this period.[189]

Most problematic, Americans are eating more of the very foods that make weight gain easy and weight loss difficult: fat-laden meat and cheese. The average American consumes 20 percent more calories today than they did in 1983, and according to the United States Department of Agriculture USDA, a significant amount of the additional calorie load is coming from increased meat consumption. In the 1950s an American consumed about 138 pounds of meat in a year. Today that figure has climbed to 222 pounds. Add to that cheese intake, which in the same period went from about 4 pounds per year to 36 pounds per year. In 1980, the average American adult consumed 57 pounds of total fat per year. By 2005 we had reached 85 pounds of fat per year.[190]

How do we calculate whether our weight is healthy or not? I think most of us have an accurate sense of whether we are carrying excess body weight. However, there is a tool with some limitations that you can use. It is not the gold standard and does not measure excess body fat per se, but the body mass index (BMI) offers a rough sense of where one is.* The BMI is a weight-to-height ratio calculated by dividing weight in kilograms by the square of height in meters. Of course, it does not account for above average muscle mass typical in athletes or bone density, nor does it factor in racial or ethnic differences. So, it can be misleading. A BMI of 18.5 to <25 is considered within the healthy range. A BMI of 25.0 to <30 is considered overweight. A BMI of 30.0 or higher indicates obesity.

One reason that excess body weight poses a risk to cognitive health is that fat cells produce inflammatory molecules. So being overweight results in chronic, systemic inflammation that can advance the pathology of neurodegenerative and other diseases.[191] Also, 80 percent of obese individuals are insulin resistant, a threat to the brain we will examine in the next chapter.[192]

---

* BMI can't determine the proportions of fat and lean body mass nor can it determine the location of fat. More precise measurements are obtained through bioelectrical impedance, hydrostatic (under water) weighing, and fat caliper analysis.

A study of 2,200 subjects aged 32-62 found that elevated body weight was linked to lower cognitive scores when tested, and greater cognitive decline five years later.[193]

BEING OVERWEIGHT OR OBESE SHRINKS THE BRAIN FASTER

Another serious problem associated with being overweight is reduced blood flow to the brain.[194] This reduced circulation slowly chokes off oxygen and nutrients from neurons and other cells, which then die off, resulting in a loss of brain mass (brain shrinkage). Excess body fat prevents arteries from expanding to increase blood flow.[195] It also produces inflammatory agents that can enter the brain and boost inflammation, which may increase the risk of Alzheimer's by restricting blood flow and damaging neurons.

In the largest study of its kind, researchers used structural MRI to look at the brains of 9,652 living people and confirmed that as body-weight increases, particularly around the waist, the brain shrinks.[196] Additional imaging studies found that midlife obesity results in loss of total brain volume as well as a reduction in size of the hippocampus, setting the stage for dementia later on.[197] Obesity also specifically causes inflammation in the hippocampus, which may result in damage to and death of neurons in this region.

While everyone will experience some degree of brain shrinkage over time, scientists in Australia have discovered that overweight people are at a greater disadvantage because they have a smaller hippocampus to begin with when compared to those who maintain a healthier bodyweight.[198] And over the years it gets smaller more quickly than in those who maintain a healthy bodyweight. Overweight and obese people are losing brain matter—neurons and synapses—faster than those who maintain a healthier body weight.[199] A study found that *obese individuals have brains that are in effect ten years older than the brains of those who maintain a healthful bodyweight.*[200]

As one becomes overweight, the risk of sleep apnea, a breathing disorder that afflicts people during sleep, increases. With weight gain comes an accumulation of fat in the neck area, including the soft tissue of the mouth and throat. During sleep, the tongue and throat muscles relax, and the soft tissue can cause the airway to become blocked, depriving the brain of adequate oxygen and damaging brain cells.[201]

The more overweight a person is at age 50, the earlier the onset of Alzheimer's tends to be. Using 1,394 volunteers from the Baltimore Longitudinal Study of Aging, Dr. Mahav Thambisetty and colleagues recently showed that midlife obesity could predict when AD would strike. *For each unit increase in the subject's BMI, Alzheimer's disease could be expected to manifest seven months earlier.* [202] Using brain scans while subjects were alive and autopsies at death, the researchers also found that a higher BMI was consistent with the presence of more neurofibrillary tangles and amyloid plaques. [203]

THE TERRIBLE TRIFECTA

While obesity, high blood pressure, and elevated total cholesterol are all independent risk factors for AD, their combined effect is even more potent. Researchers who tracked 1,400 people for up to 20 years found that when individuals had all three of these conditions, they had a six-fold higher risk of developing AD.[204]

SUSTAINED WEIGHT LOSS IS ACHIEVABLE

The positive news is there is a reliable and sustainable way to lose unhealthy bodyweight—but it's not through one of those franchised weight-loss centers you constantly see advertised. Even when calorie consumption is the same, a small study found a plant-based diet results in twice the weight loss as a meat-based diet.[205] In a study that included over 60,000 subjects, researchers found that as more animal-derived foods were added to the diet, bodyweight increased. BMI was lowest for those who avoided all animal products in their diet. For individuals who included eggs and dairy with an otherwise plant-centered diet, BMI was also higher. With the addition of fish, the BMI was higher still. Those who ate meat, dairy, eggs, and fish had the highest BMI of all.[206]

One reason that plant-based nutrition is helpful in maintaining a healthful body weight is that meat and dairy products are calorie dense, whereas plant foods tend to be calorie dilute. One can eat a hearty plant-based meal and feel satisfied and full while consuming significantly fewer calories. Moreover, a study showed that as severely overweight individuals adopt a diet that is rich in plant foods their brain structure improves, as does their attention and memory.[207]

OF COURSE, EXERCISE IS AN IMPORTANT ALLY IN THE EFFORT TO ACHIEVE AND MAINTAIN A HEALTHY BODYWEIGHT.

Although it may seem a tired refrain to some, when you peel away all the marketing gimmicks and games that make up so many commercialized weight-loss programs, the combination of daily exercise and a healthful diet with appropriate caloric intake is the most effective and sustainable way to maintain a healthy weight. Diet and exercise also have been shown to quickly improve insulin sensitivity and even reverse the next risk factor we will look at, diabetes.

8

DIABETES

According to the Center for Disease Control (CDC), which has designated the disease a pandemic, 34 million Americans suffer from diabetes. Almost all of us know someone who has diabetes. The CDC estimates that by 2050 one in three Americans will have developed the disease. One in three! In recent decades, the cost to individual sufferers, their families, and society in general has skyrocketed. A study released by the American Diabetes Association in 2018 showed that the direct and indirect costs of diabetes totaled *327 billion dollars* in the year 2017. The cost in lost production lone was $90 billion, with a further $237 billion in direct medical costs.[208]

Diabetes is a disease characterized by persistent, elevated levels of blood sugar and insulin. It is associated with accelerated brain aging and cognitive impairment, and there is a strong and consistent association between diabetes and risk of Alzheimer's. A diagnosis of diabetes early in life doubles the risk for an Alzheimer's diagnosis later on.[209] Remarkably, more than 80 percent of Alzheimer's patients have either type II diabetes or abnormal serum glucose levels. Diabetes also increases the risk of stroke and heart attack. It can cause peripheral neuropathy, which in turn can lead to limb amputation. And it can result in blindness. Diabetes is truly a frightening disease.

There are two types of diabetes. Type 1 is an autoimmune disease that is irreversible and requires lifetime insulin therapy. It is a rare condition, and in this book we won't be discussing type 1.

Type 2 diabetes, which accounts for 90 to 95 percent of cases in the United States, was once called adult-onset diabetes, but in recent years it has become more common in young people, including teenagers and even younger children. In addition to the over 34 million people who have type 2 diabetes, approximately 88 million more are considered to have prediabetes, a serious condition in which blood sugar levels are above normal though not yet high enough for a diagnosis of diabetes. Tragically, more than 80 percent of people with prediabetes don't even know they have it.

It's obvious that diabetes is a very serious and growing danger for tens of millions of people. What has caused the explosion in the number of cases over the past 30 years? Two changes in lifestyle and behavior have driven the numbers higher: first, an ever-increasing consumption of meat and cheese and sugary drinks and snacks; and second, a sharp decline in physical activity. Many people are eating worse and exercising less, a deadly combination.

The spread of diabetes around the world has resembled a pandemic, but diabetes is not contagious. Fortunately, type 2 diabetes is usually reversible if people make lifestyle changes. As you can probably guess, that means eating better and exercising more. A plant-based diet rich in fresh fruits, legumes, vegetables and whole grains, plus avoiding those sugary drinks and snacks, has been shown to be effective in helping to bring down high levels of blood sugar and restore insulin sensitivity. Combine this with an exercise program (consult your doctor before beginning one) and you can prevent diabetes from crippling or even shortening your life.

WHAT HAPPENS IN DIABETES

To understand diabetes, it helps to understand insulin, a hormone produced in the pancreas. One of its jobs is to usher glucose (blood sugar) from our blood into our muscle cells. Insulin does this by contacting special receptors on cells. If the receptors do not work—a state called *insulin resistance*—the cells ignore the insulin. As a result, glucose, the cell's fuel, can't get in. This leaves cells in danger of dysfunction. Since glucose is unable to enter the muscle cells, the level of glucose in the blood rises. In response, the pancreas makes more insulin to try to overcome the resistance. Over time, the insulin-producing cells of the pancreas can become exhausted, impaired, or even die off.

DIABETES AND THE BRAIN

Although discussions about diabetes generally focus on its effects on muscle cells, it has many serious impacts on the brain. The brain requires a great deal of energy to function, so it must have an ample supply of glucose as fuel. Like insulin resistance in the muscles, insulin resistance can occur in the brain, and not just with obesity and diabetes.

Insulin plays several critical roles in brain health, including regulating learning, short- and long-term memory, protecting neurons, adjusting the strength of neurotransmissions, and supporting synapse functions.[210]

Insulin receptors, distributed in several areas of the brain, are highly concentrated in the hippocampus and cerebral cortex, areas which degenerate early in Alzheimer's disease.[211]

Using PET scans, scientists can see how effectively the brain is metabolizing glucose. In both diabetes and Alzheimer's disease, it's apparent that glucose metabolism becomes impaired.[212] So brain cells are deprived of the fuel they need.

With insulin resistance and diabetes a cascade of destructive events occurs in the brain.[213] First, insulin resistance causes neuroinflammation in the brain, damages brain blood vessels, and thereby reduces blood flow (and oxygen) to the brain and induces oxidative stress, and increases the chance of a stroke.[214] With elevated glucose levels the production and depositing of amyloid and the production of tau tangles is increased.[215]

This is a barrage of trouble for the brain that is detrimental to the ability of neurons to function and significantly heightens the chance of cognitive impairment. A ten-year prospective study of women found that elevated insulin levels were predictive of the rate of cognitive decline. The higher the fasting insulin levels the poorer their memory and cognitive function.[216]

Moreover, elevated blood sugar levels frequently lead to sleep disturbances. With disrupted sleep comes an impairment of the critical brain waste removal operation, the glymphatic system, which takes

place while we sleep and removes amyloid protein and other metabolic waste that can gum up brain function.[217] (More about the role
of sleep later.)

With these pathological changes, memory problems are aggravated
and there is accelerated shrinkage of the hippocampus.[218] When given
neuropsychological tests, those with type 2 diabetes almost universally
show impaired cognitive performance with memory and ability to
learn.[219]

In a study that followed more than 2,000 people for nearly seven years,
researchers found that, even in people *without* diabetes, small increases
in insulin resistance led to a significant increase in risk for dementia in
the future.[220] In another study of more than 5,000 participants over a
ten-year period, researchers found that the higher blood sugar levels
were, the earlier cognitive decline set in.[221] Over a 5-year period, older
adults with diabetes suffered cognitive decline at twice the rate as adults
free of the disease.[222]

HOW DIABETES AFFECTS THE BRAIN	
Increases Neuroinflammation	Accelerates Brain Shrinkage
Increases Oxidative Stress	Decreases Antioxidant Levels
Damages Blood Vessels	Raises Blood Pressure
Deprives Brain Cells of Fuel	Impairs Cognition
Promotes beta-amyloid deposits	

WHAT CAUSES DIABETES IN THE FIRST PLACE?

Type 2 diabetes is the result of a series of events taking place over a period
of many years. Most glaringly, there is a strong association between type
2 diabetes and excess bodyweight.[223] Nearly 90 percent of diabetics are
overweight or obese.[224]

Core to the diabetes problem are the foods we eat. Evidence points to
excessive dietary fat, particularly the saturated fat chiefly found in meat
and dairy products, as highly effective at causing insulin resistance.[225]

When there's too much saturated fat in the diet fat particles build up in muscle cells and block the action of insulin, preventing blood sugar (glucose) from entering cells.[226] These tiny particles of fat that accumulate in the cells are referred to as *intramyocellular lipid*, and can begin accumulating years before there are overt symptoms of diabetes.

Then the vicious cycle begins. The glucose not going into cells will be converted into fat for storage and the fat can begin to accumulate in the liver. The pancreas, meanwhile, releases more insulin into the body to try to overcome resistance and get the glucose into the muscle cells. With more insulin released, more fat gets deposited in the liver. Now chock-full of fat, the liver itself may become insulin resistant.

The buildup of fat in the liver may become so substantial that it causes fatty liver disease (FLD), a condition becoming so prevalent that experts suggest it will affect 50 percent of Americans by 2030.[227] All that fat in the liver then spills over and accumulates in the pancreas cells which then begin having trouble producing the insulin we need. It is saturated fat that is particularly toxic to the insulin-producing *beta cells* of the pancreas.[228]

To summarize: The cascade to diabetes starts with a high saturated fat diet which leads to fat-laden muscle cells, which in turn leads to insulin resistance. Insulin resistance leads to a fatty liver, which leads to a fat-laden pancreas, which leads to damage and dysfunction of insulin-producing cells, and finally, diabetes.

In a joint study from Harvard University and Universitat Rovira i Virgili in Spain, 3,349 participants were tracked for nearly five years. Participants who consumed high levels of saturated fat doubled their risk of developing diabetes over the course of the study compared to those who ate modest amounts. [229]

It's important to keep in mind that one need not have a formal diagnosis of diabetes to have a higher risk of cognitive decline. All it takes is some degree of insulin resistance, which may now affect nearly half the US population.[230] With the resistance comes slowed or lower levels of insulin metabolism in neurons, which may be followed by some degree of cognitive impairment.

DO YOU HAVE PREDIABETES?

Your answers to the following six questions will give you a sense of whether you are likely to be pre-diabetic. Are you male? If so, mark one point on a piece of paper. If you are over the age of 40, add one point; over 50, add two points; over 60, add three points. Do you exercise regularly? If not, add one point. Do any members of your family have diabetes? If so, add one point. Do you have high blood pressure? If so, add another point. If you are a bit overweight, add one point; moderately overweight, add two points; severely overweight, add three points. If you have five or more points, the likelihood that you are pre-diabetic is high and you should see a doctor for a proper diagnosis.

CAN DIABETES BE PREVENTED AND REVERSED?

Dietary intervention can prevent, improve, and even reverse the disease.[231] Essential to healing the body is rooting out the excess saturated fat in the diet. A plant-centered diet reduces total fat and saturated fat and is very effective in helping restore insulin sensitivity.

Back in 1979 scientists found that by placing diabetics on a plant-based diet, their condition improved markedly. Insulin requirements were slashed by 60 percent, and 50 percent of the participants improved so dramatically they were able to stop their insulin therapy.[232] These improvements occurred in just over two weeks and in the absence of any exercise program.

Additionally, several studies found that when participants at risk of developing type 2 diabetes restricted their saturated fat intake, risk was lowered by 50 percent.[233] Adding exercise to the equation further enhances insulin sensitivity and thereby lowers risk.[234]

In addition to substantially reducing saturated fat intake, a plant-based diet also increases the intake of dietary fiber. The presence of higher levels of fiber, particularly the soluble form found in legumes, vegetables and fruits, creates a gel-like substance in the stomach which slows digestion and the absorption of sugars and fats and significantly improves blood glucose control.

Of all foods, meat has the strongest association with risk for type 2 diabetes.[235] A review of 12 major studies showed that the more meat men and women ate, the greater their risk of developing diabetes.[236] In addition to red meat, eating processed meat and fish have both been associated with a greater risk of diabetes.[237] In a study of 18,835 people who were followed for nearly 12 years, researchers determined that for every 50 grams (about the size of the palm of your hand) of meat consumed a day, the risk of diabetes increased by eight percent.[238]

In the Adventist Health Study-2 more than 60,000 subjects were divided into four groups according to what foods they ate: a vegan group (no animal products); vegetarian group (with eggs and milk); "pescatarian" group (vegetarians who ate fish); and omnivores, who ate a conventional diet. Two years later the researchers checked on the participants. The vegans were least at risk for diabetes. Risk went up substantially as eggs, dairy, and fish were added, with the greatest risk found in the omnivores.[239] While vegetarians have a substantially reduced risk of developing diabetes, vegans (those who avoid meat, poultry, fish, and dairy products) reduce their risk by almost 80 percent.[240]

A team of researchers looking at the effectiveness of a plant-based diet reviewed the findings of 11 prior studies. They found that participants who avoided foods derived from animals experienced significant positive changes in blood sugar balance. Participants also saw cholesterol levels drop, blood pressure go down, and some were able to reduce or even eliminate their diabetes medications in just six months.[241]

A plant-centered diet can be helpful both to prevent and to treat diabetes.[242] The American Academy of Nutrition and Dietetics and the American Diabetes Association (ADA) both endorse a plant-based diet for people with diabetes. The ADA states: "Plant-based eating patterns combined with exercise have been found to improve diabetes control and reduce the need for medication in intervention trials as far back as 1976."

This wisdom actually dates back at least to 1930, when physicians writing in the *Journal of the Canadian Medical Association* discussed the effectiveness of a plant-based diet in treating type 2 diabetes.[243] They published this nutritional wisdom again in 1935.[244] Yet here we are, 87 years later, and this information is still not well known in medicine.

YES, EXERCISE IS A MAJOR FACTOR

Dietary changes alone are powerfully effective for both preventing and treating diabetes. Adding exercise to the equation offers the best chance for long-term success. There's no question that inactivity advances insulin resistance. When we exercise, certain molecules are produced that enhance insulin sensitivity. A single session of moderate intensity aerobic exercise has been shown to enhance insulin action, increasing glucose uptake by 40 percent.[245] There's a dose-response effect. So longer sessions and greater exercise intensity result in greater insulin sensitivity.[246] Robust aerobic exercise also helps promote glucose metabolism in the brain, which simply means that your brain cells can make energy and perform their functions.[247] Combined, diet and exercise can be more effective at managing diabetes than insulin therapy alone.[248]

Conversely, just sitting in front of the TV a few hours a day increases insulin resistance and the risk of developing diabetes. In a study that tracked over 3,000 participants, scientists learned that for each hour spent watching TV, risk of developing diabetes increased by 3.4 percent.[249] Clearly, we need to move our bodies if we wish to keep diabetes at bay!

Insulin resistance and type II diabetes are preventable and reversible. As such, these are Alzheimer's risk factors that can be taken out of play.

9

HIGH SATURATED FAT INTAKE

W E KNOW THAT diets high in saturated fat speed up cognitive decline[250] and substantially increase risk for Alzheimer's disease.[251] Despite their concern over the risk for dementia, Americans are consuming more saturated fat now than ever before.[252]

In terms of Alzheimer's disease risk factors, there is little that excessive saturated fat does not make worse. In the last chapter we learned about the potent role saturated fat plays in elevating the risk of diabetes. We also learned about saturated fat's role in raising cholesterol levels. Higher cholesterol levels are associated with greater risk of AD. In addition, too much saturated fat also increases oxidative stress and inflammation, boosts production of amyloid protein, hampers clearance of amyloid protein from the brain, increases blood pressure, and promotes clogged arteries.[253]

The Chicago Health and Aging Project, a longitudinal study of aging and dementia with 6,000 subjects from three neighborhoods in Chicago, found that people who consumed the most daily saturated fat had more than three times the risk of developing AD than those who ate the least.[254] Several other studies have shown the same thing—a higher intake of saturated fat is linked with a two- to three-fold increase in the risk of dementia.[255] Yet a diet rich in saturated fat does more than increase risk for AD. A four-year study of more than 6,000 dementia-free women found that those who consumed the most saturated fat showed a decline in cognition equivalent to six years of aging.[256]

Excess saturated fat also suppresses the production of brain-derived neurotrophic factor (BDNF).[257] BDNF, which we will look at more closely later, is involved in the production, survival, growth, and maintenance of neurons; it promotes brain plasticity; and it plays a role in memory formation.[258] Suffice it to say for now that when it comes to protecting brain function, BDNF is an important ally.

In one study, participants were placed on diets composed of either low or high levels of saturated fat, but the same number of calories. In those placed on the high saturated fat diet, levels of amyloid protein in cerebrospinal fluid rose. Those on the low saturated fat diet saw levels of amyloid protein drop. This change occurred in just four weeks. The researchers who conducted the study noted that the higher levels of saturated fat hampered the body's ability to clear amyloid from the brain, possibly increasing the likelihood that it would then be deposited as plaques and thereby damage neurons.[259]

HIGH SATURATED FAT FOODS REDUCE BLOOD FLOW TO THE BRAIN

In another study, Vincent Lee and colleagues at the University of Calgary measured the blood flow in 20 otherwise healthy university students. The students were then fed two popular fast-food breakfast sandwiches composed of eggs, ham, and cheese on a bun. The sandwiches contained a substantial load of saturated fat.

The researchers then measured the flow in the subject's blood vessels. Within two hours of eating this meal, the students experienced a 15 to 20 percent reduction in blood flow.[260] Their blood had become more viscous. Perhaps this is why cognitive function has been shown to be temporarily compromised after just one meal high in saturated fat.[261]

MORE FAT, LESS BRAIN TALK

A saturated fat-laden diet can also compromise the ability of neurons to talk to one another by interfering with the release of neurotransmitters.[262] As more saturated fat is incorporated into cell membranes, they become less fluid and more rigid, the neurotransmitters cannot move as they should, and the cell itself cannot acquire sufficient oxygen and nutrients.[263] This blocked communication can lead to dysfunction in neurons and, eventually, their death.

The top sources of saturated fat in the American diet are cheese, pizza, other dairy products, and meat.[264] Dramatically reducing and ideally eliminating foods rich in saturated fat will help restore blood flow to the brain, lower cholesterol levels, and improve insulin sensitivity. The reduction in saturated fat will also slash levels of inflammation and oxidative stress, and foster more effective brain waste removal. There are so many benefits to avoiding a pepperoni pizza that it's a *no brainer*.

10
TRANS FAT
A FAT TO FORGET

JUST OVER 100 YEARS ago, Dr. Wilhelm Normann filed a patent for his novel process of converting liquid vegetable oils into solid fat. It's called hydrogenation and from it were born trans fats. Normann could not possibly have imagined the public health disaster his innovation would bring. Trans fats deserve all the bad press they've received. Even a moderate intake of this worst of all fats has been shown to triple the risk for AD; for those who consume the greatest levels of these man-made fats, the risk can be five times higher.[265]

Hydrogenated oils are a food manufacturer's dream because they extend the life of processed baked goods and give them a particularly rich mouthfeel, like butter. In packaged foods, the following ingredient terms indicate the presence of trans fat: hydrogenated oil, partially hydrogenated oil, margarine, shortening, and vegetable shortening.

FOODS CONTAINING TRANS FATS			
Biscuits	Butter-like spreads	Cake mixes	Chips
Chicken nuggets	Cookies	Cookie mixes	Some flour tortillas
French fries	Frosting	Pizza crust (commercial)	Gravy mixes
Instant soup	Margarine	Non-dairy creamers	Roasted nuts
Onion rings	Pie crust	Vegetable shortening	Tempura

And trans fats are in many commonly eaten foods—not just those that contain hydrogenated oils. They are found in donuts, French fries, fried onion rings, and many commercially available pastries, pies and baked goods, nondairy creamers, fast foods, microwave popcorn, as well as just about anything fried or battered.

A study conducted by the CDC showed that even vigilant Americans may be eating more trans fats than they think. In its survey of 4,300 common packaged foods, the CDC found that 84 percent of those containing trans fats stated "0 trans fats" on the packing. Food manufacturers get away with this because, unconscionably, the FDA permits the misleading "0 trans fats" claim if a food contains .5 grams or less per serving.[266] By specifying a smaller serving size, many more food products can get away with this deceptive practice. Moreover, the FDA has conceded that it withdrew a proposal that would require food manufacturers to place a footnote on their products' ingredient labels that would read, "Intake of trans fat should be as low as possible." Given the very serious threat trans fats pose to consumer health, it seems reasonable advice from the government agency whose job is to protect us from unhealthful foods and drugs. Yet the FDA was persuaded to change its mind. "We received very negative comments on the wording of this footnote," they say in their online report.[267] Therefore, they dropped the idea. Perhaps you can imagine from whom those comments came.

DECEPTIVE AND DEADLY

From the perspective of Alzheimer's disease risk, trans fats are highly troublesome in several ways. They clog up blood vessels and restrict blood flow to the brain,[268] promote inflammation,[269] damage the lining of blood vessels, promote oxidative stress and insulin resistance.[270]

Trans fats also get integrated into brain cell membranes and adversely affect memory by interfering with the ability of brain cells to produce energy and to communicate with neighboring cells. So lots of trans fats means less energy for the brain and compromised brain function. And we know where that leads—right toward cognitive decline and, potentially, Alzheimer's disease. French fries or any other trans-fat—containing food just aren't worth the danger.

AND WAIT, IT GETS WORSE

At Oregon Health and Science University, Dr. Gene Bowman and colleagues took blood samples from elderly subjects in the Oregon Brain Aging Study to see what kinds of fats were in their blood. Then they gave them cognitive assessment tests and performed MRI scans of their brains. Not only did the subjects who had the most trans fats in their blood perform more poorly on the cognition tests, they also had the smallest brains. Accelerated shrinking of the brain is a known feature of Alzheimer's disease.

There is nothing good to say about trans fats and their effect on our health. In addition to the risk they pose to brain health, trans fats are also a major risk factor for cardiovascular disease and diabetes. Since the Institute of Medicine states that there is no safe intake level for trans fats, this is not something to think about reducing or limiting to special occasions—your goal should be to get rid of trans fats entirely.

11

ELEVATED HOMOCYSTEINE

HOMOCYSTEINE WAS A hot topic in public health in the 1990s, when its relationship to the risk of heart disease and stroke was discovered. Soon enough homocysteine fell off the radar screen, but its threat to health is no less serious today—not only to cardiovascular health, but to brain health.

Homocysteine is an amino acid normally created when the protein we eat is metabolized. It's derived from the breakdown of methionine, an amino acid concentrated in animal products. If we consume animal-based foods and our diet is deficient in leafy greens and legumes, homocysteine will likely rise. Evidence shows that higher homocysteine levels are predictive of cognitive decline and indicate an elevated risk of Alzheimer's.[271] Reports indicate about a doubling of risk of dementia in those who have elevated homocysteine levels.[272]

Writing in the *New England Journal of Medicine*, researchers reported that in a study of more than 1,000 subjects, homocysteine levels were measured at baseline and then again in eight years. People who had the highest homocysteine levels at the start of the study were twice as likely to develop AD compared with those who had the lowest levels.[273]

Even without an Alzheimer's diagnosis, as homocysteine levels rise, cognitive function is impaired. There are a couple of reasons why this may be so. First, elevated homocysteine promotes oxidative stress.[274] It's also associated with accelerated shrinking of the brain.[275] In a ten-year study that used both MRI and autopsy, people who maintained the highest levels of homocysteine had up to three times the amount of brain atrophy compared to those with the lowest homocysteine levels.[276]

In another study, nearly 2,200 men and women took a cognitive exam and had their blood levels of homocysteine, folate, and vitamin B12 measured. Six years later the participants repeated the process. If homocysteine levels had risen over the six-year period, cognitive test performance declined. But if homocysteine levels had dropped, there was a notable improvement in those participants' test performance.[277]

In one study, a supplement containing B6/B12/folic acid was shown to cut homocysteine levels and reduce brain shrinkage markedly. In this randomized controlled trial neither the subjects nor the scientists knew who was receiving the B vitamins and who was receiving a placebo. At the start, the subjects had their homocysteine levels measured and their brain volume determined. At the end of a two-year period, both were measured again. The subjects who took the supplement saw a 22.5 percent drop in homocysteine levels and a 30 percent reduction of shrinkage compared to the placebo group.[278]

HOW TO KEEP HEALTHY LEVELS OF HOMOCYSTEINE

Elevated homocysteine may indicate a deficiency of vitamins B12, B6, or folate. In the case of preserving brain volume and cognitive function, a B-complex vitamin supplement is a prudent strategy. Yet it is also worth noting that elevated homocysteine is associated with the Western diet—rich in fatty meats and dairy and sorely lacking in the foods that help keep homocysteine in check. Foods that contain folate and vitamin B6—broccoli, black beans, spinach, asparagus, pistachios, pinto beans, leafy greens, beets, and avocado—also contain many other protective compounds that are important to cognitive health. They are rich in antioxidants and anti-inflammatory compounds and thus should be our first line of defense. Vitamin B12 is found in many fortified non-dairy beverages, but if you a choose to eat a diet free of animal products be sure to obtain the vitamin through a supplement.

Homocysteine levels can be checked through a simple blood test that ideally is included with your annual physical. Normal homocysteine levels range between 5–15 micromoles/liter.

12

FOODS THAT RAISE AD RISK

ACCORDING TO THE most comprehensive study available, the greatest risk for chronic diseases is found in what we eat.[279] In fact, diet-driven diseases are the leading killers in the US.[280] Yet people are invariably surprised to learn that diet can play a role in their risk of Alzheimer's.

As you have already read, many of the major risk factors for AD, including cardiovascular disease, diabetes, high blood pressure, trans fat, and obesity, are tightly linked to our food choices. The standard American diet—known, after all, as SAD—appears to contribute mightily to cognitive decline and greatly heighten the risk of Alzheimer's.[281]

Beginning in the last half of the 20th century, Asia saw a dramatic rise in chronic degenerative diseases—including Alzheimer's. Why were people previously protected from chronic disease now at much higher risk? Major changes in lifestyle, especially diet, were the culprits.

In Japan, for example, where people previously enjoyed one of the longest life expectancies in the world, the consumption of meat rose sevenfold and consumption of other animal products rose fourfold between 1960 and 1985.[282] In that same period, alcohol consumption quadrupled and the consumption of rice, a staple of the Japanese diet, dropped by nearly 50 percent.[283] Not only did rates of heart disease and cancer begin to climb in this period, but the incidence of Alzheimer's disease also rose sevenfold.[284]

Virtually anywhere one looks in the world this pattern occurs. As nations become increasingly urbanized and more wealth is generated, people tend to adopt a Western diet rich in meat, dairy, trans fats, salt, sugar, along with higher alcohol consumption. Invariably, this change is followed by climbing rates of disabling diseases they were formerly protected from, including diseases of the brain.

Yet too many people have failed to respond to this connection. Every day, 68 million Americans consume food from McDonald's—most of which is full of trans fat, excessive sodium, saturated fat, and cholesterol—the very things that contribute to the risk of dementia. This kind of food is also devoid of the nutrients that are protective.[285] Nearly the entire US population fails to meet the basic recommended intake of various nutrients to prevent disease. For whole grains, 99 percent of us fail to make the cut. For fiber, 97 percent of us miss the boat. For leafy greens intake, as well as legumes consumption, 96 percent do not eat what is required, while 88 percent of us do not eat enough vegetables and 79 percent don't meet the recommended intake for fruits.[286]

THE WESTERN DIET CAUSES SYSTEMIC INFLAMMATION

There is ample evidence that a diet centered upon animal products raises levels of systemic inflammation both because of an absence of anti-inflammatory elements and the presence of pro-inflammatory ones. Studies have shown that as the level of fat in the diet rises, so do indicators of neuroinflammation in the brain. As inflammation rises, neurons become dysfunctional, synapses become impaired, and ultimately neurons may be lost.[287] Also, systemic inflammation impairs the flow of cerebrospinal fluid (CSF), which can disrupt the removal of metabolic waste—including beta-amyloid—from the brain.

Tanzanians offer another example of the benefits of a plant-based diet versus the Western diet. A period of rapid urbanization is occurring in Tanzania and many other parts of Africa where residents are moving from the countryside into expanding cities. A research team from Radboud Medical Center in the Netherlands found that Tanzanians who remain in the countryside and maintain a traditional diet generally have low levels of inflammation.[288] But their urban-dwelling counterparts who have settled in cities like Moshi, for example, and begun eating higher levels of foods rich in saturated fat and cholesterol, as well as processed convenience foods, have markedly increased levels of inflammation. The traditional diet of rural Tanzanians is rich in whole grains, fruits, and vegetables—foods, as we have seen, that are low in saturated fat, contain no cholesterol, and are rich in flavonoids and other protective substances that help keep inflammation levels under control.

If you are presently following a conventional Western diet, don't despair. Adopting a plant-based diet can significantly reduce levels of inflammation in just four weeks.[289]

THE WESTERN DIET SHRINKS THE BRAIN

As we have seen, some loss in brain volume appears inevitable with age. However, in Alzheimer's the loss is premature and dramatic, particularly in the hippocampus.

It turns out that the foods we eat are strongly associated with the size of our brain. Those whose diets are rich in plant foods have significantly greater brain volume.[290]

A team of researchers decided to look at the role of diet in the loss of brain volume over time. They divided 2,500 participants into groups by diet. Then they used MRI technology to measure the volume of each subject's hippocampus. Four years later, the researchers re-imaged the participants' brains to measure changes in hippocampal volume. *Those whose diets were centered upon burgers, roasted meat, chips, soft drinks, and sausage lost the greatest brain volume over the four-year time period.* By contrast, those who followed a diet rich in fresh fruits, vegetables, and especially leafy greens, had the least amount of brain shrinkage.[291]

So, we can preserve brain volume by making smart dietary choices.

I suspect that if scientists were to produce MRI images of the brains of the centenarians (those who live to be 100 or more) of Okinawa they would find similarly or better retained brain volume. The Okinawans typically eat seven different (inflammation-fighting) fruits and vegetables a day. And not only do many of them live to age 100, almost two-thirds of Okinawa's residents are functioning well cognitively and living independently at age 97.[292]

DON'T BE A MEATHEAD

In the 1970s sitcom *All in the Family*, Archie Bunker nicknamed his son-in-law "Meathead" because he felt he was incapable of understanding the truths of life as Archie saw them. Archie was no student of epidemiology, but his insult shines a light on the connection between meat consumption and brain function. Today, scores of studies affirm that a diet centered upon meat is risky when it comes to brain health and function.[293] In one such study of Alzheimer's risk and dietary choices covering 12 countries, meat consumption was shown to pose the highest risk, followed by the consumption of eggs and fish.[294]

Remember Dr. Ellsworth Wareham from Chapter 5? In addition to dodging the number-one killer of Americans, cardiovascular disease, he was still mentally sharp at age 104. The doctor was emphatic that in addition to his high level of daily physical activity, his plant-based diet was responsible for his remarkable mental acuity.

After epidemiologist Dr. William B. Grant and colleagues compared dietary choices with rates of Alzheimer's in ten countries, he stated, "Mounting evidence from ecological and observational studies, as well as studies of mechanisms, indicates that the Western dietary pattern—especially the large amount of meat in that diet—is strongly associated with risk of developing Alzheimer's disease and several other chronic diseases."[295]

Because they are known for their healthy lifestyle and the fact that, on average, they live 10 years longer than the average American, Seventh Day Adventists are often recruited to participate in studies on nutrition. Many, but not all, Seventh Day Adventists follow a diet free of meat, poultry, and fish, and some avoid dairy products as well. A team of researchers decided to look at whether there is any difference in risk of developing AD between Adventists who eat meat and those who avoid it. They discovered that Adventist meat-eaters were up to three times more likely to develop AD compared to their vegetarian counterparts.[296]

In another study of individuals with and without AD, researchers gathered information about the foods the individuals consumed most frequently. Those who had developed AD had a high intake of meat, butter, high-fat dairy products, eggs, and refined sugars. The individuals who remained free of Alzheimer's disease had a high intake of grains and vegetables.[297] Starting to see a pattern here?

Let's look more closely at the problems with meat as the centerpiece of a person's diet. To start with, meat boosts inflammation levels and risk of metabolic syndrome, which is a cluster of several of the serious concerns we looked at earlier: high blood pressure, insulin resistance, excess body fat, and elevated cholesterol levels.[298] A meat-centered diet is also a high-fat diet, and fat is easily oxidized, leading to the production of more free radicals. However, I want to share several other reasons why meat consumption may boost the risk of Alzheimer's disease. Get ready for more long words we may not use in conversation—but may be lifesaving to understand.

INTRODUCING NITROSAMINES AND POLYAROMATIC HYDROCARBONS

Nitrosamines are a class of chemicals that include nitrates and nitrites. These substances are used as preservatives and color stabilizers in processed (luncheon) meats, bacon, sausage, smoked/salted fish, some cheese, and certain beers. Although these compounds have long been known to be human carcinogens, the FDA continues to permit their use in the food supply. [299]

Recent research has found that nitrosamine intake is associated with Alzheimer's disease and other neurodegenerative diseases.[300] Exposure to nitrosamines not only causes impairment of a cell's ability to make energy, but also causes oxidative stress and insulin resistance,[301] disrupts the production of neurotransmitters, and causes DNA damage.[302]

Polyaromatic hydrocarbons (PAH) are carcinogenic compounds formed in beef, pork, chicken, and fish during high-temperature cooking, such as pan frying or open-flame grilling, or in smoking. PAHs cause oxidative stress, increase inflammation, and are associated with a higher risk of obesity.[303]

AGES

Another bad actor that can be elevated by the Western diet is advanced-glycation end-products (AGEs), also known as glycotoxins. Like the production of free radicals, the production of AGEs is a normal part of metabolism that our body can manage. However, when levels become highly elevated in the body, AGEs can take on a pathogenic role.

These compounds promote inflammation, oxidative stress, and arterial stiffness, and are associated with atherosclerosis, diabetes, and Alzheimer's disease.[304] AGEs have been found at elevated levels in the Alzheimer's brain, both in amyloid plaques and tau tangles and may even stimulate beta-amyloid production.[305] In experiments with healthy humans, a higher intake of AGEs shows an increase in markers for oxidative stress and inflammation. Conversely, when AGE-rich foods are restricted, markers for inflammation and oxidative stress go down.[306]

Generally, AGEs are highest in high-fat, high protein foods of animal origin, aged cheese, processed vegetable oils (we'll return to oils a bit later), and spreads rich in fat, including butter, margarine, cream cheese, and mayonnaise. Levels of AGEs increase with grilling, broiling, roasting, and frying.[307] They are lowest in fruits, vegetables, legumes and whole grains. The formation of additional AGEs can be further reduced when acidic marinades that include lemon and vinegar are used in cooking.

SATURATED FAT

Let's take another look at saturated fat. As we know, a meat- and dairy-centered diet is high in saturated fat, which promotes oxidative stress and inflammation, insulin resistance, and arterial plaque. As noted, a higher intake of saturated fat throughout adulthood is associated with poorer cognitive function, impaired memory, and a significantly greater likelihood of developing dementia.[308]

Harvard researchers looked at the relationship between dietary fat intake and the risk of AD by studying 6,000 elderly participants in the Women's Health Study. They found that saturated fat specifically was associated with poorer overall cognition and verbal memory. The women who consumed the most saturated fat were 60 to 70 percent more likely to perform worse on cognitive tests when measured four years later.[309] *The researchers concluded that the women who consumed the least saturated fat had brain function comparable to women six years younger.*

IRON

Another concern with a meat-entered diet is iron. I can imagine you may be thinking to yourself, *wait a second, iron is important, and many people are deficient!* I recall as a child hearing repeatedly how important iron is for a strong and healthy body. Popeye, the cartoon character, drove the point home. He'd demonstrate that his heroic, extraordinary strength was the direct result of the iron he gained from consuming cans of spinach. In fact, Popeye is credited with increasing US spinach sales by 33 percent during the 1930s, largely due to equating iron with muscular strength. The fact that spinach is not even a substantial source of iron did not matter. The association was formed. Popeye was, in fact, heroic—at marketing.

There are two sides to the "iron coin." It is an essential component of hemoglobin, which enables the transport of oxygen in blood, and it's also involved in the health and maintenance of cells and many other processes. Yet because it's highly reactive and prone to oxidation, too much iron can easily boost oxidative stress and damage to cells. Elevated iron in the brain is a feature of Alzheimer's and other neurological diseases. As far back as 1953 the accumulation of iron in the Alzheimer's brain was noted.[310] It's been shown that increased levels of iron correlate with the rate of cognitive decline in dementia. When iron accumulates in the brain it can damage the fats in brain cell membranes, mitochondria, and oxidize cholesterol and encourage it to clog up arteries.

The body can better regulate the absorption of non-heme iron, the type of iron found in plants, to prevent overload. When iron levels are low, it allows more to be absorbed. When iron levels are sufficient, it reduces absorption. However, heme iron, the predominant type of iron found in meat (blood), is not well regulated, is readily absorbed, and can accumulate to an unhealthful level in the body.

A team of researchers conducted a study to see if subjects with Alzheimer's fared any better with less iron in their bodies. They divided their subjects into two groups. One would receive no intervention while the other would receive a chelating agent twice daily, five days a week, for 24 months.[311] The chelation agent is a molecule that bonds with and holds on to iron (or other heavy metals), helping the body to excrete excesses. The subjects who received no treatment deteriorated twice as fast as the subjects who received the chelation therapy.[312] Noteworthy is that Parkinson's patients given chelation therapy to reduce iron levels in the early stages of the disease have shown improvement in motor activity.[313]

Although some degree of iron accumulation seems inevitable with age, the point here is that, given the serious destructive potential of iron overload, it seems prudent to take whatever steps we can to avoid the accumulation of excess iron.

With a plant-based diet you can easily meet your iron requirements with less of a concern for iron-overload. Other steps to help avoid iron excess? Avoiding cooking in cast-iron pans because food will absorb iron from the cooking surface. Unless you have been directed by your physician to do otherwise, if you take supplements choose iron-free products.

SUMMARY OF RISKS PRESENTED BY A MEAT-CENTERED DIET

Multiple studies, including those that followed hundreds of thousands of subjects for up to 24 years, have reported that diets that derive protein from animal products are associated with an increased risk for cancer, cardiovascular disease, and overall mortality.[314] Meat-based diets contain saturated fat and cholesterol, both of which contribute to raising blood cholesterol levels. As we saw in Chapter 5, high blood cholesterol is associated with greater risk for AD pathology. Meat promotes inflammation, is low in protective antioxidants, devoid of protective fiber, and tends to have higher concentrations of environmental contaminants such as pesticides, dioxin, and phthalates. If you are determined to protect your brain health, let alone your cardiovascular health, I hope you will keep in mind these serious concerns.

BE WARY OF DAIRY

Although the once popular notion that humans need the milk of cows to achieve and sustain bone health has fallen out of favor, for many the dairy habit is still deeply ingrained.

If you think about it, consuming the milk of a cow is truly odd behavior. In addition to humans, 5,400 mammalian species make milk for their offspring. In every case, milk is nutritionally unique to meet the needs of the species.

Because milk drinking appears to be a gateway to numerous health problems, it's critical to extinguish the milk-drinking-equals-fracture-resistant-bones myth so we can look at the bigger picture of concerns. Worldwide, the highest rates of bone fracture tend to be in nations where the *most* dairy and calcium is consumed.

Dubbed "the world's most influential nutritionist" by the *Boston Globe*, Walter Willett, M.D., MPH, D.PH., has shared his researched opinion about the usefulness of drinking milk. Dr. Willett has published over 2,000 original research papers and reviews, and serves as the chair of the Department of Nutrition at Harvard's School of Public Health. He cautions, "Consuming plenty of dairy products is being portrayed as a key way to prevent osteoporosis and broken bones. But not only does this fail to fit the bill as a proven prevention strategy, it doesn't even come close." He also states, "Dairy products shouldn't occupy a prominent place in our diet, nor should they be the centerpiece of the national strategy to prevent osteoporosis."[315]

One of the most provocative studies of milk drinking and bone health came from one of the largest examinations of risk for chronic disease in women. Starting in 1976 and ongoing today, the Harvard Nurses Health Study is in its third generation. Study number one involved 78,000 nurses aged 34 to 59. These subjects provided a detailed report of the foods they ate regularly. Then they were followed for 12 years to see who suffered bone fractures. The women who consumed three or more glasses of milk per day had no less risk of fracture than those who drank little or no milk.[316]

Aside from the bone health factor, there are other concerns associated with drinking cow's milk. In one study of 61,433 women and 45,339 men who were tracked for between 11 and 20 years, those who drank milk had higher levels of blood markers for oxidative stress and inflammation. With higher intakes of milk, the men in the study were found to have a higher risk of death in the study period.[317] The greater risk of death could be related to the fact that dairy is the number-one source of artery-clogging saturated fat in the human diet. Cow's milk is the primary source of d-galactose, a compound that has been shown to promote oxidative stress and chronic inflammation, may pose a risk to neuron health, and is believed to advance aging and generally shorten life span.[318] Several studies have found an association between milk drinking and a higher risk of Parkinson's disease and metastatic prostate cancer.[319]

On its website the EPA states, "Milk fat is likely to be among the highest dietary sources of exposure to persistent, bioaccumulative, and toxic (PBT) contaminants," and goes on to note 11 chemicals that have been found in milk above prescribed limits.[320] We should do everything possible to avoid exposure to such substances.

When I speak of milk, I'm also referring to all the products made from it, including butter, cream, yogurt, ice cream, and, of course, irresistible (and seemingly addictive) cheese. Americans are particularly big cheese consumers, with most of us taking in 36 pounds of the stuff a year. What, no grilled cheese sandwiches? I realize that some people find parting ways with cheese to be a major challenge. A lifetime of cheeseburgers, mac n' cheese, grilled cheese sandwiches, and cheese pizzas can leave one wondering how they will possibly navigate the culinary terrain ahead. A key motivator is remaining cognizant of how unhealthful cheese is for you. But there are healthier options to help wean you away. If it is any consolation, I have served non-dairy grilled cheese sandwiches to the most ardent cheese lovers who never suspected they weren't eating the real thing. I'll discuss this more later.

EGGS ARE NOT ALL THEY'RE CRACKED UP TO BE

Eggs are the most concentrated sources of dietary cholesterol, with about 187mg in a large egg. That's more cholesterol than contained in a fast-food double cheeseburger. The official word on egg consumption has changed from decade to decade, leaving many confused. Since Americans are eating significantly more eggs than they did just five years ago, let's clear the air. Can anyone tell us definitively whether eggs are friend or foe?

Why has the status of eggs in the American diet been unclear for so long? Some blame goes to the findings of conflicting short-term studies. Some may also go to the egg industry. According to the United Egg Producers, there's an estimated 328 million hens at work laying eggs for Americans. Each hen lays about 290 eggs per year. This produces about 79 billion dozen eggs annually.

For years, federal dietary guidelines suggested that a person not exceed 300 mg of cholesterol a day. That left little room for eggs in a prudent diet. The average American now eats 289 eggs per year—33 more eggs than they did in 2015, the year that the U.S. Dietary Guidelines loosened up on cholesterol recommendations, and more eggs than we have in decades. [321]

First, in some but not all people, eating an egg raises their bad (LDL) blood cholesterol levels by about five points. Should those of us whose blood cholesterol levels are not affected by eating eggs consume them with abandon? Not according to the *Harvard University Health Letter*. It recently advised, "No more than three eggs per week is wise if you have diabetes, are at high risk for heart disease from other causes (such as smoking), or already have heart disease."[322] This would apply to the 34 million Americans with diabetes and, according to the American Heart Association, the 48 percent of American adults with some form of cardiovascular disease.[323]

In 2019, a new study looked more closely at the results of six previously published studies and examined the effect of egg consumption in 30,000 Americans. The study was prospective, meaning it looked at the health outcomes in people over time, from 10 to 30 years. The results? Eating just half an egg a day raised one's risk of suffering a heart attack, stroke, or early death by 6 percent to 8 percent when compared to those who ate no eggs at all. An egg a day raised the risk to 12 percent. Two eggs per day amounted to a 24 percent increased risk.[324]

Studies have shown that eggs are routinely found to contain up to nine pesticide residues, which are concentrated in the yolk.[325] Let's remember what the National Institute of Medicine has already advised; individuals should "eat as little cholesterol as possible."[326] The good news is that it's possible to eat zero cholesterol since our body manufactures all the cholesterol it needs.

If you enjoy baking and wonder how you will do so without eggs, you will be pleased to know that there are egg substitutes, such as Bob's Red Mill Egg Replacer, for just this purpose. More about this later.

A FISHY STORY

Inevitably, you have encountered articles asserting that eating fish is essential to a healthful diet. The standard claim is that eating fish will protect you from cardiovascular disease (heart attacks, strokes, and other heart irregularities) and improve brain function. The question of whether today's catch is healthful to consume is an important and widely misunderstood topic.

Today, fish consumption worldwide is at an all-time high. In 2018, 94 million tons of sea life —greater than the weight of the entire human population—was removed from the world's oceans.[327] Yet *USA Today* and many other sources suggest that Americans should eat even more.[328] Both the widespread belief in the dietary necessity of fish and the assumption of its inherent health and safety need to be examined.

The heavy public promotion of fish, particularly salmon, may have its roots in the 1970s research on the Greenland Eskimos, who had a relatively low incidence of cardiovascular disease. The idea that eating fish might be protective derived from the fact that cold-water fatty fish contain essential omega-3 fats. Omega-3 fats are polyunsaturated fats that go by the tongue-twisting names *alpha-linolenic acid* (ALA), which is found in plant foods; and *eicosapentaenoic acid* (EPA) and *docosahex-aenoic acid* (DHA), which are found in fish and shellfish. DHA is one of the building blocks of brain tissue, protects neurons, and is important to the health of cell membranes throughout the body.[329] It was theorized that these fats help reduce the risk of arterial plaque, blood clots, and stroke, and might also possibly lower blood pressure.

The theory that fish eating might reduce the risk of negative cardiovascular events quickly got traction, and soon the American Heart Association was recommending fish consumption two times per week. The truth, however, is that the research findings were inconsistent. While some studies showed a benefit, more showed no benefit.

To clear up the confusion, a 2006 meta-analysis distilled the findings of 48 prior studies and concluded there was no clear cardiovascular benefit from eating fish. Six years later, another meta-analysis of 14 prior randomized, double-blind, placebo-controlled studies (the gold standard of studies) involving over 20,000 patients with cardiovascular disease reported that there was "no significant preventive effect" for stroke, heart attack, or heart failure from eating fish.[330] The authors of a more recent study concluded: "Omega-3 PUFA (polyunsaturated fatty acid) supplementation was not associated with a lower risk of all-cause mortality, cardiac death, sudden death, myocardial infarction, or stroke."[331]

It is important to remember that cardiovascular disease is not caused by a lack of fish oil in the diet. Rather, it's caused chiefly by a diet rich in artery-clogging saturated fat, trans fats, cholesterol, lack of physical activity, and smoking. So it may be unreasonable to expect that adding fish to the diet will ameliorate the problems caused by these risk factors.

Heavy Metal is More Than Rock and Roll

But does fish consumption nonetheless protect or improve cognitive function? In her San Francisco practice, Dr. Jane Hightower studied her own patients who frequently consumed fish, and her findings were distressing. The patients paid a heavy price, one that underscores the current danger of eating fish: heavy metal poisoning. (More on Dr. Hightower's findings in Chapter 16). Among the most common and dangerous of these metals is methylmercury, a potent neurotoxin that also poses a risk to the lungs, kidneys, and immune system. More than 80 percent of the US population's exposure to mercury comes from seafood, and 40 percent of it comes from just fresh fish and canned tuna.[332]

A similar finding to what Dr. Hightower discovered in her patients came from health-conscious corporate executives residing in Florida. These individuals generally consumed three to four servings of fish *per month*. Forty-three percent of those tested had mercury levels that exceeded the EPA suggested limit. While some did show a cognitive edge over non-fish-eating counterparts, that benefit disappeared as their mercury levels rose. The more fish these individuals ate per week, the higher their levels of mercury. Compared to matched individuals with low levels of mercury, those who had the highest mercury levels suffered nearly a 5 percent reduction in brain function.[333] And virtually all fish have measurable levels of mercury.[334]

A study from Harvard researchers found that mercury levels in fish are rising. For example, mercury levels in samples of Atlantic bluefin tuna rose 3.6 percent per year between 2012 and 2017.[335] According to the United Nations Environment Program, global mercury emissions rose 20 percent between 2010 and 2015, so one can expect mercury accumulation in fish and the environment in general to continue to rise. Worsening the problem, in 2020 the United States Federal Government elected to further loosen regulation on industrial mercury releases.[336] And, in addition to mercury, the heavy metals arsenic, cadmium, and lead are also frequently present in fish.

Poisonous Companions

Metals are not the only contaminant in fish. The world's oceans have truly become the great invisible dumping ground. Each year, the cruise and cargo ship industries discharge an estimated 80 million gallons of oil bilge water and untreated human waste into the oceans. In 2020, University of South Florida researchers tested more than 2,000 fish from the Gulf of Mexico and found oil contamination in the flesh of every single one.[337] Then there's the poorly regulated effluent from mining operations, some of which may release up to 160,000 tons of toxic sludge into the ocean through discharge pipes or offshore dumping *every day*.[338] The long list of pollutants found in fish today includes antibiotics, arsenic, cadmium, pesticides, flame retardants, lead, PCBs, prescription drugs, formaldehyde, solvents, dioxin, and a substantial amount of microplastics.[339]

What? Plastic? I'm afraid so. According to the United Nations, eight million metric tons of plastic (equivalent to the weight of nearly 90 aircraft carriers) is discarded into the world's oceans annually, adding to the 150 million tons and 15 trillion pieces estimated to already be in the sea.[340] At this rate, it's estimated that by 2050 the seas could contain more plastic than fish.[341] In the ocean water, this plastic has a degradation rate of hundreds of years. As this pollution breaks down, it forms a new hazard called microplastics. Reports of the growing problem of microplastics found in fish and shellfish suggest heavy consumers could ingest tens of thousands of pieces of microplastic per year by eating fish.[342] When the plastic particles get small enough, they can cross the membrane of tissues and enter the cells of fish and, presumably, of those who eat them. Scientists evaluating this problem have suggested that humans who consume these microplastics may be at risk of inflammation, damage to internal organs, compromised immune system function, and blood clots.[343]

Leading researchers believe there's a very real risk that eating microplastic elevates your exposure to other dangerous compounds because the plastic acts like a sponge for pesticides, flame retardants, PCBs, and other neurotoxic pollutants that accumulate in the ocean. Some have called ocean-borne microplastics a Trojan horse of sorts because once the plastic is ingested by fish or humans and further degraded it releases the pollutants that have adhered to it.[344]

One study reported that the levels of the brain toxin called toxaphene, the pesticide dieldrin, and polychlorinated biphenyls (PCBs) found in farmed salmon sold in Scotland, Norway, the Faroe Islands, and European markets qualified for the EPA's most strict consumption advisory of less than one-half meal of salmon per month.[345] The report further stated that in the USA, "consumption of farmed Atlantic salmon must be effectively eliminated, and consumption of wild salmon must be restricted generally to less than one meal per month." Wild Pacific salmon had the most generous advisory of one meal per week, most salmon consumed in the US is the Atlantic farmed variety.[346]

The largest assessment of contaminants in farmed salmon included 700 salmon samples acquired from supermarkets in 16 large cities in the US and Europe as well as from salmon farm operations in Scotland, Norway, Chile, Canada, Maine, and Washington State. This study looked at levels of contaminants including mirex, DDT, endrin, dieldrin, cis-nonachlor, t-nonachlor, chlordane, heptachlor epoxide, lindane, hexachlorobenzene, toxaphene, PCBs, and dioxins (all things you hope never to ingest) and found "levels of certain contaminants were sufficiently high to trigger stringent consumption advice for farmed salmon from all locations, and for some species of wild Pacific salmon." Chinook salmon from Alaska was the most contaminated of all wild salmon tested.[347] These advisories are developed by considering the risk associated with single pollutants, such as PCBs or mercury. Yet no advisory board can estimate the risk posed to you from consuming fish that contains five or 10 different contaminants. The reason is that there are no studies that have looked at the health effects of consuming a cocktail of toxins together.

Fish on Drugs

Worldwide, river-caught and lake-caught fish are exposed to increasing concentrations of pharmaceutical and illicit drugs, including cocaine, which may remain in the fish.[348] For example, in a study of freshwater shrimp caught at 15 different sites in England, all samples tested positive for cocaine.[349] The Chinook salmon from the Puget Sound tested positive for not only cocaine but the cholesterol-lowering drug Lipitor, the notorious opioid Oxycontin, Valium, and the antidepressant Prozac.[350] The drugs accumulate in fish brains, muscles, gills, skin, and other tissues.[351]

The CDC recently confirmed that wild-caught Alaskan salmon were found to be infected with larvae of the Japanese tapeworm, which, once in the body, can grow to six feet in length. Although they usually confine themselves to the intestinal tract, in 2019 one was removed from a woman's brain.[352] The risk of exposure to tapeworm is highest when consuming undercooked or raw (sushi) fish.

Farmed Fish: A Chemical Arms Race

According to the National Oceanic and Atmospheric Administration, to meet the insatiable demand for salmon alone, 70 percent of the species consumed worldwide today is now derived from aquaculture or fish-farming. The problem is that farmed fish contain ten times the level of toxic pollutants found in wild fish. It is important for consumers—and those who continue to tout salmon consumption—to understand the fish farming industry is in a monumental struggle with nature to produce fish in a most unnatural habitat. Whether in Scotland, Norway, or Canada, fish farmers are learning that containing millions of migratory and carnivorous fish in confined spaces where they must swim amidst their own waste and contend with rampant parasites, pollution, and disease, makes for an exceedingly unhealthy product, not to mention a growing environmental disaster. Moreover, the fish themselves are increasingly sick with pancreatic disease and Infectious Salmon Anemia virus.[353]

Thus, to the question of whether farmed fish are any safer to eat, the answer is no.

The fish farming industry's primary nightmare is an infestation of blood sucking *Lepeophtheirus salmonis,* or salmon lice, which attach to the fish, causing lesions and secondary infections. In a Sisyphean attempt to control this rapidly spreading problem, farmers are using increasingly toxic pesticides and antibiotics to battle the lice and infections. As the parasites and bacteria continue to develop resistance, fish farmers are turning to increasingly stronger chemicals and veterinary drugs.[354] In some fish farms the use of toxic chemicals has risen 1,000 percent in just ten years.[355] This has led one expert to refer to the fish pens where salmon are raised as "toxic toilets." In the Spring of 2020, the Scottish EPA authorized aquaculture operations to increase their use of two pesticides due to the impact of COVID-19 on staffing their operations.[356]

Also problematic to fish consumers is that the FDA only inspects 2 percent of the seafood the U.S. imports, with 90 percent of the seafood eaten in the U.S. sourced from outside the country.[357] In a study that examined 27 samples of the most popular fish purchased from supermarkets in Arizona and California, investigators detected five different antibiotic drugs in farmed salmon, tilapia, catfish, swai, and shrimp.[358]

Yet even with strong evidence that fish eating does not protect one from cardiovascular disease, health writers continue to promote fish consumption, now shifting the focus to the benefits to brain function. The author of the publication *Brain Food: The Surprising Science of Eating for Cognitive Power,* recommends three servings of salmon and tuna *per week*—three times the amount that caused the drop in cognitive function and large intake of mercury noted in the Florida fish-eaters. And as of January 5, 2019, the popular website WebMD was advising readers to eat fish "a few times a week." Promoters of the South Beach Diet suggest fish be consumed two to three times weekly.[359] Yet Today.com takes the booby prize for telling readers, "For most individuals it's fine to eat fish every day."[360] This is not advice likely followed by members of The Mercury Policy Project, who reported that some tuna they tested have had mercury levels nearly four times the average level reported by the FDA.[361]

Eating just one 7-ounce serving of swordfish and tuna per week (canned tuna serving size would be 1.5 cans) was shown to quadruple blood mercury levels in consumers within just 14 weeks.[362]

While federal guidelines have for years led the public to believe that mercury exposure from eating fish was safe in limited amounts, these guidelines have long been influenced by the fishing industry and are not reliable as a guide for protecting your brain.[363]

If there are any benefits to an occasional piece of fish in the diet, it appears to be obviated by the widespread and growing presence of numerous dangerous contaminants. No amount of mercury, let alone the plethora of other pollutants, should be consumed if it can be avoided. And, quite simply, fish of any kind is not required for good health anyway.

The Fish Oil Foil

Whether because they don't enjoy the taste of fish or because they have come to understand how seriously polluted fish flesh is, many people have taken to a daily ritual of swallowing pills containing fish oil. So many that the fish oil industry has ballooned to a $30 billion a year enterprise, leading some researchers to ask if the fish oil supplementation story is nothing but a fish tale. These supplements are well known for causing bad breath, belching, flatulence, nausea, and diarrhea; they frequently contain fewer EFAs than stated on the packaging; and they are sometimes rancid. All of them—including those that are molecularly distilled—contain measurable levels of mercury.[364] Some scientists have proposed that long-term use of fish oil supplements may lead to fatty liver disease.[365] But do they offer any benefit? In 2013 a meta-analysis of 14 previously published double-blind-placebo studies found no benefit to the user.[366] Then came the largest to date study of fish oil supplements, a meta-analysis involving 79 studies and over 112,000 people. The study found there is "good evidence that taking long-chain omega-3 (fish oil, EPA, or DHA) supplements does not benefit heart health or reduce our risk of stroke or death from any cause. The most trustworthy studies consistently showed little or no effect of long-chain omega-3 fats on cardiovascular health."[367] In short, skip the fish oil, too.

Non-Fish to the Rescue

With all that said, we do need the omega-3 fats in our diet. Our brain needs DHA for maintenance and proper brain function as do cells throughout the body. There is evidence that people whose DHA levels are at a particular threshold show slower mental decline with age, less brain shrinkage, and better retain brain structural integrity over time.[368]

So how do we get these fats if we are not eating fish? The body uses a plant-sourced omega-3 fat, alpha linolenic acid (ALA), to synthesize the long-chain omega-3 fats, EPA and DHA. Vegetables and legumes are a source of small amounts of ALA and foods with higher levels of ALA include chia seeds, edamame, flax seeds, hemp seeds, pumpkin seeds, and walnuts.

However, the synthesis of these essential fats from ALA can be hampered by a high intake of oils rich in omega-6 like safflower oil, sunflower oil and corn oil (found in many processed foods), saturated fat, trans fats, and alcohol. And the body may be less efficient at this synthesis as we age.[369] So what's a good back-up plan? Seek DHA and EPA from the same place that fish derive these fats: algae.[370]

As a form of insurance, a supplement made from lab-grown microalgae, lab-cultivated to be free of harmful environmental contaminants, can provide a bioequivalent form of the DHA and EPA derived from fish.[371] Algae-oil supplements were tested in a study where participants received either salmon or algae-oil capsules. Both resulted in the same increase in blood levels of DHA.[372]

In summary, we are fortunate that fish are not required for human health, because today's catch may be the most contaminated food one can eat.

THE NOT-SO-SWEET FACTS OF LIFE

According to the World Health Organization, the average American consumes about 165 pounds of refined sugars a year, or about 24 teaspoons of added sugar per day—more than ever before and more than any other people on the planet.[373] Although we generally associate sugary foods and drinks with good feelings, in addition to the key role added sugar plays in the worldwide epidemic of obesity, sugar's potential to wreak havoc in our brains is a genuine concern.[374]

Other than its influence on flavor, our attraction to sugar may be related to its activation of opiate receptors in the brain. Research suggests that each time we stimulate the opiate receptors in this way we modify brain chemistry and reinforce a pathway of neurons, a neuropathway, that can lead to cravings and feelings of withdrawal when sugar is avoided. Sugar also promotes the release of cytokines, molecules that lead to inflammation, free radical production in the brain, and that compromise communication between neurons. Neuroscientist Amy Reichelt found that as the quantity of sugary foods one eats goes up, neuroinflammation increases, neurogenesis may be suppressed, and cognitive function becomes compromised. Dr. Richard Stevenson, a professor at Macquarie University in Australia, conducted research on the impact of sugary foods on brain function and came to a similar conclusion, suggesting the adverse impact is most focused on the hippocampus.

Dr. Fernando Gomez-Pinilla, a professor of neurosurgery at the David Geffen School of Medicine at UCLA and member of the university's Brain Research Institute, has also studied the effects of sugar on the brain. He believes that because sugar decreases synaptic activity, interferes with communication between neurons, and interferes with insulin function, eating a high-sugar diet may alter the brain's ability to learn and make new memories.[375]

Unwittingly, the more sugar people pack in their diet, the more trouble they may be causing for their brains in the long term.

Artificial sweeteners may help with calories but are no better for the brain; they can act as excitotoxins that overexert brain cells and lead to their death. This may be why their use has been associated with an increased risk of dementia.[376]

For most people, the primary sources of refined sugar intake today are sweetened beverages—colas (containing ten teaspoons of sugar), sports drinks, energy drinks (a typical one contains 13 teaspoons of sugar), specialty coffees and teas, and alcoholic beverages.[377] However, be aware that added sugars are also found in 68 percent of the food products sold in supermarkets today.[378] You might be surprised to learn that sugar is frequently added to most sandwich bread, processed meats, baked beans, barbeque sauce, bottled fruit juice, ketchup, pasta sauce, peanut butter, salad dressing, soups, crackers, vitamin water, and some dairy products. Mostly you can find this out by simply reading the label. We already know that breakfast cereals are highly sugared, except for a few such as Shredded Wheat, Kashi 7, and Three Wishes Grain Free cereal.

Aside from cane sugar, a major player is high fructose corn syrup (HFCS). Because U.S. Government farm subsidies make it extremely cheap, this sweetener (also called fructose syrup), of which Americans now eat 63 pounds a year, remains the darling of manufacturers of processed junk foods. Scientists have found that this substance is more damaging to memory than table sugar.[379]

When shopping for packaged foods, be on the lookout for disguised refined sugar as well as artificial sweeteners.[380] Whether natural or artificial, the words to watch out for on nutrition labels include Aspartame, agave nectar, beet sugar, cane juice crystals, coconut sugar, corn syrup, corn syrup solids, dextran, dextrose, Equal, evaporated cane juice, Florida crystals, fructose, galactose, high fructose corn syrup, honey, invert sugar, maltodextrin, malted barley, maltose, molasses, Necta Sweet, Nutrasweet, rice syrup, Splenda, sucanat, sucrose, Sweet & Low, turbinado sugar, and Twin Sweet.

A lesser-known sweetening agent with no known negative side effects is derived from monk fruit (also known as swingle fruit), which is native to southeast Asia. The skin and seeds are removed, and the meat of the fruit is pressed into a juice. The juice is further refined to remove the fructose and retain an antioxidant known as mogrosides that gives the sensation of sweetness. Unlike cane sugar and many other common sweeteners, monk fruit sweeteners provide zero calories and do not raise blood sugar levels.[381] Approved by the FDA back in 2010 and available in many other countries, monk fruit as a sweetening agent is becoming increasingly well known in the U.S.

PROCESSED VEGETABLE OILS ARE NOT HEALTH FOOD

Prior to the 20th century, refined vegetable oils were not available. They now account for about 20 percent of calories consumed.[382] Yet if you ask most people how much oil they add to their diet, chances are they would tell you very little. In a way, they don't have to: oil is added anyway. Refined vegetable oils are ubiquitous in the American diet. Most processed foods, including salad dressings, chips, cookies, crackers, granola bars, pasta sauces, mayonnaise, fried foods, broth, energy bars, contain refined, degraded, and unhealthful oils.

Why are oils employed with such abandon? Partly because they help food processors make appealing products. But the more important answer is that some oils have been sold to Americans as health food and so we don't view them as problematic when we see them listed on ingredient labels. We have essentially been told, "Look, they are derived from plants, they contain no cholesterol, and they are, with a few exceptions, low in saturated fat. So, they're not a bad choice."

Given their pervasiveness in the American diet, the truth about vegetable oils is tough for many people to face but this is one subject you want to be clear about. To begin with, oils really work against you if you desire to maintain a healthy bodyweight. That's because each tablespoon of oil packs 120 calories. For a bit of perspective, if you weighed 125 pounds, you would need to exercise vigorously with weights for a half an hour or run just over a mile to burn up those calories. Yet, there is more than calories to be concerned about.

Almost invariably, oils are extracted with industrial petroleum-based agents. The most common product used is a flammable solvent called hexane, classified as a neurotoxin by the CDC.[383] Because hexane is considered a "processing agent" and not a food ingredient, oil producers are not required to disclose its presence to consumers.

Additionally, vegetable oils are routinely bleached, degummed, deodorized, and processed at temperatures that lead to oxidation, and ... hold on, the production of your new worst enemy, trans fats.[384] An additional concern is that much of canola, corn, and soy oils sold in the U.S. and added to packaged foods are made from crops that have been genetically modified to withstand heavy applications of the herbicide Roundup. Therefore, they are likely to be tainted with residues of this this controversial weed killer.

All vegetable oils are highly sensitive to oxygen, light, and heat, which accelerate their degradation. Many oils are now packaged in clear plastic bottles, and the oil can leach a group of plasticizer chemicals called phthalates from the bottle.[385] Some plasticizers are associated with a thickening of the walls of the arteries that reach the brain, are neurotoxic, interfere with neurogenesis, and hamper nerve transmission at synapses.[386] Every effort should be made to avoid plasticizers in your food!

Refined oils made from safflower, sunflower, peanut, corn, and soy, which are particularly good at promoting inflammation, are used in more manufactured foods today than ever before.

We amplify the problems when we expose oils to heat in sautéing, baking, broiling, and frying. Heat rapidly degrades vegetable oil, causing it to react with oxygen, and produces a few new problematic compounds. The first is toxin is called acrolein and is associated with protein mis-folding.[387] Heated oils also produce chemicals called aldehydes that are linked to Alzheimer's, cancer, and Parkinson's disease.[388] Finally, heating vegetable oils raises levels of Advanced-Glycation End-products (AGEs), those problematic compounds we learned about earlier that increase inflammation, oxidative stress, and arterial stiffness.[389]

Of all common vegetable oils, genuine extra virgin olive is the least problematic because it is not refined, high heat processed, deodorized, bleached, or treated with solvents. After all, olive oil is prized for its aroma, variable color, and characteristic flavor. Because it has not been refined, it also contains antioxidants, including vitamin E, carotenoids, and phenolic compounds which may help combat free-radicals and inflammation. Here's the bad news: In far too many cases, the olive oil you think you are buying is not what you get.

Counterfeit olive oil is a thriving business. Experts at the University of California Davis Olive Center estimate that 69 percent of olive oil on supermarket shelves is fake. Others suggest it may be as much as 80 percent. In one of the university's reviews, 186 extra virgin olive oil samples were analyzed using standards established by the International Olive Council. Seventy-three of the samples derived from the five biggest selling brands of imported olive oils were deemed counterfeit. These products were oxidized, of inferior quality (not extra virgin), or simply not olive oil, but instead a blend of cheap refined vegetable oils disguised with coloring and aroma agents.[390] The National Consumers League tested 11 different olive oils from a variety of supermarkets and found six of them, despite being labeled "extra virgin," did not meet the extra virgin quality standards for which they were so labeled.

Here are some things to keep in mind when buying olive oil. Seek out extra-virgin olive oil. This designation means the oil is produced from the first press of the olives using no heat or extraction chemicals. It will have the highest content of beneficial ingredients. Because you don't want oil sitting around for months degrading, purchase oil in small bottles. Select oil that is in darkened glass that protects the oil from light. Avoid plastic bottles entirely. Because conventional olive groves are often sprayed with as many as 20 different pesticides, residues of which have been detected in oil, choose a product that carries the USDA organic seal.[391] Remember, all oil is 100 percent fat—one tablespoon of olive oil yields 14 grams of fat. As with all oils, olive oil is vulnerable to degradation from exposure to heat, oxygen, and light. Many people have been misled to believe that cooking with olive oil is healthful. Olive oil has a low smoking point, is degraded by heat, and should not be used in cooking. As an oil begins to release smoke it's a sign that nutrients in the oil are degrading and toxic compounds that promote inflammation and oxidative stress are being produced. I encourage you to try steaming, baking, and using low-sodium vegetable broth to prepare foods instead.

TRANS FATS

As we saw earlier, trans fats are a nutritional nightmare. They are a virulent enemy of the brain and raise the risk of Alzheimer's. There is no known safe level to consume. I advise avoiding them at all costs.

A simple rule is that anything fried—whether at home or in a restaurant deep fryer—is going to contain trans fats. This means it is wise to avoid fried chicken, French fries, onion rings, battered and fried vegetables (tempura), fish, and donuts. I know that for many readers the sight of French fries on the no-fly list may be deeply worrying. After all, according to the USDA, for Americans, potatoes fashioned into fries, chips, tots, and hash browns—plus the ketchup they are frequently eaten with—constitute two-thirds of their total vegetable intake. In addition, commercially made cookies, cakes, pastries, as well as popular stick and tub margarines almost invariably contain trans fats, even if undisclosed on the label.

Trans fats are also found in packaged foods that are labeled with the ingredients or *partially hydrogenated oil*. Remember, due to lax regulation by the FDA, even the non-dairy spreads that claim "0 trans fats per serving" on the label may contain trans fats.

SALT

In Chapter 6 we looked closely at the role of dietary sodium in raising blood pressure, a major risk factor for dementia. High salt intake reduces nitric oxide, a compound important to the relaxation of blood vessels and enhancing blood flow.

In addition to stiffening blood vessels and raising blood pressure, excess sodium derived from salt promotes free radicals and increases inflammation.

Although we tend to use the words sodium and salt interchangeably, they are not the same thing. Table salt is composed of 40 percent sodium and 60 percent chloride. The guideline below shows approximate levels of sodium in a measure of table salt as well as the definition of sodium terms on food packaging.

Quantity of Sodium in Measures of Table Salt

- ¼ teaspoon salt = 575 mg sodium

- ½ teaspoon salt = 1,150 mg sodium

- ¾ teaspoon salt = 1,725 mg sodium

- 1 teaspoon salt = 2,300 mg sodium

- 1 tablespoon salt = 6,976 mg sodium

Meaning of Sodium Terms on Packaging

- Sodium-free – Less than 5 mg of sodium per serving

- Very low sodium – 35 mg or less per serving

- Low sodium – 140 mg or less per serving

Today, most people are so accustomed to consuming salt-laden food that they have little understanding of how regularly they exceed a healthful sodium level. To get an idea of how easily you can exceed the official recommended daily limit of 2,300 mg sodium, look at the table below that lists the sodium levels of popular fast foods. The 2,300 mg/day guideline for sodium is not ideal—it's merely what the government believes average people may be willing to strive for.

SODIUM LEVELS OF POPULAR FAST FOOD[392]	
McDonald's Big Breakfast	2,260 mg
Taco Bell Volcano Nachos	1,670 mg
Starbucks Turkey & Swiss	1,140 mg
Subway Spicy Italian (ft. long)	3,200 mg
KFC's Variety Big Boy Meal	3,000 mg
Popeye's Chicken Po Boy	2,120 mg
Dominoes Mac 'N Cheese	1,760 mg
Chipotle Burrito (Pork, cheese, sour cream, guacamole)	2,650 mg
Wendy's Baja Salad	1,975 mg
Coke (12 oz)	55 mg

By far the largest contributors of sodium to the diet are meat dishes and restaurant food (especially fast food, as seen above). The second largest contributor: canned and packaged foods.

The good news is that even if your diet is now high in sodium, by switching to a low-sodium, plant-based diet and refraining from adding salt at the table or in cooking, you can reduce the stiffness of your blood vessels in as little as two weeks.[393]

A FEW LAST WORDS ON RISK FACTORS

Clearly, cardiovascular disease, high blood pressure, diabetes, obesity, high homocysteine levels, and a diet rich in saturated fats and trans fats significantly increase chances of impairing brain function and ultimately suffering from AD. Yet we can keep our brains sharp and reduce our risk of Alzheimer's by making lifestyle changes that tackle all these problems. Is there any reason not to?

In the next chapters we are going to examine emerging risk factors that get far less attention from public health authorities, but a growing body of evidence indicates absolutely warrant our attention. I understand that the depth and scope of the material that follows could feel overwhelming at times, but I highly encourage you to stay engaged and not skim over the material. In a few cases the late-breaking research findings show that we have previously overlooked factors that appear to be a significant contributor to risk for cognitive decline and Alzheimer's. All these risk factors will also be addressed in the lifestyle plan presented in Part IV.

PART III

EMERGING RISK FACTORS

13
ALCOHOL AND BRAIN DAMAGE

Many adults like to wind down at the end of the day with a glass of wine, a pint of beer, or a tumbler of scotch. Why not, right? It can be relaxing and most of us have heard that moderate drinking might lower the risk of cardiovascular disease.

Whether used at celebrations, in socializing, or to take the edge off, alcohol is deeply woven into our society. For some, alcohol is also deeply entangled in their lives, causing a range of negative health outcomes. And for some, alcohol may be adversely affecting our brain health more than we realize.

A growing body of evidence indicates we have overlooked (or perhaps even resisted accepting) alcohol's role as a potent contributor to risk for dementia. We should take a closer look because Americans—especially women—are drinking more alcohol than ever before.[394] The most recent data, which took population growth into account, shows that between 1999 and 2017 the number of US deaths tied to alcohol increased by 51 percent overall and by 85 percent for women.[395]

The average American drinks ten alcoholic drinks per week, or 500 drinks per year; 24 million Americans aged 18 and older consume up to 36 drinks per week, or 1872 per year; and 30 million Americans binge drink at least once a week.[396] (For men, binge drinking is defined as consuming five or more drinks in two hours; for women, it's four or more drinks in two hours.)

RETHINKING ALCOHOL AND BRAIN HEALTH

A ten-year study of 500,000 men upended years of advice that moderate drinking is protective for cardiovascular health. Moreover, the findings suggest that we have substantially underestimated the role that alcohol plays in our risk for dementia.[397] The study found that even moderate alcohol intake, as little as one drink a day, increases blood pressure, which as a result may raise the risk for stroke by 10 to 15 percent. The authors emphasized that they *found no protective effect for alcohol consumption*. Other researchers have reported the same finding: *there is no limit within which alcohol does not cause damage to the structure and function of the brain*.[398]

WHAT ALCOHOL DOES TO THE BRAIN

Over time, alcohol ingestion changes both the brain's function and physical shape. It begins by increasing inflammation, first in the gut and then systemically, eventually causing neuroinflammation in the brain.[399] Alcohol promotes oxidative stress, attacks the hippocampus, interferes with the absorption and utilization of vitamin B1, B12, and folic acid, and raises homocysteine levels.[400] Alcohol also interferes with the brain's ability to clear itself of beta amyloid, the protein that forms the hallmark brain plaques seen in Alzheimer's disease.[401] Alcohol disrupts nerve cell communication in the hippocampus and thereby interferes with the brain's ability to form new long-term memories.

So what does all this mean? For one thing, when people joke about their excessive drinking by lamenting, "I really killed some brain cells," they may be depressingly accurate.

Drinkers understand a night of alcohol consumption is dehydrating to the body. But it is correspondingly dehydrating for the brain. That hangover headache? It's caused by dehydration shrinking the dura, the membrane that encases the entire brain

In her research in the VA Boston Healthcare System and as assistant professor at Harvard Medical School, neuropsychologist Catherine Brawn Fortier has documented the adverse effects of alcohol on the brain. Using MRI scans, she found that the more people drink, the more damage they do to their frontal cortex, the region of the brain that involves planning, complex cognitive behavior, personality expression, decision making, and moderation of social behavior.[402]

As is commonly known, alcohol also damages the liver. Fortier believes the liver's cells become less effective at preventing the elements ammonia and manganese from entering the brain, where they wreak havoc on neurons. In this regard, drinking after age 50 seems to have a heightened impact on the brain. More damage can occur when alcohol is metabolized, as it produces a chemical called *acetaldehyde*. This substance is highly toxic to brain cells and a known carcinogen.[403]

ALCOHOL SHRINKS THE BRAIN

Let's consider in more detail the fact that the brain shrinks in proportion to the amount of alcohol consumed. A loss in brain volume is caused by a loss of brain cells. Even moderate alcohol consumption shrinks brain volume at an accelerated rate.[404] While we all lose a degree of brain volume as we age, accelerated brain loss is a hallmark in dementia.

Researchers performed MRI brain scans on 1,839 subjects aged 34 to 88. They classified them as nondrinkers, former drinkers, low drinkers, moderate drinkers, and high drinkers. Then they re-scanned their brains over the next several years. They found that the more alcohol people consumed, the more substantial their loss of brain volume.[405]

A research team from Oxford University looked at data from a 30-year study of 10,000 participants who underwent brain-imaging studies using MRI. They found that in those who consumed four or more drinks daily, the risk of shrinkage of the hippocampus was six times higher than in those who drank less. Even moderate drinkers had three times the risk of hippocampal shrinkage.[406] Other studies have confirmed that even light drinkers suffer brain shrinkage when compared to those who abstain from alcohol.[407]

ALCOHOL USE DISORDER AND EARLY-ONSET DEMENTIA

Another study looked at alcohol use among 4,414 female veterans over the age of 55, from 2004 to 2015. Half the women were diagnosed with alcohol use disorder (AUD)*. All were free of dementia at the start of the study. In the women with AUD the risk of developing dementia was more than three times higher than in those without.[408]

In 2018, the largest study ever conducted on alcohol use and brain health examined medical records from one million hospital cases in France that involved dementia. It was determined that alcohol use was directly related to more than one-third of the 57,000 cases of early-onset dementia.[409] "We concluded that alcohol use disorders were the most significant modifiable risk factor for dementia onset and remained so after controlling for 30 possible or potential risk factors," said the lead author of the study, Dr. Michael Schwarzinger. Ultimately, the study reported that alcohol use disorders are associated with triple the risk of all types of dementia. Liquor, wine, and beer have the same deleterious effect on the brain, so it does not matter what type of alcoholic beverage one consumes.

Although the effects of alcohol consumption may manifest insidiously, leading one to believe that no damage is occurring, the effects are real and measurable. Even with moderate drinking, the changes taking place in the brain may be subtle and nearly undetectable until outward changes in memory function become evident.

It's time we stop soft-pedaling the risks from alcohol consumption and refrain from promoting "moderate consumption" to ward off cardiovascular disease. There are plenty of non-harmful ways to do that, such as jettisoning the primary causes of cardiovascular disease—a diet rich in saturated fat, trans fat, and cholesterol—and getting at least 150 minutes of robust exercise per week.

As was the case with the risk from smoking in the 1970s, the good news is that influential public health organizations, including the American Cancer Society (ACS), are heeding the wakeup call from the latest research, and are no longer promoting moderate alcohol consumption. In its June 2020 revised guidelines, the ACS states that it's best simply not to consume alcohol at all.[410]

*Alcohol use disorder is considered a long-term brain disease characterized by an inability to stop or control alcohol use despite negative social, employment and health consequences.

Finally, there is a rapidly growing market for non-alcoholic beverages, including beer, wine, and spirits. For example, the gin maker Gordon's has launched an alcohol-free spirit made from botanicals. Ariel is a producer of non-alcoholic chardonnay and cabernet wines, Chateau de Fleur offers a non-alcoholic sparkling wine, and some leading beer producers, such as Sam Adams and Becks, offer alcohol-free beer.

14

INSOMNIA AND ALZHEIMER'S

Two years ago I endured a bout of insomnia at a most inopportune time—I was preparing to ascend Mt. Kilimanjaro in Tanzania. The night before my nine-day trek, I checked into a small motel in Moshi, Tanzania, that had been selected by the guide company that was to lead me up the mountain. Two hours after falling asleep I was awakened by a rooster crowing next door.

As it turned out, a resident of the apartment building raised chickens in an open-air coop atop the building. Incredibly, the bird resumed crowing each time I was on the verge of dozing off again. As I noted the time and considered that at sunrise I was to embark on the most physically challenging event of my life, I became increasingly anxious. I opened my window and called out to the rooster as though it might sympathize with my plight, and then pleaded with the front desk staff to call the neighbor, but all to no avail. After two hours the rooster suddenly ceased his crowing, but by then I was so worked up over the little time that remained for me to fall asleep that rest remained impossible.

I became focused on my lack of rest and worried that my insomnia might recur on the mountain. In a classic example of a self-fulfilling prophecy, it did just that. Each night I slept worse than the last, taking even greater agitation to my tent at night until, after four long days of trekking with little or no sleep, I wondered whether I might need to be evacuated off the mountain. Thankfully, a doctor I was climbing with had brought medications for a variety of conditions and kindly helped me break the spell by giving me a sleeping aid.

It turns out that my four-day bout with insomnia is far more common than I had imagined; every year an estimated 60 million Americans struggle with one or more experiences of insomnia.[411]

Have you ever heard anyone express pride in how little they sleep, as though it were a badge of courage? Our culture of productivity gives us the message that a lack of adequate sleep is evidence one is working hard and getting a great deal accomplished. It almost seems as if some people believe only slackers sleep.

A rapidly growing body of evidence indicates insufficient sleep disrupts an essential brain maintenance process, triggering a cascade of events that eventually raises the risk of Alzheimer's disease.[412] Insufficient sleep may also markedly increase the risk for depression.

Insomnia, the inability to fall or stay asleep, is not only surprisingly common in the USA, but the problem seems to be worsening. Only recently has science permitted us to understand why sleep is so critically important, not just for feeling and performing well in life but to facilitate essential brain cleansing processes.

We all know how good we feel when we sleep well, and how a day can be ruined when we don't. New research shows that our distress is based on more than simply feeling fatigued. Insufficient sleep disrupts a very important process that may protect cognitive resilience and help prevent us from succumbing to neurological disease. Conditions like obstructive sleep apnea also deprive the brain of sufficient oxygen and blood flow, elevate blood pressure, and promote oxidative stress, and may thereby further accentuate the risk of dementia over time.[413]

Some sleep researchers now believe that inadequate sleep over one's lifetime is significantly predictive that one will develop Alzheimer's pathology in their brain. One reason is that amyloid protein levels are regulated by the sleep-wake cycle.[414] During wake periods, amyloid levels are highest. They drop when we sleep. With sleep deprivation, amyloid levels increase and clearance of the protein decreases.[415]

In a study from the University of Wisconsin–Madison, scientists recruited male and female subjects with an average age of 63 who were cognitively healthy. Each participant was assessed for sleep quality, and then a spinal fluid sample was taken from them. The subjects who reported the poorest quality and quantity of sleep had a greater number of markers for the presence of amyloid and tau proteins, as well as markers indicating inflammation and brain cell damage.[416]

One study found a 51 percent increase in the level of tau protein (not tau tangles) in people who had been deprived of one night's sleep compared to those who had a solid night's sleep.[417] Not only does sleep deprivation lead to higher levels of tau as measured in cerebrospinal fluid, and increase the chances that it will accumulate, but it also encourages established tau tangles to spread in the brain.[418]

By using special imaging technology, researchers from the Johns Hopkins Bloomberg School of Health took pictures of and measured deposits of plaques in the brain over time relative to subjects' sleep quality and duration. The highest level of amyloid plaque accumulation was seen in subjects who had the shortest periods of sleep and the most disrupted sleep.[419] This less-sleep/more-plaque relationship has been shown in both humans and animals.[420]

At UCLA, researchers showed that a single night of sleep deprivation resulted in significantly elevated levels of amyloid protein in the hippocampus of human subjects. The scientists also noted that the relationship between amyloid and sleep deprivation is bi-directional, since the accumulation of amyloid not only results from insufficient sleep, but can also impair sleep.[421]

Lack of adequate sleep can also raise blood pressure[422] and cortisol levels,[423] impede neurogenesis, and increase insulin resistance.[424] As one is increasingly deprived of sleep, the brain's ability to use glucose is hampered and therefore neurons may be deprived of fuel.

ESSENTIAL BRAIN CLEANSING OCCURS WHEN WE SLEEP

Although it was unclear why until recently, all species have a biological need for sleep. Dr. Maiken Nedergaard, co-director of the Center for Translational Neuromedicine at the University of Rochester Medical Center, together with her team of researchers discovered that during deep sleep the body clears waste from the brain. In the space between your brain and your skull is about five ounces of clear liquid called cerebrospinal fluid (CSF). In addition to cushioning the brain and transporting nutrients, CSF clears waste from the brain. The body uses CSF and a system of "pipes" that parallel blood vessels in the brain to flush waste products out of the interstitial space and to clear them from the brain and spinal cord.[425] This includes amyloid protein,[426] tau, and other potentially neurotoxic metabolic waste that accumulates while we are awake.[427]

When the brain enters what is called slow-wave (deep) sleep, pulses of CSF flush through the brain at 20-second intervals to remove the toxins. With lack of or poor-quality sleep, this waste-removal process is hampered, limiting the brain's ability to clear neurotoxic waste products associated with Alzheimer's. While some of this waste removal goes on during waking hours, it's ten times greater while we sleep because brain cells shrink by about 60 percent at that time and allow for the more efficient removal of toxins.[428]

The brain waste removal process is also enhanced after robust exercise. So the better our sleep and the more we exercise, the more we will help protect the brain from waste that impairs its function.

SLEEP CREATES AND PROTECTS MEMORIES

Sleep is essential for the creation of memories.[429] While we are in deep sleep, the brain consolidates and encodes memories from the preceding day into long-term storage.[430] Thus, inadequate sleep can impede the brain's ability to learn and to recall information later.[431]

NEW NEURONS GROW WHILE WE SLEEP

It's during sleep that scientists believe we can grow new brain cells in the hippocampus. To facilitate this, levels of the stress hormone cortisol, a growth inhibitor, are reduced. Levels of melatonin, growth hormone, and our friend brain-derived neurotrophic factor (BDNF), all of which are believed to support neurogenesis, are increased.[432] So, the belief is that with reduced sleep comes inhibition of neurogenesis.[433] University of Warwick sleep research has found that brain function and brain volume of children is also affected by sleep duration.[434] The less sleep the poorer their cognitive performance and the smaller their brain volume.

SLEEP AND DEPRESSION RISK

Both the time one goes to sleep and the time one rises seem to have an influence on the risk for depression. A study that included over 32,000 nurses found that those who were early risers had a 27 percent reduced risk of a major depressive episode in the following four-year period when compared to those who slept in.[435] Sleep researchers have also found that for each hour earlier one's sleep midpoint (the halfway point between sleep and wake times) is, the risk of depression is reduced by 23 percent. So, if a person who normally goes to bed at 11:00 pm shifts to a 10:00 pm sleep time, they may enjoy a considerably reduced risk for depression even when sleep duration remains the same. It's not entirely clear what factors lead to this improvement, but it may be related to aligning more closely with a natural circadian rhythm. Night owls who watch TV late in the evening or are exposed to other technology such as computers, tablets, phones, etc., may be stimulating their brain in a way that keeps them operating outside of their natural circadian rhythm. As we will see in future chapters, getting in synch with our natural circadian rhythm may require we adjust our exposure to technology and more specifically light, as well as adjust the time we eat dinner.

Impacts of Poor Sleep
- Increased blood pressure
- Increased cortisol levels
- Increased insulin resistance
- Increased amyloid deposits
- Suppressed neurogenesis
- Suppressed BDNF levels
- Disruption in memory formation

In Chapter 30 we will look at a comprehensive list of strategies that are truly effective at helping one attain deep and restful sleep. Surprisingly, one strategy involves choosing the right foods. The good news is that the foods that best protect the brain and reduce risk of cognitive decline are also the ones that support quality sleep.

15

CHECK YOUR HEARING

EVERYDAY CHOICES YOU make now could irreversibly diminish your hearing and place you at an elevated risk of developing dementia. If you think you are too young to be concerned about your hearing, think again.

I grew up riding mini-bikes and go carts. In my teens, I used a chain saw and a lawn mower on landscaping jobs. As an adult, I went to concerts and car races. When the first portable personal cassette player, the Sony Walkman, came out in 1979, the unit's headphones became my cranial appendage. Never did it occur to me that engaging in these activities might be risking my hearing, not to mention my future cognitive health. Yet before age 50 I was diagnosed with hearing loss, and today I endure persistent tinnitus or ringing in my ears. Now I go to great lengths to protect the hearing I have left, and there's good reason you should do the same.

According to the World Health Organization, hearing loss—even in teens—is on the rise worldwide and with profound consequences. Tinnitus, or ringing in the ears, is a symptom of damage to one's hearing and will affect one in five American adults in their lifetime. For the 48 million Americans who suffer from it, hearing loss may do more than compromise quality of life and lead to social isolation. Depending on its severity, it may also raise the risk of future dementia two to fivefold.[436] Those with untreated hearing loss also tend to experience cognitive decline earlier than individuals with normal hearing. A study by scientists at Johns Hopkins University enrolled 639 adults who were considered cognitively healthy but had various amounts of hearing loss. The subjects were followed for 12 to 18 years. Compared to a person with normal hearing, those who had even mild hearing loss at the start of the study had double the risk they would develop dementia. Subjects with moderate hearing loss at the start of the study were three times as likely as those with normal hearing to develop dementia. Individuals with severe hearing loss were five times as likely to develop dementia.[437]

HOW DOES HEARING LOSS LEAD TO DEMENTIA?

Using sophisticated brain imaging technology, scientists have found hearing loss causes the brain to shrink at an accelerated rate, especially in the region called the auditory cortex. Without stimulation through sound processing, this part of the brain diminishes over time, just as a muscle will shrink from disuse. Experts theorize that with loss of hearing the brain endures a greater "cognitive load," meaning it must work much harder to decipher sounds and make sense of language. This can result in stress or "brain fatigue." Further, some neuroscientists believe that when the brain must direct more resources to deciphering sounds, it detracts from the resources used to consolidate and encode new memories. Finally, hearing loss often causes an individual to become socially isolated, and socially withdrawn people are at greater risk of dementia. This may be because without a strong social network people are at greater risk of becoming depressed, and depression itself is a known risk factor for Alzheimer's disease.

The good news is that treating hearing loss not only helps with hearing, but it also helps with brain health, too. Unfortunately, only about 20 percent of Americans with hearing loss get diagnosed and treated, and those who are treated wait, on average, seven years before seeking care. Some struggle with or even hide their hearing loss rather than admit that they are having trouble. Even after they get assessed, they may wait an additional 10 years before they get fitted with a hearing aid. Dr. Timothy Teague, an audiologist, notes that many patients feel ashamed or embarrassed to wear hearing aids due to the social stigma of hearing loss. One study found that 23 percent of subjects had yet to use their hearing aid two years after purchasing it, probably in part because of social stigma.[438]

Don't wait. Delaying treatment for hearing loss means missing a critical window for minimizing negative brain changes and preserving cognitive health. Evidence shows that hearing aids, cochlear implants, or neuroprosthetic hearing devices can improve cognitive function and mental and emotional health, increase frequency and quality of social engagement, and raise self-esteem.

Researchers at the University of Melbourne assessed 100 adults aged 62–82 for degrees of hearing loss, cognitive function, speech perception, level of physical activity, sense of loneliness, and mood.[439] Each was then fitted with hearing aids. After 18 months, 97 percent of participants experienced significant improvements in cognitive health, including their ability to plan, organize, and initiate tasks. They also showed improvements in working memory, which is used for reasoning and decision-making.

In a study of patients receiving cochlear implants, 81 percent of participants showed improved cognition after one year.[440] There was also a significant reduction in the number of participants testing positive for depression compared to the number who tested positive prior to surgery.

IT'S NEVER TOO SOON TO PROTECT YOUR HEARING

Contrary to common belief, hearing loss can occur relatively early in life. For example, a surprising one in five American teens is estimated to have already suffered some degree of hearing loss, primarily due to playing loud music through earbuds.[441] According to Dr. Gary Curhan of Harvard-affiliated Brigham and Women's Hospital in Boston, despite years of widespread warnings about the use of such listening devices, the problem, especially in teens, is worsening.

Another relatively young group affected by hearing loss is members of the military. About half a million military veterans who served in the Iraq and Afghanistan wars are receiving disability compensation or treatment for hearing loss related to their service.[442] The Veterans Administration says an additional two million suffer from tinnitus. For soldiers, the risk comes primarily from aircraft, artillery, missiles, improvised explosive devices (IEDs), noise from tactical vehicles, and small-arms fire, all of which can damage the auditory sensing part of the brain. Also, head trauma from shrapnel and blast shock waves generated by rocket propelled grenades (RPGs) and land mines can cause damage to the central auditory cortex in the brain or rupture the membrane of the cochlea, the spiral-shaped cavity of the inner ear that converts sound vibrations into nerve impulses.

HOW DOES LOUD NOISE CAUSE HEARING LOSS?

Hearing loss begins with damage to tiny auditory hair cells in a part of the ear called the cochlea. These cells convert sound into electrical impulses that get transmitted to the brain. Loud sounds can overburden the hair cells to a point at which they can no longer send information to the brain, and they die. Although a single loud sound can cause instant and permanent hearing loss, for most people the loss is gradual, cumulative, and, for a period, imperceptible. Three factors determine whether a noise poses a risk: the level of a sound, the proximity of the sound, and the duration of the sound. Generally, the closer we are to the source of the sound, the longer we are exposed to the sound, and the louder the sound, the greater the risk to our hearing.

OTHER CAUSES OF HEARING LOSS

Some hearing loss and tinnitus, both temporary and permanent, can be triggered by prescription drugs such as quinine, chloroquine, and hydroxychloroquine. Most commonly these medications are used pro-phylactically against malaria. However, they are also used off-label to treat lupus. Hydroxychloroquine was temporarily approved for emer-gency treatment of COVID-19 in 2020, even though its efficacy for this purpose was (correctly) called into question. The class of antibiotics known as aminoglycosides are also associated with hearing loss, as are platinum-based chemotherapy drugs. All drugs prescribed for erectile dysfunction are now required to carry a warning about the risk of sud-den sensorineural hearing loss (SSHL), an emergency condition which can lead to permanent hearing loss, as is a drug called Revatio, used for rare hypertension of the pulmonary arteries, because it also contains the active ingredient used in Viagra. Some over-the-counter pain relievers (NSAIDs), when taken in doses of 8–10 per day, may cause reversible hearing loss in some individuals. In addition to medications, illnesses such as meningitis, shingles, and even diabetes can lead to hearing loss. But most hearing loss is caused by exposure to loud noise.

PROTECT IT OR LOSE IT

Commonly used home appliances and tools may exceed a safe decibel level and could place your hearing at risk if you do not use appropriate protection. Even running a hair dryer at high speed every day may be gradually diminishing your hearing. Likewise, a carpenter may think nothing of using a Skil saw on the job, but the noise it produces far exceeds the safe limit for preserving hearing. If you live in a city, you may have grown accustomed to the frequent passing of emergency vehicles. Yet their sirens can pose a serious threat to your hearing. The blender I use for my daily smoothies is effective and convenient, but it's also very loud and obviously exceeds a safe decibel level. To protect the precious hearing I have left, I wear industrial earmuffs when I operate the blender or other loud equipment and tools.

ARE MOVIE THEATERS TOO LOUD?

For years it seemed to me that the sound in movie theaters was getting increasingly louder. Turns out I'm not alone in this perception. Theater sound systems have become increasingly sophisticated and elaborate over the last couple of decades, with speakers and subwoofers behind the screen, speakers lining the right and left walls, and speakers in the back wall. Moviegoers are literally enveloped by sound. While these sound systems achieve their intended effect of heightening the sense of realism and engaging the moviegoer more fully, the American Hearing Research Foundation believes there is legitimate concern that they may be contributing to hearing loss. Sound levels in theaters have been measured at 98 to 133 decibels, greater than the sound produced by a passing train or a jet taking off.[443] Even dialogue sequences have been measured at 85 decibels. (85dB is considered the safe upper limit.) In 2020 growing complaints led federal lawmakers to introduce legislation that would regulate sound levels in theaters. Not surprisingly, the Motion Picture Association of America did not welcome the bill and claims it would violate the First Amendment right to freedom of speech.

HOW LOUD IS TOO LOUD?

Generally, sounds above 85dB are harmful, but proximity and duration may make lower decibel sounds harmful as well. Sounds over 120dB can cause immediate and permanent damage to hearing. A whisper is about 30dB. A normal conversation is about 60dB. Following is a reference list for things that may expose you to unsafe sound levels.

Audio headphones (85–110dB)

Racing cars (up to 140dB)

Concerts, sporting events, movie theaters (94–120dB)

Emergency vehicle sirens (120–130dB)

Fireworks (140–160dB)

Food processors, blenders (88dB or greater)

Gunshots (140dB)

Hammering (20–140dB)

Hairdryers (90dB)

Highway traffic (70–80dB at a distance of 50 feet)

Lawnmowers, leaf blowers, and other gardening equipment (95–115dB)

Shop machinery/power tools (80–110dB)

Vacuum cleaners (75+dB)

Skill saw (100dB)

Subway trains (80-100dB)

The best thing to do is avoid risky sound environments altogether. Otherwise, always use appropriate ear protection, such as foam earplugs or headphones, around excessively loud noise. In the absence of such devices, cover your ears with your fingers until the sound has subsided. I keep individually wrapped foam ear plugs in my car and coat pockets so that I always have them on hand should I find myself near sound levels that pose a threat.

There are several free apps, such as the National Institute for Occupational Safety and Health Sound Level Meter, Decibel X, and Too Noisy Pro that let your smartphone measure sound levels in theaters, concerts, restaurants, and other locations.

The telltale signs of hearing loss include frequently asking other to repeat what they have said, turning the television up to hear broadcasts, and ringing in the ears (tinnitus). Even without signs of hearing loss, adults should get their hearing checked every ten years until age 50 and every three years after that. Remember, the sooner loss is confirmed, the sooner you can get treated and protect your cognitive health and your quality of life.

In 2021 the FDA moved to make hearing aids available on an over-the-counter basis. This means one will be soon able to obtain them without needing an exam, prescription, and fitting. The move is expected to bring down the cost for the devices which are seldom covered by health insurance. This is great news for the 37 million Americans who are experiencing hearing loss, some of whom may not have sought treatment due to high cost and limited access to healthcare.

16
MEDDLING WITH METALS

FOR THOUSANDS OF YEARS humans have known that ingesting certain metals harms the brain, yet aside from a successful lead awareness campaign, relatively little attention has been given to educating the public about the risk of exposure to other metals.

Five metals have been associated with risk of cognitive impairment and Alzheimer's: mercury, aluminum, copper, iron, and lead. Most of us are unwittingly exposed to all five by some of the foods we eat, beverages we drink, and to a lesser degree by some products we use.

MERCURY

Of the five metals, mercury has a particularly nasty effect on the brain. It's an undisputed neurotoxin that promotes oxidative stress,[444] depletes glutathione levels,[445] inhibits the production of neurotransmitters,[446] interferes with the function of critical enzymes and, ultimately, damages and kills brain cells.[447]

There's also evidence that in utero exposure to mercury during critical stages of development can predispose a person to developing neurodegenerative disease later in life.[448] In short, mercury is a serious threat to neurological health and every effort should be made to avoid exposure to it.

Although volcanoes and forest fires can release mercury into the air, the bulk of the mercury produced comes from coal-fired power plants, the burning of other fossil fuels, mining, and some manufacturing processes. The coal industry generates about 70 percent of all mercury emissions. This makes it particularly concerning when politicians who have little or no understanding of the science related to coal burning and mercury continue to promote coal dependency in order to win votes in coal-producing regions.[449] The result is that the public has yet to see advisories that accurately and honestly disclose how pervasive and risky the problem of mercury has become.

Once in the brain, mercury stimulates an immune response, including activation of microglia;[450] triggers inflammation; and stimulates free-radical production.[451] Mercury also boosts the production of amyloid protein, and as we know by now, these issues all increase the risk of AD.[452]

From a regulatory standpoint, we're only just beginning to understand how widespread and serious the worldwide problem of mercury poisoning is. A 2018 study that tested more than 1,000 women in 25 countries on six continents revealed that 36 percent had mercury levels that exceeded the EPA health advisory level.[453]

The USA emits about 158 tons of mercury into the environment each year.[454] The mercury is released into the air as inorganic mercury and ends up in rivers, lakes, wetlands, and the ocean. Then certain anaerobic bacteria act on the mercury to convert it to methyl mercury, the form that's found in fish and shellfish. This is the most toxic form of mercury, and it's readily integrated into our body tissues.

MERCURY IN FISH

In the past 200 years, the level of mercury in the first 300 feet of ocean water has tripled,[455] and, as we've already learned, the levels of mercury found in fish continue to climb each year.[456] Through a process called biomagnification, wherein smaller fish are eaten by bigger fish, mercury levels build up in the flesh of fish over time. Some, such as swordfish, shark, tilefish, king mackerel, grouper, tuna, lobster, and marlin, have exceptionally high levels. Fish are so reliably contaminated with the metal it's been estimated that over 85 percent of the mercury you will ingest will come from the seafood you eat.[457] Fresh water fish are just as problematic. Thirty-nine states now have advisories cautioning citizens against eating fish from their lakes and rivers.[458]

A CDC study, for example, found that among women who had eaten three or more servings of fish in the prior 30 days, mercury levels in their bodies were almost four times those of women who ate no fish.[459] People who eat fresh fish and canned tuna two to three times a week have in their bodies up to 400 percent of the mercury levels considered acceptable by the EPA.[460]

WHAT HAPPENS WHEN WE INGEST TOO MUCH MERCURY?

In the 1950s in Minamata, Japan, a startling outbreak of what the locals called "cat-dancing disease" occurred. Residents of this fishing village began exhibiting slurred speech, numb fingers, loss of coordination, partial paralysis, diminished hearing, difficulty swallowing, tremors, and an inability to maintain balance. Ultimately, thousands of residents were affected, some losing their ability to perform relatively simple tasks such as buttoning their shirts or putting on their sandals.[461] Many from the local cat population, which also fed on fish from nearby waters, ended up in convulsions from mercury poisoning. To the locals it looked as though the cats were dancing. This tragedy occurred because a local factory was discharging mercury-laden waste into the waters which subsequently contaminated the local fish population.

While this kind of acute poisoning results in obvious and dramatic symptoms, the average person's exposure to mercury today occurs at subtler levels that too frequently escape detection.

Based at California Pacific Medical Center in San Francisco, Dr. Jane Hightower noted that many of her affluent clientele—doctors, lawyers, bankers, and CEOs—frequently included fish in their diet because of the purported health benefits. When she heard about neurological symptoms in people with high mercury levels, she decided to conduct a study of her own patients, some of whom exhibited these symptoms.[462]

What Dr. Hightower found was reported in the *New England Journal of Medicine* and surprised many health professionals around the world. It turned out that 89 percent of patients she tested had blood mercury levels above the standard of five parts per billion (PPB) set by the EPA and National Academy of Sciences. Specifically, 63 patients had mercury levels in their blood twice that level; 19 patients had mercury levels four times that level; and four patients had mercury levels ten times the EPA limit. One patient, a woman who had been suffering from various symptoms for years, was found to have blood mercury levels 15 times the EPA standard.[463]

A child in the study, who customarily ate two cans of tuna fish a week, had lost her ability to tie her shoes, suffered diminished verbal skills, and was lethargic. Her blood mercury levels were at 13 PPB, well over twice the EPA standard.

All patients included in the study were suffering from symptoms indicative of heavy-metal poisoning, including fatigue, headache, joint pain, poor concentration, and failing memory.

"They think they're doing the right thing by eating swordfish, sea bass, halibut, and Ahi tuna steaks," said Dr. Hightower, "but [these fish species] just happen to have the highest content of mercury sold in restaurants and grocery stores."[464]

San Francisco's affluent aren't the only ones suffering heavy-metal poisoning from eating seafood. A study suggests that 10 percent of high-school children in Hong Kong now suffer from mercury poisoning brought about by their steady diet of fish.[465] Given the findings of Dr. Hightower's study, it's likely that if we were to take blood samples from others who make fish a regular part of their diet, we'd find widespread mercury poisoning.

MERCURY IN DENTAL FILLINGS

While fish consumption is by far the greatest source of exposure, it is not the only way we are exposed to mercury. Dental amalgams, or silver fillings, are another major source of mercury exposure.[466] These kinds of fillings were standard in dentistry for decades. Only recently have other options become available.

If you have multiple amalgam fillings in your mouth, you are exposed to mercury vapor and may have as much as ten times the average level of mercury in your saliva and feces when tested. The good news is that by having your mercury fillings replaced by composite fillings, you can eliminate this source of mercury exposure. However, make sure you go to a dentist experienced in environmental dentistry and in metal filling replacement; specific protocols must be followed so as not to expose you (and the dental office staff) to more mercury during the removal procedure.

ALUMINUM

While there is evidence showing an association between aluminum and AD, a causal relationship has yet to be demonstrated. However, there is no debate over the neurotoxicity of aluminum.[467]

Have you ever heard of *the precautionary principle*? It's the idea that one should avoid exposure to potentially toxic substances or practices even if the risk hasn't yet been proven. And it applies to possible aluminum ingestion from our food and water supplies.[468]

Research into the connection between aluminum and Alzheimer's has focused on four compelling points: that aluminum is an undisputed neurotoxin;[469] that it crosses the blood–brain barrier and thus gets into the brain;[470] that it has been found deposited in the brain plaques of AD patients;[471] that aluminum exposure in animals leads to brain inflammation[472] and increased amyloid proteins.[473]

Aluminum is also known to activate microglia, which results in prolonged states of inflammation of the brain that can last up to a year. Aluminum also interferes with the production of glutathione, a critical brain antioxidant.[474]

What remains under consideration is whether the aluminum found at higher levels in people with dementia, and specifically Alzheimer's, is the cause of damage or if the metal has an affinity for the tangles and plaques where it accumulates. This is an important distinction but by no means a reason to delay minimizing exposure to aluminum.

The most recent study to examine the risk from aluminum accumulation measured levels of the metal in brain samples of 12 subjects who were diagnosed with AD. The scientists reported that the concentrations of aluminum were "extremely high," and higher than all previous measurements of brain aluminum.[475]

Numerous studies, including population studies conducted in Canada, England, France, Norway, and Wales have shown an association between high concentrations of aluminum in drinking water and an increased risk of cognitive decline and Alzheimer's disease.[476]

HOW ARE WE EXPOSED TO ALUMINUM?

Aluminum is the most abundant metal in the earth's crust. We ingest aluminum through some prepared foods, municipal drinking water, and over-the-counter medications.

Antacid medications, for example, can be a significant source of aluminum exposure. In one study, individuals who were taking antacids containing 470 mg of aluminum multiple times daily were found to have significantly elevated aluminum concentrations in their brain tissue after ten days of taking the medications.[477] Those with compromised kidney function will tend to absorb more of the aluminum from such exposure. Aluminum-containing antacids taken with orange juice will significantly increase the amount of aluminum that is absorbed. If you use antacids, look for products that are aluminum-free, such as Rolaids or Tums.[478]

Calcium supplements have also been found to be contaminated by aluminum. Since calcium supplements are also frequently contaminated with lead, those taking them may wish to reconsider their use.

Elevated aluminum levels in foods largely come from certain preservatives and anti-caking, leavening, and coloring agents. Commercially prepared foods sold in restaurants and bakeries are more likely to contain such ingredients, but there are some at your favorite grocer that you may have never suspected. For example, unless the packaging declares otherwise, most baking powder contains added aluminum. The USA maintains very weak standards for preventing aluminum exposure through diet. Our suggested tolerance level is seven times higher than both the World Health Organization and the European Food Safety Authority tolerance limit.

One of the highest sources of aluminum among foods is pancake mix. One study found that a single serving of pancakes made from a mix contained 180 mg of aluminum.[479] It's there as an anti-caking agent as sodium aluminum phosphate. These pancake mixes, cake and muffin mixes, and baking powder itself, as well as the cheese on frozen pizzas, non-dairy creamers, and single serving salt packets are the primary sources of dietary aluminum.

Another way that aluminum gets into our food is through aluminum foil. When foil is used to cook or prepare foods, aluminum can migrate into the foods at levels the WHO finds concerning. This is particularly so if the foods are acidic or spicy.[480]

Tea is also recognized as an efficient accumulator of aluminum.[481] Because much of the aluminum is bound to the tea leaves, our absorption of aluminum from the beverage is thought to be limited. Hibiscus teas have a higher amount of aluminum and therefore there is a higher absorption rate from these teas when compared to black and green teas.[482]

The aluminum that is used in antiperspirants can be absorbed through the skin and enter the bloodstream. Typically, aluminum is not used in regular deodorant, but be sure to read the labels. Look for "aluminum chloralhydrate" or "aluminum zirconium tetrachlorohydrex GLY."

ALUMINUM IN DRINKING WATER

One source of aluminum that is frequently overlooked is drinking water.[483] Aluminum salts (aluminum sulphate and polyaluminum chloride) are used as coagulants to purify municipal water in many cities. They effectively cause impurities, such as bacteria and other particulates, to clump together, which makes them easier to remove through sedimentation and filtration.

However, small residues of aluminum remain in the water and this may be risky for humans over time. At the very least, we should remove it with an activated carbon or reverse-osmosis filtration system at home.[484] Water treatment facilities are moving toward aluminum-free binders so that over time this may be one less source of exposure.

An additional source of aluminum may be the pots and pans many of us use for cooking.[485] The best option is pans with an aluminum core (for heat conductivity) and a stainless cladding cooking surface. Finally, if you are fond of drinking beverages from aluminum cans you may be absorbing small quantities of aluminum from them as well. Studies have shown that the longer the beverage is stored in the can the higher the aluminum content may be.[486] This is especially the case with soft drinks because their acid content erodes the aluminum from the can wall.

COPPER

Copper is an essential dietary element, involved in the production of red blood cells, nerve function, immune function, and supporting cell respiration. However, we need only a very small amount. While findings are mixed about copper's possible role in contributing to Alzheimer's risk, and experts continue to debate the matter, a meta-analysis that reviewed the results of 26 published studies on the subject found that Alzheimer's patients did have higher levels of serum copper than control subjects who were cognitively healthy.[487] Also, researchers have found that those with high copper levels who also eat a diet rich in saturated fat and trans-fat experience dramatically greater cognitive decline over time.

For reasons unknown, in Alzheimer's disease the regulation of copper levels becomes compromised. This is also the case in Parkinson's disease and Amyotrophic Lateral Sclerosis (ALS). Excessive copper not only can promote free radicals and oxidative stress, but it can also impede the removal of amyloid protein and encourage it to clump together into plaques. [488] Further, when tested, both adults and children who have higher levels of copper in their blood tend to perform more poorly when it comes to memory, attention, and learning. [489]

You have probably seen the verdigris that copper gutters, downspouts, and roof flashing take on when they become oxidized. Before 1982, pennies were made from 95 percent copper so you could see the oxidation in them as well.

HOW ARE WE EXPOSED TO COPPER?

Since our daily need for copper is so small (0.9 mg) most people have no problem meeting that requirement through diet. However, one's copper intake can creep up to unhealthy levels through supplements, water pipes, and some foods. Most multivitamins have historically and unnecessarily included copper and iron. However, manufacturers are beginning to offer formulas free of these elements. Read labels to know for certain what you are ingesting.

Often, water pipes and brass faucet fittings in homes (and offices) are composed of copper. With age, the metal leaches into the water we drink and cook with, and the more acidic your water is to begin with, the more effectively it corrodes pipes and leaches copper. Copper can and should be filtered from drinking water using an activated carbon or reverse osmosis filtration system.

Meats, particularly liver and veal, are high in accumulated copper, as are oysters. A typical portion of liver contains nearly 15 times the daily value for copper. There is some evidence that the adverse effect of high copper levels may be exacerbated by a diet rich in saturated fat and trans fats.[490]

While copper regulation in the body is still somewhat of a mystery, it seems prudent that we look to avoid exposure to excess copper that might place us at greater risk.

IRON

As with other elements essential to human health, excess iron can wreak havoc in the body and mind. Too much iron intake presents a health threat, including liver damage, joint damage, and heightened risk of heart disease. High iron levels are associated with poorer cognitive function and may increase risk of developing AD.

Iron in healthy amounts is critical for the formation of hemoglobin, the protein in red blood cells that carries oxygen from the lungs throughout the body, and to the maintenance of cell function.

If we take in too much vitamin C through supplementation, any excess gets excreted in the urine. However, the body does not excrete excess iron. With age, iron continues to build up in the body—most significantly after menopause in women.[491] That said, giving blood lowers iron levels markedly.[492]

With age, iron accumulates in the hippocampus and in an area called the substantia nigra, where Parkinson's disease is focused.[493] Tests in both Alzheimer's and Parkinson's patients frequently confirm excessive iron in these brain regions. Iron also is known to accumulate in amyloid plaques.[494]

Iron was first declared a risk factor for Alzheimer's in 1950. At that time researchers conducting autopsy studies found that the brains of people who had died from AD had high levels of iron. More recently, pathology studies and MRI studies have linked iron accumulation with risk for Alzheimer's disease.[495]

In one study, researchers screened subjects who were cognitively normal, those who had mild cognitive impairment, and those with AD. They measured levels of ferritin (a protein that stores iron) in their cerebrospinal fluid as an indicator of iron levels in the brain. During the following seven years, all subjects were given cognitive tests and had MRI scans to monitor changes in brain volume. In all three groups, those with the higher levels of iron showed the most cognitive decline and brain shrinkage, and were more likely to progress to AD.[496]

How might iron contribute to neurodegenerative disease? Iron oxidizes very easily.[497] In vitro studies have shown that as excess iron accumulates and oxidative stress develops, neurons can be damaged and killed.[498]

Dr. George Bartzokis, a professor of psychiatry at the Semel Institute for Neuroscience and Human Behavior at UCLA, and his colleagues have used MRIs to confirm that as higher levels of iron accumulate in the brain, more damage is seen in the hippocampus region. With 31 Alzheimer's patients and 68 healthy subjects, Bartzokis's team measured iron levels in the brain and found that the more iron accumulated in the hippocampus, the more tissue damage was apparent. Excessive brain iron was seen in the AD patients but not in the healthy subjects.[499]

Dr. Bartzokis's hypothesis is that in some people iron accumulation in the brain first damages myelin, a substance that insulates nerve fibers like the plastic coating on electrical wire. With damage to the myelin, communication between the neurons is disrupted, leading to neuron dysfunction, plaque formation, and eventually, cell death.

Elevated levels of iron in cerebrospinal fluid are also predictive of how rapidly one will transition from MCI to AD.[500]

HOW ARE WE EXPOSED TO IRON?

How might our lifestyle choices contribute to risk of iron overload? There are two primary routes: diet and supplements. Meats contain two types of iron: heme and non-heme. Heme iron is easily absorbed, even if your iron levels are sufficient. Plants, such as legumes and leafy greens, contain only non-heme iron which the body can better regulate. With non-heme iron, if you are low in iron, your body will absorb more from plant sources. If you already have sufficient iron levels, the body will absorb less. In short, if your diet is centered upon meat, it may push you toward iron overload more easily.[501]

The second common source of iron is vitamin-mineral supplements. Although supplement manufacturers have begun to offer iron-free formulas, for decades there was an assumption that everyone could benefit from the presence of iron in their supplement. Many people who already had sufficient iron levels were taking this additional dose, unaware of the risk it posed. Another source of iron is fortified breakfast cereals. Their iron content can range from between 3.6 milligrams to 18 milligrams per serving. Be sure to read the labels.

There's a widespread belief that as a matter of course humans, particularly menstruating women, are likely to be iron deficient and need iron supplementation. Iron deficiency is seen in two percent of adult men and 9-12 percent of white women and may be as high as 20 percent in Black and Mexican-American women.[502] In the Framingham Heart Study, 1,000 participants aged 68 to 93 had their iron levels measured. Only three percent had a deficiency, but 13 percent had high, unhealthful levels of iron.

Some people have hereditary conditions such as hemochromatosis and thalassemia intermedia, which cause them to absorb excessive iron, but most people with elevated iron levels develop this condition due a meat-centered diet, unnecessary supplementation, or environmental exposure. The Iron Disorders Institute estimates 16 million Americans have elevated iron levels.[503]

Other sources of iron include cast-iron pans, old iron water pipes (though rare), and drinking water. My recommendation is that you toss the cast-iron pans and replace them with a stainless-clad variety.

Occupations that can lead to significant iron exposure include welders, sheet metal workers, plumbers, auto mechanics, and steel workers.

A simple blood test can measure iron levels, specifically serum ferritin (the iron-storage protein) levels. Ferritin levels may range from 12 to 300 nanograms per milliliter of blood (ng/ml) for males and 12 to 150 ng/ml for females. The ideal range is 50 to 150 ng/ml. It may be wise to avoid iron supplements unless your healthcare provider has prescribed them specifically to treat a deficiency.

LEAD

In the first century AD Emperor Nero's physician, Dioscorides, cautioned that "lead makes the mind give way."[504] Even the ancients knew that the accumulation of lead could cause psychosis. Nonetheless, it was used extensively in aqueducts and as a wine sweetener.

In more recent times, much of the attention to lead's toxicity has focused on exposure in children. We know that even at low levels lead exposure can be toxic to the developing brain. In fact, there has been no threshold established below which lead does not cause damage. Still, in a 2019 Harvard University study, dangerous levels of lead were found in the drinking water of nearly 50 percent of schools in the US.[505] An elementary school in Maine had lead contamination at 15 times the EPA limit. Although this survey was focused on water at schools, the municipal water that reaches schools is the same water that reaches homes.

Lead can affect both the peripheral nervous system and the central nervous system, and exposure to it can cause the loss of the myelin coating on nerves and damage to nerve fibers.[506] Lead crosses the blood–brain barrier and increases its permeability,[507] causes oxidative stress,[508] interferes with the production of neurotransmitters,[509] interferes with synaptic function, and causes amyloid proteins to clump together. It mostly finds its way to the hippocampus and cerebellum, where it's been found in high concentrations.[510]

Lead exposure has been shown to affect visual-spatial and visual-motor function, language, information-processing speed, executive function, and verbal and visual memory.[511] A nine-year study of lead exposure showed how it can affect cognitive health over time. In more than 1,000 subjects, lead concentrations in both blood and bone were measured. The subjects were divided into four groups based upon the total lead burden they carried, with each group representing a progressively higher exposure. The subjects were then given a battery of cognitive tests. Nine years later they were tested again. As the researchers tested the four distinct groups, they found that members within each distinct quartile, with their progressively higher lead exposures, showed mental deficits equal to five additional years of cognitive aging.[512] Group one showed cognitive aging of five additional years, group two showed ten additional years of cognitive aging, group three showed 15 years of additional cognitive aging, and so on. The more lead they had in the body, the more compromised was their cognitive health.

There is an emerging theory called Latent Early-Life Associated Regulation or LEARn. This theory suggests early-life exposures can predispose an individual for diseases in adulthood. In the case of lead, brief exposures to lead at the fetal stage result in epigenetic changes—a temporary rise in proteins involved in AD and then an overproduction of amyloid protein later in adult life.[513] So, just as is the case with mercury, early exposure to lead may predispose us to Alzheimer's later in life.

HOW ARE WE EXPOSED TO LEAD?

Lead exposure occurs through lead-containing paint, older water pipes that leach lead into drinking water, imported toys, artificial turf, pottery painted with lead-containing glaze, leaded crystal glassware, lead solder in imported food cans, and cosmetics such as lipstick. Fish and shellfish are also frequently contaminated with lead.

Analyses of many different chocolate products show that lead contamination, largely absorbed from the manufacturing machinery used to process chocolate, is a widespread concern. Many samples exceed the acceptable levels established by regulators, and chocolate is consistently among the foods with the highest levels when tested.[514]

Calcium supplements, reported to be taken daily by 25 percent of the US female population, are a frequent source of lead contamination. The lead has accumulated in the bone, seashells, and coral from which calcium supplements are made. In a survey of 70 different brands of calcium supplements tested, researchers found that while lead contamination was low in some brands, in 25 percent of samples levels were in excess of the FDA's provisional "tolerable" daily intake of lead.[515] In another survey that included 136 brands of calcium supplements, two-thirds exceeded the California state standard for acceptable lead levels.[516]

SOURCES OF LEAD	
lipstick	old water pipes
leaded crystal glassware	imported canned foods
lead solder used in welding	chocolate
calcium supplements	lead dust from old paint
folk medicines	firearms / ammunition
bottled water	imported dried fruits

The warnings are clear. We should be concerned about overexposure to these metals—or any exposure to lead—and work to minimize them in our diet and in our environment. There is no reason to allow them to possibly become additional risk factors for dementia.

17

PESTICIDES

POISON BY ANOTHER NAME

Pesticides by design are toxins. Another word you could use for them would be *poisons*. It is now well understood that they can contribute to the risk of developing a neurological disease, yet for a long time, people didn't understand the extent of their danger to human health. I want to be sure that you understand the serious threat pesticides pose to your brain health, so I have devoted considerable space to the topic.

I understand that what I share in this chapter can be disheartening to read and that there may be a part of you that wishes to skip ahead and avoid learning more bad news. I hope you will persevere! As difficult as it is at times to learn what a mess we've made of our planet, the better informed you are the more effective you will be at making choices that protect you and your family.

When I was a child, my family had a pool in our backyard. We lived in Southern California, the climate was warm, and my five siblings and I took advantage of every opportunity to swim.

Once out of the pool, however, we were frequently pestered by horseflies and bees, and, if it was late in the afternoon, mosquitos. To contend with the pests, we always had a can of Raid insect spray nearby. The slogan inscribed on it was classic: "The only good bug is a dead bug." Of course, that's untrue anyway.

Not only did we spray bugs that dared approach us, but we also periodically "fogged" the air around us, unwittingly enveloping ourselves in a cloud of poison. I can still recall the acrid odor that the spray produced.

Some ingredients then routinely used in consumer insecticides, such as DDT and Chlordane, have long since been banned due to their known toxicity. This is a good thing—there are no more kids dancing around in clouds of DDT before jumping into a pool—but, sadly, the new generation of home insecticides is just as dangerous.

Pesticides are introduced into the environment annually through applications to schools, homes, parks, roadsides, and crops. Pesticides are in the air we breathe,[517] the tap water we drink,[518] the rain that falls upon us, the soil in which we grow our food,[519] and on or in the food itself.[520] Even the fog that settles onto our communities is laced with pesticides.[521]

Ninety-seven percent of all North American rivers and streams are now contaminated with pesticides.[522] They're in umbilical cord blood, amniotic fluid, and breast milk, so the next generation is not only bathed in pesticides for nine months before birth, but they also encounter pesticides in the first meal their mother gives them.[523]

Do you use pesticides in your home? Some 85 percent of American households use three to four different pesticide products regularly, and according to the EPA 4.4 billion pesticide applications are made in family homes, yards and gardens every year.[524]

When I was in my twenties, I moved to an apartment complex in Ft. Worth, Texas, where I did my undergraduate study. Before moving there, I might have seen three cockroaches in my life. As anyone who has spent time in Texas will confirm, roaches are not just present in abundance, they are exceptionally large and seem to find their way into everything. As was required by the property manager, each month an exterminator would enter and "treat" all resident apartments.

Because I was attending school at the time, I seldom was home to see what they did. On one occasion, I happened to come back to my apartment to find the door ajar. Inside was the exterminator, clad in elbow high rubber gloves, rubber boots, goggles, and a respirator. Strapped to his back was a large plastic tank that fed a rubber hose and a metallic dispensing wand in his hand. He gave me a perfunctory greeting and went back to work. As I sorted through a stack of papers on my countertop, I watched him with one eye as he released the liquid in a stream where my carpet met the baseboards, then in closets, and under the kitchen and bathroom sink cabinets. Suddenly, the incongruence of what the two of us were wearing stuck me. He was clad in gear to protect his health, while I was in shorts, a t-shirt, and sandals. Why did he need all that protection but I, apparently, needed none? Do people know what kinds of risks they're taking when they use pesticides in and around their homes? I certainly had no understanding of what I was exposed to in my apartment in Texas.

The American Optometric Association estimates that 40 to 50 percent of homeowners who use retail pesticide products are likely to have little understanding of the toxicity simply because the disclosure labels are written in such small print, and are difficult to understand, too. It's foolish to think we could unleash this far-reaching payload of poison into the environment and not experience a human health toll.

PESTICIDES AND THE BRAIN

Given the ubiquity of pesticides in our society, there has been relatively limited research to determine what types of health hazards pesticides pose to humans. But evidence is mounting that over time these poisons may have a devastating effect on the human nervous system.[525]

Pesticide exposure is now linked to neurological problems,[526] mild cognitive impairment,[527] ALS,[529] Parkinson's disease,[530] and Alzheimer's disease.[531] While most pesticide formulas have never been adequately tested for toxicity in human subjects, a number of these compounds, such as maneb, a fungicide, and paraquat an herbicide, have been proven to reliably caused brain damage in animals used in research.[532]

The most common class of pesticides we use is called organophosphates. They damage the brain by inhibiting a neurotransmitter that enables communication between brain cells. Organophosphates also promote free radicals and oxidative stress, encourage the accumulation of amyloid protein, and trigger inflammation and apoptosis, a form of cell self-destruction.[533]

A well-regarded scientist from Harvard Medical School, Dr. David Bellinger, along with Philip Landrigan, dean of global health studies at Mt. Sinai School of Medicine, believe we may be in the midst of a silent pandemic, and that the chemicals in pesticides are slowly and insidiously poisoning our brains.[534]

Whether the issue is lowered IQs, ADHD, skyrocketing rates of autism and behavioral disorders, AD, Parkinson's disease, or other neurological disease, the dramatic rise in incidence is undeniable, and other scientists share Landrigan's and Bellinger's concern that pesticides may be a critical and largely overlooked player. Dr. Warren Porter, an environmental toxicologist at the University of Wisconsin–Madison, shares their concern. He points out that registrations for pesticides with the EPA do not include testing for neurological or epigenetic effects. Formulations (a list of all ingredients contained in a pesticide) are considered proprietary and therefore kept secret. The data that we do have is provided directly from the chemical manufacturers and thus unlikely to include any adverse finding that would place sales of these products at risk. Yet Porter's own research has shown that combinations of agricultural chemicals commonly found in groundwater do have an impact on the brain.

I have sometimes wondered if pesticides played a role in my grandmother Mollie's Alzheimer's disease. She spent her adult life living in the corn and soy belt of the Midwest where, for decades, the drinking water that millions rely upon has been routinely contaminated by the controversial weed killer Atrazine, and other poisons as well. Europe long ago imposed a ban on Atrazine because it makes its way into groundwater so easily. Yet in the USA 76 million pounds of this substance are sprayed annually on crop fields, predominantly those growing corn.

In 2021 the EPA authorized the use of a pesticide, aldicarb, on Florida citrus crops. Aldicarb is so toxic that it has been banned for use on citrus crops in 100 countries under the Rotterdam Convention.[535] Designated by the World Health Organization as "extremely toxic" Aldicarb is a known neurotoxin that plants can absorb from the soil and accumulate in their leaves and fruit.[536]

PESTICIDES AND ALZHEIMER'S DISEASE

The association between pesticide exposure and the risk of developing AD has been well researched. In a study of 17,942 subjects, those who lived closest to agricultural areas where intensive pesticide use occurred had twice the risk of developing Alzheimer's compared to those living in areas with low exposure.[537]

A six-year prospective study of 1,507 subjects in France exposed to pesticides in their work found that they were at 2.39 times higher risk of later developing AD.[538] In a five-year longitudinal Canadian study of occupational exposure to pesticides, subjects were 4.35 times more likely to develop AD.[539]

In another study reported in *JAMA Neurology*, scientists from Rutgers University, Emory University, and the University of Texas Southwestern Medical Center took blood samples from both Alzheimer's patients and from healthy, elderly individuals used as controls. Then they measured the level of DDE, the breakdown product of DDT, in their blood. The scientists found that in those with AD, levels of DDE in the blood were almost four times higher than in those who remained free of Alzheimer's.[540] Those who had both high levels of DDE and carried the APOE4 gene were the most severely cognitively impaired.

It's remarkable that although the USA banned DDT in 1972, it is still found in the food chain with beef, poultry,[541] and dairy products[542] most heavily affected. China and India still produce approximately 5,000 tons of DDT annually, and when it is used around agricultural products, it may end up in foods imported into the USA.[543] A 2014 study found that 75 to 80 percent of all blood samples obtained from the Center for Disease Control and Prevention contain measurable levels of DDT.[544] So we are not free of DDT yet, even in the 21st century.

Studies have also consistently shown a link between exposure to insecticides, herbicides, and fungicides and the risk of developing Parkinson's disease.[545] For years scientists have known that they can cause symptoms of PD to develop in animals exposed to the fungicide maneb[546] and the herbicide paraquat.[547] In the US, four million pounds of paraquat are used annually in the farming of soy, corn, and cotton, and as you might guess, it's found in many sources of drinking water.[548]

We should not be surprised that pesticides are detrimental to the health of the brain and that exposure to them has been associated with a higher risk for AD. Many pesticide classes are designed to damage the nervous system of living creatures.[549] They do so by blocking a certain enzyme (cholinesterase), which controls a certain neurotransmitter (acetylcholine). In humans, this causes neurons in the brain to fire uncontrollably and die.[550]

Exposure to pesticides also produces free radicals, which damage the mitochondria of neuronal cells.[551] This promotes inflammation, which in turn results in more free-radical production and more damage to neurons. It also depletes an important antioxidant, glutathione, which our body uses to fight oxidative stress. Making matters worse, the toxicity not only is amplified through repeated exposure, but the compounds also accumulate in our bodies.

ROUNDUP AND GLYPHOSATE

In 1987, Roundup was 17th on the list of commonly used herbicides. With the introduction of "Roundup Ready" crops, including corn, soy, canola, alfalfa, and sugar beets, which are genetically engineered to tolerate the weed killer and survive, the chemical became the bestselling herbicide in the world.

Because farmers need not worry about damaging their genetically engineered crops, they use the chemical liberally to fight weeds. There have been two major consequences. First, weeds treated with Roundup developed resistance to the chemical. Second, the farmers' response has been to apply more Roundup. Also, wheat farmers planting non–genetically modified crops have discovered they can use Roundup as a desiccant (drying agent) just before harvest. The result is that even non-GMO wheat and much of the supply of oats is now frequently tainted with glyphosate (the active ingredient in Roundup) residues.

According to a handful of recent tests conducted in the US and abroad, these factors have led to widespread contamination by glyphosate of many foods found in grocery stores. The highest levels are seen in non-organic wheat, conventional oats, and soy, as well as the foods made from these crops. This includes bread, pasta, crackers, beer, wine, corn chips, granola and granola bars, breakfast cereals, as well as many other snack foods. Glyphosate was present in all California wines tested, European beers,[552] and a host of popular foods including Cheerios, Ritz crackers, Special K cereal, Triscuit crackers,[553] and Ben & Jerry's ice cream.[554] Nestle discovered high levels of glyphosate in its coffee beans.[555]

The levels of glyphosate in human blood samples have climbed more than 1,000 percent in the last 20 years,[556] and it's now detected in the urine of 92 percent of Americans tested.[557] Later on, I will tell you how you can slash the level of glyphosate you are ingesting.

In recent years, Roundup has made headlines worldwide after multimillion-dollar jury awards related to its reported relationship to non-Hodgkin's lymphoma. However, glyphosate is just one of many ingredients in Roundup and because the formula for the product is considered proprietary, no adequate research has been conducted that would permit scientists to fully understand the broader risks it may pose. We know nothing about how it may affect gene expression in humans; given that it is detectable in the urine of most Americans today, we certainly should. Some research, however, suggests glyphosate itself may be a neurotoxin—that is, may poison neurons.[558]

HOW EXPOSURE HAPPENS

One common way we're exposed to pesticides is through our diets. Despite the growing body of evidence indicating these poisons are taking a toll on the health of humans, more pesticides are applied to food crops today than ever before. Moreover, American farmers routinely apply 85 different pesticides that, due to their known toxicity, have been banned in France, Italy, Spain, the United Kingdom, China, and Brazil.[559] In a process that has been called the circle of poison, pesticides that have been banned in the USA are still permitted to be exported to developing countries where they are used on crops the USA then imports back to the US market.[560] Up to fifty percent of fresh fruits and one-third of fresh vegetables sold in US supermarkets are now imported from other countries.

The USDA Pesticide Data Program indicates that today's conventionally grown spinach is treated with up to 54 different pesticides, 11 of which are known neurotoxins; conventionally grown strawberries are treated with up to 45 different pesticide products, seven of which are known neurotoxins. Potatoes, especially the Russets used predominantly to produce French fries, are treated with a plethora of chemicals to produce a blemish-free product demanded by the world's biggest fast-food chains. As a result, when tested, they may contain residues of up to 35 different pesticides, herbicides, and fungicides, seven of which are neurotoxins.[561]

To understand the degree to which typical supermarket-bought foods are contaminated with pesticides, scientists collected and analyzed more than 300 samples of 31 different foods from a supermarket in Dallas, Texas. Every food sample they looked at contained residues of multiple pesticide chemicals, including the 50-years-ago-banned DDT. Unless you are shopping for certified organically grown products, foods found in your supermarket may carry a similar level of contamination.[562]

The federal government has sat for decades on strong evidence that commonly used pesticides—routinely applied in our homes, schools, and churches as well as on athletic fields, roadsides, airplanes, golf courses, and parks, and on our foods—place us at risk for health effects such as brain damage, reproductive damage, birth defects, infertility, suppression of the immune system, and cancer. Even the Toxic Substances Control Act of 1976, intended to protect Americans, is 43 years old now and lacks adequate safeguards to truly protect us.

The recent case of one pesticide under review is a clear example of how difficult it is to get the EPA to act in the interest of American citizens. For 40 years, scientists have known about the neurotoxicity and troubling effects on the brains of children exposed to chlorpyrifos. Finally, in 2000, the EPA banned the use of the pesticide in households. Yet it took another 21 years before the EPA banned its use in agriculture. Since 1975, the US government has managed to ban just six toxic chemicals out of the 85,000 that have been approved for use without adequate testing for safety.[563]

The European Union has taken a different approach to regulating pesticides. A fundamental tenet of the EU's governing policies related to food safety, human health, and the environment is the *precautionary principle* I mentioned before. The principle dictates that if a chemical is suspected of having the potential to cause harm, and there is a lack of scientific consensus affirming it does *not*, it is assumed to be unsafe. The burden of proof will fall on the manufacturer of the chemical to prove otherwise. Too bad the same logic does not hold sway in the US Clearly, protecting ourselves is up to us alone. We can't count on regulating agencies to do it for us.

I know that it's deeply disheartening to learn how we have contaminated our soil, air, rivers, lakes, and of course food with toxic pesticides. There's no question about it: a comprehensive strategy to protect our brains should include the avoidance of all toxic pesticides. Do not buy them, apply them, or have others apply them in your home or workplace, or anywhere else you spend time. Choose organically produced foods, beverages, herbs, and spices every time you have the option to do so. Later I'll share more details on how to protect yourself and your family.

18

A TOXIC CATCH

I N MARCH 2019 more than a dozen dolphins were found stranded on beaches in Florida and Massachusetts. This sort of thing had been seen before—fish, turtles, whales, and dolphins have all been found beached around the world. However, University of Miami marine biologists investigating the case made a surprising and unsettling discovery. Under autopsy the dolphin brains revealed the hallmark amyloid plaques and tau tangles seen in the brains of humans diagnosed with Alzheimer's. Accompanying those plaques and tangles was mercury and a substance called BMAA.

A possible threat to human brain health, BMAA (beta-methylami-no-L-alanine) is a non-protein amino-acid. It first came to the attention of science in 1944, when the US recaptured the island of Guam from the Japanese, who had occupied it during the two prior years. As US forces began to reestablish themselves on the island, army physicians noticed that the native inhabitants of the island, the Chamorro, suffered from an exceptionally high rate of neurological disease. Nearly every household on the island had an afflicted member. At the time the incidence of neurological disease in Guam was 100 times the incidence worldwide.[564]

The Chamorro named the condition that afflicted them *lytico-bodig* which means paralysis-dementia. Because they suffered from a constellation of symptoms that were seen in Alzheimer's, ALS, and Parkinson's disease, the condition was called amyotrophic lateral sclerosis-parkinson-ism-dementia-complex (ALS-PDC)—a mouthful, indeed. Behind the mouthful was a mystery: What could be responsible for such a dramatic rate of neurological disease in such a remote area?

139

After careful consideration, neurologists who came to study residents of the island noted two things about the Chamorro: They made their own tortillas from flour derived from the seeds of the cycad trees, and they commonly ate a native fruit bat called the Mariana flying fox. The bats were stewed in coconut milk and eaten in their entirety—wings, brains, bones, and skin.

It wasn't until 12 years later that noted plant biochemist Arthur Bell, of the Kew Royal Botanic Gardens, tested the cycad plant seeds and discovered the presence of BMAA, which proved to be a neurotoxin.

Initial tests showed that BMAA damaged neurons as well as caused convulsions in rats and chicks and shaking and paralysis in macaques.[565] It turned out that the flying fox had a penchant for cycad seeds and foraged for them. When ethnobotanist Dr. Paul Alan Cox and his colleague Sandra Banack tested skin samples from the bats, they found they had 10,000 times as much BMAA accumulated in their flesh as was found in the cyanobacteria itself.[566] Clearly, the BMAA toxin had been biomagnified over time in the bat's flesh.

Such high levels of a known neurotoxin were now considered a prime suspect in the staggering rates of neurological disease among the Chamorro. After testing the brain tissue of both those who died of ALS-PDC on Guam as well as two people who died from Alzheimer's in Canada, the team discovered BMAA in the brains of both. But they found none in the brain tissue samples of people who died of other illnesses.[567]

Neurologist Deborah Mash, founder and then director of the University of Miami's Brain Endowment Bank, one of the largest repositories of brains from people who died from Alzheimer's Parkinson's and ALS, decided to look at stored brain samples to see if she could detect BMAA. Mash found the substance in some brain samples from those who died from Alzheimer's and ALS, further affirming the suspicion that it might play a role.[568]

In 2016, scientists showed that BMAA-laced fruit fed to vervet monkeys for 140 days caused the hallmark features of Alzheimer's—plaques and tangles—to develop in their brains, further supporting the hypothesis that BMAA may be a trigger for neurological disease in humans.[569] Additional research showed that the neurons in the hippocampus region of the brain were particularly sensitive to BMAA assaults when tested in vitro.[570] BMAA has also been linked to protein misfolding and clumping, neuroinflammation and the suppression of certain enzymes.[571]

The prevailing theory is that after one is exposed to BMAA it crosses the blood-brain barrier. The substance then accumulates in neurons by directly incorporating itself into the protein chain by substituting itself for the amino acid L-serine, resulting in a faulty protein sequence. The protein then assumes an altered shape and is no longer able to do its job, leading to protein misfolding, clumping, and, eventually, cell death.[572]

So how is something isolated on the island of Guam found in the brains of people in Canada and Florida? As it turns out, a strain of cyanobacteria (sometimes called blue-green algae) that was found on the root and seed of the cycad produces BMAA. Ecologist Dr. Aspassia Chatziefthimiou of Weil Medical College at Cornell University studies BMAA in the lab and has hypothesized that cyanobacteria may produce the toxin as a means of communication, perhaps signaling changes in their environment.

The same BMAA-producing cyanobacteria found in Guam proliferates all over the world. In fact, cyanobacteria are the oldest organism known to inhabit Earth. Fossil records indicate that bacteria were present 3.5 billion years ago and were the first producers of oxygen.[573] They are found in oceans and freshwater, the Arabian Desert, the Antarctic, Europe, North America, and Australia.

Cyanobacteria can be a dominant presence in the growing incidence of algae blooms found in seawater near nutrient-dense runoff, such as in the Gulf of Mexico. Picture fertilizers from agriculture, suburban lawns, and golf courses flowing into the ocean via rivers and streams, fueling these algae blooms. Many such bodies of water now have expansive, recurring, and sometimes persistent cyanobacteria blooms.[574]

When BMAA is present in the proliferating algae blooms what might this portend for sea life? In 2010 that question was answered when fish and shellfish in Florida Bay, including lobster, shrimp, crab, mussels, porpoise, and large-mouth bass, were found to contain significant levels of BMAA.[575] In 2015, scientists found BMAA in seafood from four continents, including muscles, scallops, crab, and lobster.[576] In 2020,

BMAA was detected in about half of the seafood that was tested from markets in Stockholm, including oysters, mussels, shrimp, plaice, char and herring.[577] BMAA has also been found in freshwater-caught fish in Nebraska including bass, bluegill, carp, catfish, and walleye.[578]

Because they take on the toxin payload of those they eat, it was assumed that predator fish may have even higher levels of BMAA if tested. The ultimate predator, of course, is the shark. Staggeringly, an estimated 100 million sharks are killed annually worldwide, both by destructive fishing practices that trap them and also when they are caught momentarily, have their dorsal and pectoral fins sliced off and are thrown back into the ocean. Commanding up to $400 a kilo, the fins are used to make shark-fin soup (a long-standing Chinese favorite) and certain supplements.[579] Customers who buy the soup typically subscribe to the folklore that says it "nourishes" blood and "energizes" internal organs, and promotes virility and longevity.[580] For others, the soup is the Rolex of cuisine, a symbol of wealth and prosperity. Demand for the soup continues to rise due to China's rapid economic growth. Although evidence supporting health claims made for them are nonexistent, and a lengthy list of side effects have been reported by users, at the time of this writing costly supplements made from shark fins are legally sold at such places as GNC stores and through Amazon.com.

Researchers from the University of Miami Medical School discovered that shark fins are a concentrated source of BMAA.[581] Levels detected in shark fins are in some cases at the same concentration as those found in the brains of people who died from AD and ALS.[582]

After testing the most popular shark fin supplements, researchers found that 15 out of 16 brands contained BMAA.[583] BMAA has also been found in blue-green algae supplements.[584] Advertisements for these supplements often claim that they are vitamin and antioxidant-rich superfoods.

Not only does BMAA appear to be an independent risk factor, but Marquette University's Dr. Doug Lobner, a professor of biomedical sciences, has shown that mercury and BMAA work synergistically to damage brain cells. A very low level of mercury may not be enough to kill neurons, but when combined with BMAA, it completes the task.[585] Adding just two milligrams of mercury to 100 milligrams of BMAA multiplies the neurotoxin's power by five times.[586] So, you may get a double-whammy impact by eating fish that is contaminated with mercury and happens to be carrying BMAA in its flesh.[587]

WARMER OCEANS AND LAKES = MORE BMAA

As the climate continues to heat up, warmer waters mix with increasing amounts of nutrient runoff from fertilizers from agricultural operations, animal waste, and municipal sewage, and cyanobacteria-containing algae blooms are becoming increasingly prevalent and more persistent in both the ocean and in freshwater bodies the world over.[588] We have all seen stories in the news about popular vacation spots temporarily unsafe for swimming because of an algae bloom.

In 2016 in Salt Lake City, Utah, officials reported an unprecedented bloom of cyanobacteria in Utah Lake they attributed to the discharge of treated wastewater and infiltration of nitrogen and phosphorus from fertilizers.[589] At the time of this writing, New Jersey reported that its largest body of fresh water, Lake Hopatcong, popular with swimmers and water skiers, was infiltrated with the largest bloom of cyanobacteria ever recorded.[590] Thankfully, the state took measures to warn the public that the water presented a serious health hazard.

The possibility that BMAA could act as a trigger for neurological disease in humans remains controversial.[591] There is no definitive evidence that it does. However, the findings reported above are substantial, concerning, and warrant caution. Currently, there are no public warnings about the potential risk of exposure to BMAA from eating fish, shellfish, supplements, or protein powders made with blue-green algae.[592]

DOMOIC ACID

A mass poisoning of seabirds in North Monterey, California, in 1961 captured the imagination of master storyteller Alfred Hitchcock, who spun the real-life events into his classic 1963 horror film, *The Birds*. The

Santa Cruz Sentinel reported "thousands of birds floundering in streets" and residents witnessed disoriented birds flying into windows, regurgitating fish, and dying.[593] Although the birds never directly attacked residents, their disoriented state led them to swoop aggressively, appearing as though they were aiming for people.

It turned out that the birds were poisoned with a second ocean-borne neurotoxin called domoic acid (DA). It, too, comes from algae blooms. This toxin accumulates in sea life; therefore, like BMAA, you may be exposed to it through consumption of seafood.

The scientific community first learned about the human threat of DA when in 1987 more than 100 people on Prince Edward Island, Canada, became ill and a few died from eating mussels contaminated with the toxin.[594] Typical symptoms from exposure to DA include gastrointestinal distress, confusion, disorientation, seizures, and in extreme cases, death. Those who do not die are left with permanent short-term memory loss.

Scientists are beginning to attribute some cases of dolphin beaching and seizures in sea lions to poisoning from domoic acid.[595] Upon autopsy of the brains of the diseased mammals, they have discovered widespread depletion of the neurons of the hippocampus.[596] It's believed that DA causes continuous firing of nerve cells until they become so overstimulated that they die.

Attention is turning away from rare acute poisonings, such as the fatalities on Prince Edward Island that occurred in 1987, to the question of whether subtle slow-moving neurological damage like that caused by BMAA is occurring in some people who eat seafood. It is especially concerning that DA is not destroyed by cooking at high temperatures or by freezing.

Regulatory bodies in the US, the European Union, Australia, and New Zealand have proposed limits on DA exposure, set significantly lower than the levels known to have caused severe illness and death in the 1987 case. However, they have done so without any certainty that a subtler form of brain damage isn't occurring with lower exposures, even in the absence of early symptoms.[597]

Given that the DA toxin has been detected in anchovies, clams, halibut, mackerel, mussels, sardines, scallops, sole, tuna, and crab, [598] and that the toxic algae blooms that harbor DA are growing both in size and duration, the opportunity for exposure appears to be increasing.[599] In 2015, the National Oceanic and Atmospheric Administration measured the largest toxic algae bloom yet, stretching from the Gulf of Alaska to the coast of Mexico.[600] Could human exposure to this brain toxin, by way of fish and shellfish, be a growing threat to cognitive health?[601]

Seafood consumption in general is rising. Clearly, the most promising way to assure that you are not exposed to BMAA or DA is to avoid consuming seafood, and to steer clear of those blue-green algae drinks and supplements.

19

A PRESCRIPTION FOR TROUBLE

THREE OTHER RISK factors have received surprisingly little attention when it comes to their potential role in contributing to the development of neurologic disorders. They are prescription medications, recreational drugs, and smoking.

ARE PRESCRIPTION DRUGS SAFE FOR YOUR BRAIN?

As consumers, we expect that prescription drugs have been thoroughly tested for safety. Unfortunately, like some street drugs, certain prescription medications pose a genuine risk of both short- and long-term cognitive impairment. Since Americans take more prescription drugs than people in any other nation, this is an area that needs urgent attention.[602]

A Commonwealth Fund survey of adults 65 and older found that 68 percent of Americans regularly take two or more prescription medications. More than half take four or more such drugs. Moreover, the use of prescription medications is on the rise, dramatically in some cases. According to the National Center for Health Statistics and the CDC, the use of cholesterol-lowering medications in those 45 and older more than tripled in a 12-year period. Are these prescription medications safe for the brain? Let's look at a few common classes of drugs to see what risks they pose.

ANTICHOLINERGIC DRUGS

Some of the most prescribed anticholinergic drugs are used for seasonal allergies (antihistamines), high blood pressure, urinary incontinence, COPD, and depression. Anticholinergic drugs block a chemical messenger called acetylcholine that is involved in a variety of bodily functions and is also an essential player in memory retention. In both prescription and over-the-counter versions, there are over 100 different such drugs on the market today. This class of drugs is associated with MCI and may heighten risk for Alzheimer's in those who are genetically predisposed.

Longer term, users of these medications were found to be more likely to develop MCI and Alzheimer's disease, as well as experience brain shrinkage.[603]

At an annual American Urological Association meeting, Dr. Gary Kay of Georgetown University School of Medicine presented the findings of his clinical trial involving two popular prescription drugs used for incontinence. One of them, he found, significantly impaired memory in users. When compared to subjects who were taking a placebo, "the effect on memory with oxybutynin ER was comparable to about 10 years of cognitive aging. In other words, we transformed these people from functioning like 67-year-olds to 77-year-olds," Dr. Kay reported.[604]

A study of more than 3,400 dementia-free participants conducted by the University of Washington evaluated participants intermittently for seven years and tracked their medication use during this time. Subjects taking anticholinergics, specifically at least ten milligrams per day of doxepin (Sinequan, a sleep and depression medication); four milligrams a day of diphenhydramine (Benadryl, for allergies or sleep); or five milligrams a day of oxybutynin (a bladder-control drug) for three years or longer were at 54 percent higher risk of developing dementia compared to individuals who used them for three months or less.[605]

The Alzheimer's Disease Neuroimaging Initiative enrolled 688 individuals with an average age of 74 who had no memory problems at the start of the study. One-third of the participants took at least one anticholinergic drug, and all were given annual cognitive tests over a period of ten years. The risk for developing MCI was 47 percent greater in the group taking anticholinergic drugs than in those taking no such drugs.[606]

It's believed that the drugs deplete the brain's stores of acetylcholine and thereby inhibit activity in the hippocampus. (I should note that newer allergy medications, including Claritin and Zyrtec, are not associated with memory loss or cognitive problem).

ANTIDEPRESSANTS (TRICYCLIC CLASS DRUGS)

A study conducted by the Olmsted Medical Center and the Mayo Clinic has reported that nearly one in four American women aged 50 to 64 is currently taking antidepressant drugs.[607] These medications are prescribed primarily for depression but may also be prescribed for anxiety, obsessive-compulsive disorder (OCD), and chronic pain. Pharmacist and author Dr. Armon B. Neel Jr. reported that roughly 35 percent of long-term users experience memory impairment and another 54 percent report problems with concentration.

The problems may be caused when the drugs block two key neurotransmitters in the brain, norepinephrine and serotonin. The drugs studied include Amitriptyline (Elavil), clomipramine (Anafranil), desipramine (Norpramin), doxepin (Sinequan), imipramine (Tofranil), nortriptyline (Pamelor), protriptyline (Vivactil) and trimipramine (Surmontil).

ANXIETY MEDICATIONS (BENZODIAZEPINES)

Although a definitive cause-and-effect relationship has not been established, one study has shown that benzodiazepines, such as lorazepam (Ativan), diazepam (Valium), and alprazolam (Xanax) are associated with a heightened risk of Alzheimer's disease when used over the long term.[608]

Used to treat anxiety, delirium, and seizures, benzodiazepine drugs can impair memory and cognition in some users and are associated with a significantly increased risk of dementia.[609] The drugs work by slowing neuron activity and they seem to interfere with the transfer of experiences from short-term to long-term memory. The greater the dose and the longer they are taken, the greater the risk. One of several studies of benzodiazepine drugs found when they were taken for three months or less no greater risk was seen; three to six months use showed a 32 percent increased risk of Alzheimer's. When taken for six months or longer the risk climbed to 84 percent.[610]

CHOLESTEROL-LOWERING MEDICATIONS

With 100 million Americans contending with high cholesterol levels, it should not come as a surprise that the cholesterol-lowering medications known as statins are among the most widely prescribed drugs in the world. Various degrees of cognitive impairment, including memory problems, have been widely reported by statin users and the FDA now cautions users of that risk. Examples include atorvastatin (Lipitor), fluvastatin (Lescol), lovastatin (Mevacor), pravastatin (Pravachol), rosuvastatin (Crestor) and simvastatin (Zocor). In most cases the impairment is reversed once statins are discontinued. However, in some cases the memory problems persist.

Some medical experts believe that statins are prescribed too often, and that a greater emphasis should be placed on giving robust dietary and lifestyle changes a chance to bring cholesterol down to safer levels.[611]

MOOD-STABILIZING MEDICATIONS

Mood-stabilizing medications are among the most widely prescribed drugs in America today. These drugs have several unwanted side effects linked to obesity, high blood pressure, elevated cholesterol, and diabetes. However, the greater concern is that such drugs, including Seroquel, Abilify, Risperdal, Geodon, and Zyprexa, have been reported to cause users to lose brain tissue at an accelerated rate.[612] The higher the doses and the longer they are taken, the more brain tissue is lost.

Additionally, mood stabilizers are frequently prescribed off-label, or for conditions for which the drug was not intended, including agitation, behavioral problems, depression, post-traumatic stress disorder, and insomnia.

A special concern is that the use of these drugs in children, which increased by 100 percent between 2001 and 2011, may pose a heightened risk because their brains are smaller, the duration of exposure to the drug is likely to be greater, and thus, presumably, the degree of brain tissue loss will be greater as well. [613]

A large study of anticholinergic drug use that looked at 284,343 U.K. adults aged 55 and older between 2004 and 2016 found that in those who took the drugs daily for at least three years, risk of dementia was raised by 50 percent.[614] The study found the strongest link with the antidepressants paroxetine and amitriptyline, the bladder control drugs oxybutynin and tolterodine, the antipsychotic drugs chlorpromazine and olanzapine, and the antiepileptic drugs oxcarbazepine and carbamazepine.

OPIOIDS

Opioid painkillers, some of which are known to be highly addictive, are another class of drugs that can cause short- and long-term memory problems, whether used under medical supervision or illicitly.[615] Examples include fentanyl (Duragesic), hydrocodone (Norco, Vicodin), hydromorphone (Dilaudid, Exalgo), morphine (Astramorph, Avinza), and oxycodone (OxyContin, Percocet).

A growing number of cases have been reported in which recreational users of opiate drugs have shown up in emergency rooms with amnesia, which in some cases lasted more than a year. Using imaging scans, doctors have found lesions on the hippocampus in these individuals.

SLEEPING AIDS

The use of sleeping medications is quite common and has been reported to result in problems with memory. An estimated one in five older adults uses such medications regularly. As part of the Health, Aging and Body Composition study, Kristine Yaffe, M.D., and Yue Leng, Ph.D., at the University of California San Francisco, looked at the risk of dementia in those using sleeping medications. They followed 3,068 dementia-free adults, aged 70 to 79, for 15 years to see who developed dementia. Participants were distinguished between those who reported taking sleep medications "never or rarely," "sometimes," "often," or "almost always." When compared to those in the "never or rarely" group, subjects from the "often" or "almost always" groups were 43 percent more likely to develop dementia.[616] Examples of drugs involved include Eszopiclone (Lunesta), Zaleplon (Sonata) and Zolpidem (Ambien).

In a separate study, non-prescription (over the counter) sleeping aids that contain diphenhydramine, such as Benadryl and Aleve PM, were shown to increase risk of dementia by 54 percent in those who took them for three years compared to those who took them for three months or less.[617]

DRUGS ASSOCIATED WITH MEMORY LOSS	
Antianxiety drugs	Antiseizure drugs
Antidepressant drugs	Antihistamine drugs
Cholesterol drugs (statins)	Opioid painkillers
Incontinence drugs	Sleeping aids

Note that the risk of cognitive impairment from medications rises in older people because their kidneys and liver function less efficiently and thus they process and excrete the drugs more slowly. Additionally, those who are taking more than one medication have the additional risk of a compounding effect from the mix of drugs. Ask your physician for a comprehensive review of the drugs you are taking to see if they are still appropriate for your conditions. If any are considered a risk to cognitive health, consider the risks versus the benefits, and ask what alternative medications may be available. If you elect to eliminate any medications, do so with the guidance of your doctor, as a sudden cessation of certain medications can be problematic.

ILLICIT DRUGS

It stands to reason that people using illicit drugs may not have the preservation of their brains as a top priority. It may also stand to reason that it never occurs to many drug users that their habit might have significant consequences when it comes to their brain health. Let's set the record straight, drug by drug.

Marijuana

Some drugs, including the now quasi-legal marijuana have been shown to alter brain structure in users, interfere with memory, and over the long term cause shrinking of the hippocampus.[618]

In a landmark study that followed 1,000 participants from adolescence to age 38, researchers found the strongest evidence to date that cannabis consumption has a permanent damaging effect on the developing brains of adolescents. Researchers gave participants IQ tests at age 13 and then again at age 38. Smoking marijuana four days or more per week as a teenager resulted in lasting damage to the brain, sufficient to reduce IQ by eight points.

Recent tests have revealed some breeds of the plant are tainted with heavy metals, including arsenic, cadmium, chromium, lead, mercury, and nickel. These metals can be absorbed through smoke inhalation, and over the long term could contribute to brain damage.[619]

It is unclear whether the physical changes in the developing brain in adolescence may lead to a higher risk of dementia later in life.[620] It's also not entirely clear what the effects are in adults. Marijuana use is one of those "Do you want to take the chance? Is it worth it?" dilemmas.

Cocaine

An estimated 21 million people worldwide use cocaine and the USA has the highest rate of abuse in the world with Americans spending $28 billion on the drug annually.[621] Whatever its pleasures, researchers at the University of Cambridge have shown that cocaine use, as confirmed by MRI, eats away at the brain, causing twice the loss of gray matter annually as seen in a same-age, non-drug user.[622] Loss of gray matter is associated with early cognitive decline including memory problems. And as we have already seen, accelerated loss of brain volume is one of the hallmarks of AD pathology.

MPPP/MPTP and the Frozen Addicts

In the early 1980s there was a sudden outbreak of young recreational drug users showing up at emergency rooms across the country with Parkinson's-like symptoms. In a short time, they would advance to what appeared to be end-stage Parkinson's. They exhibited tremors, had difficulty speaking, their bodies and limbs were twisted and rigid, their faces eventually frozen. Neurologists were dumbfounded and dubbed this tragedy the case of the "frozen addicts," a condition from which none will recover.

How could these individuals, some just teenagers, have a disease that normally struck decades later in life, and how could the disease have advanced so suddenly?

As it turned out, due to a shortage of heroin on the streets, these individuals took to cooking up batches of an illicit heroin-like drug called 1-methyl-4-phenyl-4-propionpiperidine, or MPPP. But that wasn't the end of the story. These drug users *thought* they were taking MPPP. But apparently an error in the recipe resulted in a different product, called 1-methyl-4-phenyl-1,2,5,6-tetrahydropyridine, or MPTP being created and subsequently injected by users.

Neurologists performed PET scans of the addicts' brains, and autopsies on those who died, confirmed that they had the hallmark damage seen in Parkinson's disease. The MPTP had destroyed the dopamine-producing neurons of the portion of the brain called the substantia nigra.

Further study of the effects of illicit drug use would be valuable in helping us strategize to reduce the risk of Alzheimer's.

Smoking

Would you believe that many websites report that smoking cigarettes protects against Alzheimer's?[623] The truth is just the opposite; many studies indicate that smoking poses a significant risk factor for dementia.[624]

The World Health Organization reports that smoking is associated with a significant elevation in risk for all forms of dementia, and a Kaiser Permanente study found that smoking cigarettes, particularly at midlife, raises the risk of Alzheimer's by as much as 157 percent.[625]

UCSF's Dr. Kristine Yaffe led a team of investigators that looked at the relationship between smoking and cognitive function over a 25-year period. Their study revealed that smokers may experience cognitive impairment as early as their forties, and "heavy stable" smokers were 1.5 to 2.2 times more likely to become cognitively impaired when compared to nonsmokers.[626]

Why? Cigarettes and their smoke contain some 2,000 different chemical compounds, many of which threaten brain health. One compound in particular, nicotine-derived nitrosamine ketones (NKK), triggers microglia cells in the brain which in turn leads to neuroinflammation. Smoking causes cardiovascular disease, depletes antioxidants, and causes oxidative stress in the brain as well.[627] Cigarette smoke is also a source of the neurotoxic heavy metals lead[628] and cadmium,[629] and includes formaldehyde, arsenic, and vinyl chloride. Smoking clearly isn't worth the risk.

For too long, both prescription medications and illicit drugs have not received the close examination they require for possibly contributing to cognitive decline and dementia. Talk with your doctor about any prescriptions you may be taking to be sure you are not exposing yourself to a problematic medication. There may be a safer alternative you can take. And it goes without saying that if you are using drugs recreationally, it would be wise to stop.

20

DEPRESSION AND ALZHEIMER'S DISEASE

According to the CDC, one in ten Americans take antidepressant medications. Among women in their forties and fifties, the rate is one in four.[630] About 25 million Americans have been taking such medications for at least two years. While statistics indicate that depression has become increasingly common in the USA, particularly over the past 20 years, many sufferers are unaware that a history of depression is a risk factor for Alzheimer's disease.

Globally, 350 million people report having at least one major depressive episode, which is defined as two weeks or more of symptoms that extend beyond a sense of sadness and despair to include problems with four or more of the following: sleep, eating, energy, concentration, and self-image.[631]

In a meta-analysis that evaluated the findings of 20 studies looking at depression as a risk factor for Alzheimer's, researchers found that a history of depression doubled the risk of developing the disease later in life.[632] In another study the risk of AD was 2.7 times higher in those who had a history of depression.[633] The 2020 Blue Cross Blue Shield Health of America report revealed that among those diagnosed with early-onset Alzheimer's disease between 2013 and 2017, 57 percent had filled an antidepressant medication prescription in the year prior to their diagnosis.[634]

The triggers for depression are manifold. A depressive episode can be caused by stress, grief, loss of a loved one, loss of a job, a difficult relationship, loneliness, or witnessing a traumatizing event such as an auto accident or other violent occurrence.

Depression can also be brought on by a medical condition, such as an imbalance of thyroid hormone, or as a side effect of certain prescription medications, including beta blockers, blood pressure medication, hormone replacement therapy, birth control pills, and tranquilizers.

How does depression influence risk for AD? Although the entire picture has not come into focus yet, we know that people who are depressed have elevated levels of brain inflammation.[635] And as we know, chronic, unregulated brain inflammation damages and ultimately leads to the loss of neurons and synapses.

It is also thought that depression involves changes in brain chemistry, both inside and outside the neurons themselves. For example, levels of brain-derived neurotrophic factor (BDNF), the compound that protects neurons and supports memory formation, drop in individuals who are depressed.[636]

The regions of the brain involved in depression include the amygdala, thalamus, and the hippocampus. Using imaging techniques, scientists have seen that in those who are depressed there is a loss of volume in the hippocampus.[637] It appears that the more episodes of depression one has, the greater the loss of volume in the hippocampus.

CAN DIET PLAY A ROLE IN DEPRESSION?

Research has begun to uncover a link between consuming an unhealthy diet and the risk of becoming depressed.[638] A diet high in saturated fat and refined carbohydrates is associated with an increased risk of depression,[639] whereas a diet rich in fruits, vegetables, and whole grains is associated with a reduced risk.[640] In a study of 43,000 women who were tracked from 1996 to 2008, none of the participants suffered from depression at the start of the study. The researchers found, after measuring levels of inflammation in the participants, that those who followed an inflammatory diet centered upon meat, refined grains, sugar-sweetened soft drinks, margarine, refined vegetable oils, fish, and processed foods were significantly more likely to develop depression than those who followed a diet low in those foods and rich in vegetables, including leafy greens.[641]

In a study that involved 292 employees at ten corporate sites of the Geico Insurance Company, participants were given a questionnaire at the beginning and end of the study to assess risk of depression and anxiety and to measure their productivity. During the 18-week study, participants were divided into two groups. The control group received no instructions. The intervention group received weekly instruction for following a low-fat, vegan diet. After retesting, the researchers found the vegan diet group experienced a significant reduction in depression and anxiety as well as increased levels of productivity.[642] Another study from New Zealand found similar outcomes. The more fruits and vegetables subjects ate over the course of the 21-day study, the better their mood and the greater their levels of energy.[643]

One way diet can adversely affect mood is through its influence on gut health. Gut bacteria synthesize hundreds of neurochemicals, all of which are critical to mood, memory, and healthy brain function. The balance of healthy gut bacteria needed to produce such chemicals can be compromised by a diet rich in saturated fat, refined carbohydrates, sugar and alcohol, and devoid of fiber-rich fruits, vegetables, and whole grains. We'll return to the subject of gut health in Chapter 24.

Exercise is also a helpful guardian against depression, because it too has a potent effect on brain chemistry, such as causing the release of our internal antidepressant, endorphins. Even a minimal amount of exercise can be helpful in guarding against depression. In a study of 22,000 individuals followed for 11 years, those who failed to get just one to two hours of exercise per week were 44 percent more likely to become depressed.[644] Some studies have found regular aerobic exercise to have a more favorable effect than traditional medications in warding off depression.[645]

For many, an effective aid in addressing depression is to speak with a skilled therapist who can help identify and understand feelings and thought patterns that may be involved. The best way to address depression may be a three-pronged approach: a healthful diet, consistent exercise, and talk therapy.

21
AIRBORNE POLLUTION

I GREW UP IN Los Angeles, a city well known for its frequently appalling levels of smog. The nearby mountains and proximity to the coastline make the area prone to temperature inversions which trap pollutants in stagnant air. When my family resided there in the 1960s and early '70s, the air quality was among the worst in the world. This was partly due to a lack of basic automotive emission standards. Things improved substantially after it was mandated that all new cars be equipped with a smog-reducing catalytic convertor.

I recall stepping outside our front door in the morning and looking north toward the Hollywood Sign that hangs on the face of Mount Lee in the Santa Monica Mountains. For my siblings and me, the visibility of the sign was our barometer of the day's air quality. Some days the letters looked chalky white and deceptively close. On those days it looked as though I could walk a few city blocks and touch the gargantuan letters. But on far too many days the sign was obscured by a dirty haze that dulled the letters, made them seem much farther away, and made it nearly certain that I would return from school with watery eyes and a burning sensation deep in my lungs.

The primary constituents of the haze that obscures the Hollywood Sign are tiny particles that measure 2.5 micrometers in size, commonly referred to as 2.5 PM (particulate matter). Infinitesimally small, these particles are a mere fraction of the diameter of a strand of hair, and they hang in the air of cities worldwide.

Whether in India, Mexico, China, Pakistan, or Bakersfield, California, too many cities have become known for their choking smog that not only obscures iconic tourist attractions but makes breathing difficult and contributes to a host of other problems including cardiovascular disease, stroke, and respiratory diseases that end millions of lives prematurely each year. Now a rapidly growing body of evidence indicates that 2.5 PM also makes its way into our brains, where it triggers inflammation and oxidative stress, cognitive decline, and ultimately raises our risk of Alzheimer's disease.[646]

Drawing from the Women's Health Initiative Memory Study (WHIMS), a team of researchers at the University of Southern California looked at the health records of 3,647 dementia-free women aged 65 to 79 who resided throughout the US. After following the participants for 11 years, they found that subjects who resided in areas where fine particulate air pollution exceeded federal health standards were twice as likely to develop AD. Of these women, those who were already predisposed to AD due to their genes had a 263 percent greater risk of developing the disease. The scientists believe that if these findings hold up in the general population, fine particulate matter such as that created by automobile engines and smokestack emissions may be shown to be responsible for up to 21 percent of cases of dementia.[647]

How does air pollution reach the brain? The pollution emitted from automotive traffic, factory smokestacks, and burning coal and wood is a mix of both ultrafine particulate and liquid droplets that are inhaled deeply into the lungs. There they are picked up by the blood stream and transported to the brain. Another route of entry is for the particles to migrate up the nose and into the olfactory nerves, and ultimately to the olfactory bulb inside the brain. Once in the brain, they accumulate over time, triggering the release of pro-inflammatory agents that foster long-term inflammation, promote oxidative stress, damage the cerebral blood vessels, accelerate the rate of amyloid deposits, and lead to structural changes in the brain.[648]

In London, where air quality is seriously degraded due to the high concentration of automobiles running on diesel fuel, researchers looked at a study of more than 130,000 Londoners, aged 50 to 79, and calculated their residential proximity to major roads with heavy traffic. They found those who were most exposed to the exhaust produced by vehicles were more likely to develop Alzheimer's disease over the following eight years.[649]

Canadian researchers looked at the records of 6.5 million residents of Ontario and found a similar trend. Closer proximity to heavily trafficked roads increased risk of AD. Living within 50 meters (164 feet) of a busy roadway raised the risk by 12 percent. From 50 to 100 meters (164 to 328 feet), the risk dropped to four percent. A proximity of greater than 200 meters (656 feet) showed no elevated risk.[650]

Mexico City is notorious for its noxious air, so it was a magnet for another researcher who wished to see how air pollution affects the brain. Physician and neuropathologist Lilian Caldern-Garcidueas started by looking at the brains of diseased homeless dogs. Surprisingly, she found that they had Alzheimer's-like pathological changes in their brains.

What followed was even more unsettling. Looking at autopsy reports of children—and even infants—who had died in accidents and who had breathed the same heavily polluted air for their short lives, she found amyloid protein building up in their brains as well as inflammation and loss of brain volume.[651]

While genes may play a role in making some individuals more susceptible than others, the ten large studies conducted thus far indicate the pollution we generate by burning fossil fuels at the very least hampers cognitive function and leads to early cognitive decline, and at worst is another factor that moves one in the direction of an Alzheimer's diagnosis.[652] At least 146 million Americans now live in cities that exceed safe air quality standards.

According to the American Lung Association, the 12 US cities with air most chronically polluted with 2.5 PM are:

1. Bakersfield, CA

2. Fresno-Madera-Hanford, CA

3. Visalia, CA

4. Long Beach, CA

5. San Jose-San Francisco-Oakland, CA

6. Fairbanks, AK

7. Phoenix-Mesa, AZ

8. Pittsburgh, PA

9. El Centro, CA

10. Detroit-Ann Arbor, MI

11. Cleveland-Akron, OH

12. McAllen-Edinburg, TX

Unlike all the other risks I present in this book, which are highly actionable, this is one over which we can exercise only a limited degree of control. The reality is that air pollution is a fact of life in our world. It has been produced at prodigious levels for many decades, and while some real progress has been made toward its reduction, it will continue to pose a risk for the foreseeable future. However, this is an area where, through policy and technology, we can make further big improvements. It's been estimated that cutting 2.5 PM levels by just 10 percent could slash air pollution-induced dementia by 14 to 26 percent.[653]

In the meantime, not everyone can pack up their life and move to an area known for its cleaner air. This is not to say there is nothing you can do. First, now that you understand the seriousness of breathing highly polluted air, perhaps you will be inspired to play whatever role you can in reducing your own contribution. This may include energy conservation at home, relying upon public transit, selecting a car with greater fuel efficiency or that is powered electrically, installing solar panels, carpooling, and avoiding excessive driving trips. If you live in a city that has high levels of smog, consider wearing an N95 face mask when outside for extended periods, to filter out particulate. Avoid exercising and recreating near heavy traffic areas. You may also consider using a HEPA air filtration system in your home. Costing hundreds of dollars just a few years ago, these air purifiers have become relatively small, portable, energy efficient, and more affordable than ever, with some priced under $100. Finally, support elected officials who demonstrate a desire to protect public health and advance regulations that will wean us off pollution-generating technologies and onto greener and cleaner options.

22

TRAUMATIC BRAIN INJURY

I F YOU WANT to see the results of an unchecked risk factor for brain damage, look at American football.

Former Chicago Bears quarterback Jim McMahon is the athlete who put the subject of traumatic brain injury (TBI) on the public map. In 2011 he shared his own struggles with dementia and filed suit against the National Football League (NFL). At the time of this writing, another football great, Mark Gastineau, who played for the New York Jets, revealed that he had received a double diagnosis of Alzheimer's disease and Parkinson's disease, which he attributes to his ten-season career in football.[654]

In 2005, Dr. Bennet Omalu published in the journal *Neurosurgery* details of his seminal study and discovery of chronic traumatic encephalopathy, or CTE, a condition that mirrors many of the symptoms of AD. Omalu first diagnosed the condition in former Pittsburgh Steelers center Mike Webster, as revealed in the 2015 movie *Concussion*.

Dr. Omalu's findings led to a dramatic, if brief, focus on the relationship between head trauma and brain disease. In 2014, the *New York Times* reported that the NFL was preparing to agree to a settlement with what had grown to 5,000 former players who were already suffering from, or expected to suffer from, various forms of dementia as a result of their profession. Surprisingly, the NFL further acknowledged that nearly one in three players could be expected to eventually suffer some form of brain damage and that their symptoms would become apparent at "notably younger ages" (average age 53.8 years) than those seen in the general population.[655] *Frontline* later reported the NFL's settlement amount of $1 billion to the players.[656]

Yet the prognosis for pro football players may be even worse than the NFL asserted. Researchers with the Department of Veterans Affairs and Boston University who examined the brains of 91 deceased NFL players found evidence of CTE in 96 percent of the brains examined.[657] Ultimately, professional football players, especially "speed players" who tackle and are tackled at high rates of speed, have as much as six times the risk of dying from Alzheimer's disease and ALS when compared to the US general population.[658]

Concussions are not new in the sports world. As far back as 1928 scientists knew of a concussion-induced condition that occurred in boxers, a condition that varied in its resemblance to either Alzheimer's or Parkinson's disease. They called it *punch drunk syndrome*. Yet it was not until a 1994 mortality study of NFL players that a relationship between the sport and *nervous system deaths* was noted.[659]

Today, soccer players, in particular those who "head" the ball, are becoming as concerned as some football players. Landmark research from the University of Glasgow revealed a professional soccer player has 3.5 times the risk they will develop and die from neurological disease, compared to the general public.[660]

Evidence indicates that even a single episode of TBI can increase risk of AD.[661] An analysis of 15 case-control studies showed a 50 percent increased risk for Alzheimer's disease for males who sustained just one TBI.[662]

Of course, it's not just athletes who suffer head trauma and TBI. These conditions can result from injuries sustained in other ways. The number one cause of TBI is falling and second is automobile accidents.

Researchers have seen that combat veterans who have been subjected to TBI as a result of close proximity to blasts are at elevated risk for Alzheimer's as well. This includes hundreds of thousands of veterans of the Iraq and Afghanistan wars.[663] Studies suggest that risk goes up according to the severity of the trauma. A study of 178,779 veterans found an increased risk of 2.5 times in those who experienced mild TBI without a loss of consciousness, 2.8 times if there was a loss of consciousness, and 3.8 times in severe TBI with a loss of consciousness.[664] One study found combat veterans with severe TBI (without reference to loss of consciousness) were four times more likely to develop AD compared to those who did not experience TBI.[665]

There is also evidence that with severe head trauma comes specific pathological features that would advance neurological disease. These include damage to the blood–brain barrier, bleeding in the brain, activation of microglia, accumulation of neurofibrillary tangles, and neuroinflammation.[666]

Lastly, and very worryingly, there is evidence that a history of TBI fast-forwards the onset of Alzheimer's by several years, which is very worrying indeed.[667]

Obviously, we are wise to do everything within our power to protect ourselves while participating in activities that pose a risk for head trauma. We should wear appropriate protective headgear while skiing, cycling, horseback riding, and ice-skating, among other sports. However, as the NFL studies show, even a helmet may not be sufficient to prevent TBI. To play football is to gamble with one's brain. To fight in a war has so many risks that they defy making a list, but among them is certainly proximity to explosions. Playing it safe can mean preserving your cognitive health

PART IV

THE ALZHEIMER'S REVOLUTION LIFESTYLE PLAN

23

YOUR MASTER PLAN

You ARE DUE some relief. Having learned about every known factor believed to contribute to your risk of cognitive decline and an Alzheimer's disease diagnosis, how about learning the best protections against developing Alzheimer's in the first place?

As you now know, an array of factors contributes to the risk of developing AD, so it's important to cast a wide net and employ a holistic approach to prevention. The research that has come from both the Chicago Health and Aging Project and the Rush Memory and Aging Project have underscored that the more lifestyle factors one addresses the greater the potential for prevention. There is a "dose-response" relationship between the number of actions we take and the reduction in risk. Risk declines commensurate with the number of healthful lifestyle strategies you adopt.

What I call the Alzheimer's Revolution Lifestyle is itself a first: no study to date has explored the fullest potential of protecting oneself from Alzheimer's disease by exploiting all the known risk-reduction strategies you are about to be shown.

I urge you to explore the comprehensive Alzheimer's Revolution Lifestyle approach that addresses diet, physical exercise, stress management, cognitive stimulation, social engagement, sleep hygiene, and the avoidance of known toxic substances. The benefits of the Alzheimer's Revolution Lifestyle, by the way, extend far beyond reducing the risk of neurological disease. The program is also a potent plan for reducing your risk for heart disease, stroke, high blood pressure, diabetes, obesity, osteoporosis, and even some forms of cancer. But here Alzheimer's is our focus.

As noted early in this book, researchers have suggested that if we address the primary risk factors for AD—including diabetes, obesity, high blood pressure, depression, sedentary living, smoking, and cognitive inactivity—we could slash the risk of AD by about 50 percent. Not a bad start, but it's not enough.

At a biological level, our primary goals are to minimize three serious threats: inflammation, oxidative stress, and exposure to brain damaging agents. To preserve brain cells, we also need to ensure maximum blood flow to the brain and the ability of insulin to do its job of getting fuel into cells. So, we are making choices that support healthy blood pressure and keep our blood vessels flexible and free of plaque. The foods we eat are the primary driving force behind whether we can achieve these goals and avoid developing atherosclerosis, high blood pressure, insulin resistance and diabetes, obesity, and, ultimately, Alzheimer's.

Nothing—nothing—is more important than diet. In order to prevent Alzheimer's (and several other all-to-common degenerative diseases) *the single most powerful action we can take is to address what we eat.* Yes, other factors have been proven important to helping keep one's mind healthy. I'll address each in its own chapter, but none is as critical as diet.

Unfortunately, too many medical doctors are still not well informed about the role of nutrition in disease, and often believe age-old food myths just as the patients they treat do. A major survey found that 71 percent of medical schools failed to provide their medical students with the minimum recommended 25 classroom hours of nutrition education.[668] So it is no wonder that just 14 percent of physicians surveyed felt they were trained sufficiently to be able to offer nutritional advice to their patients.[669] "It is a scandal that health professionals are not introduced to these facts above and beyond minimal information about nutritional deficiencies in biochemistry, and that these things do not appear on their examinations to become a practicing physician," says Dr. David Eisenberg, of the Harvard T.H. Chan School of Public Health.[670]

You must make the choices that will guide your path to cognitive health. Get ready, for here they come.

24
FOODS FOR THOUGHT

AT LEAST THREE times a day we have a choice to consume foods that will either protect our health, or instead advance the likelihood of disease. We can choose the typical Western diet, high in saturated fat, trans fat, cholesterol, sugar and sodium that clogs up and damages our blood vessels and restricts blood flow, robbing our brains and other organs of the oxygen and nutrients they critically need. Or, with our Alzheimer's Revolution diet, we can control inflammation, minimize oxidative stress, and prevent (and reverse) clogged blood vessels and other damage caused by the standard diet. We can also maximize our intake of protective anti-oxidants, phytochemicals, and anti-inflammatory agents; slash exposure to trans fats; and root out brain-damaging pesticides, dangerous heavy metals, and other contaminants. We can *curate a diet for health.*

The most effective way to do this is to adopt a diet built upon foods derived from plants. That means forgoing the dietary pattern associated with AD risk, one centered on meat, dairy, eggs, fish and, of course, fried foods and refined sugar.[671]

It's believed that our hunter-gatherer ancestors consumed 800 or more different plant varieties.[672] Today, few Americans get more than three servings of plant foods each day and most of us rarely venture away from a couple of favorites. The numerous protective compounds on which the body and mind thrives are primarily found in plants. Compared to those eating just one serving daily, subjects who consumed 3-4 servings of vegetables daily experienced a 40 percent reduction in cognitive decline over a 6-year follow-up period.[672]

Foods of animal origin—hamburgers, cheese, milk, chicken, bacon, fish, and so forth—are rich in saturated fat and have the highest concentration of toxic environmental contaminants. These foods bring brain-damaging chemicals such as pesticides, PCBs, dioxins, and mercury into the body, thus promoting inflammation, oxidative stress, and insulin resistance. These foods are also lacking in the protective antioxidants and phytochemicals that support good health and lower the risk of disease.[673]

Individuals who follow a plant-based diet are also at a big advantage over omnivores when it comes to lowering risk of cardiovascular disease, hypertension, obesity, and diabetes—the four big risk factors we examined in Chapters 5 through 8.[674] It's not just the saturated fat and cholesterol, the lack of fiber and the contaminants. Evidence shows that compared to plant protein, protein derived from meat generates more oxidative stress and inflammation.[675]

STRENGTHENING YOUR MICROBIOME

In recent years much attention has been paid to the importance of gut health and the link between the ten thousand different species of bacteria that reside in our small and large intestine and our level of wellness. The trillions of microorganisms, and the genetic material they contain, are collectively referred to as our *microbiome*. What are all these bacteria doing in our gut? It turns out much more than extracting nutrients from the foods we eat. About 70 percent of our immune system resides in our gut, and vitamins, hormones and neurotransmitters are synthesized there as well. Yet, not all gut bacteria are beneficial. Some are potentially pathogenic fungi, parasites, and viruses, and need to be kept in check by healthy bacteria.

Scientists have found that there is a direct link, with cross-talk between our gut and our brain referred to as the gut-brain axis.[676] It seems the idiom *I have a gut feeling* taps into a real connection between the gut flora, neurons, and the central nervous system. Some have referred to the gut as a "second brain," because of the network of over 100 million neurons that lines your gut wall. Not surprisingly, there is an association between a reduced diversity and function of gut microorganisms (dysbiosis) and gastrointestinal disorders such as leaky gut (an increased permeability of the gut wall that permits unwanted molecules to enter the bloodstream).[677] A loss of healthy microbes can also lead to inflammation, mental health problems, and a growing body of evidence connects gut health with cognitive function.[678] When the gut is in dysbiosis, emotional and cognitive health may suffer.

The health of our microbiome is influenced by a number of factors including, genes, age, health status, exercise, stress/anxiety, tobacco and alcohol use, and medications. Most influential, however, is the food we eat. To maintain bacterial diversity and best support the critical activities that occur in the gut, we must choose the right foods. Diets that are high in saturated fat and sugar and devoid of plant foods reduce diversity of gut bacteria and can promote the growth of potentially pathogenic bacteria and inflammatory conditions.[679] Fiber-rich whole grains, beans and lentils, leafy greens, fruits, vegetables and nuts and seeds support gut bacteria diversity and stability, which in turn promotes stronger immune function, better digestion, healthy cognitive function, and reduced risk of common chronic diseases.[680] In chapter 32 I'll share how exercise can positively influence the composition of gut microbes.

An increasing number of public health organizations acknowledge the scientific evidence that says a diet created from plant foods can be not just healthful but enable one to thrive. One of the most important of these organizations is the Academy of Nutrition and Dietetics, the world's largest organization of food and nutrition professionals. In an official policy paper, the Academy wrote: "Vegetarian, including vegan, diets are healthful, nutritionally adequate, and may provide health benefits for the prevention and treatment of certain diseases. These diets are appropriate for all stages of the life cycle, including pregnancy, lactation, infancy, childhood, adolescence, older adulthood, and for athletes. Vegetarians and vegans are at reduced risk of certain health conditions, including heart disease, type 2 diabetes, hypertension, breast, colorectal, and prostate cancers, and obesity."[681]

The World Health Organization (WHO) now recommends, "Households should select predominantly plant-based diets rich in a variety of vegetables and fruits, pulses or legumes, and minimally processed starchy staple foods. The evidence that such diets will prevent or delay a significant proportion of non-communicable chronic diseases is consistent." [682]

Joining the WHO in advocating a plant-based diet are the American Diabetes Association, American Association of Retired Persons (AARP), the American Cancer Society, the Mayo Clinic, and the US Department of Health and Human Services.[683] As one of America's leading health-care providers and insurers, Kaiser Permanente has a solid grasp of what health problems Americans are struggling with most and why. In its 2013 Nutrition Update for Physicians, the healthcare giant noted that "healthy eating may be best achieved with a plant-based diet," and recommended that physicians "consider recommending a plant-based diet to all their patients, especially those with high blood pressure, diabetes, cardiovascular disease, or obesity." [684]

Not only does plant-based diet lower one's chances of developing the conditions above, it strengthens the immune system and seems to offer significant protection against severe COVID-19. Researchers from Harvard-affiliated Massachusetts General Hospital wanted to investigate the association between dietary patterns and the severity and duration of COVID symptoms. They gathered dietary and demographic information from 592,000 participants in the US and the UK and found that those whose indicated they ate the most plant-rich diet had a 41 percent lower risk of developing severe COVID-19 compared to those who had the least amount of plant foods in their diet.[685]

In another study that was published in *BMJ Nutrition, Prevention & Health*, researchers asked 2,884 frontline healthcare workers in France, Italy, Germany, Spain, the United Kingdom, and the US who, due to their work, were regularly exposed to COVID-19 to fill out a 47-item food frequency questionnaire and to provide details about the severity of any COVID-19 infection they experienced. They found those who reported following a strict plant-based diet were 73 percent less likely to develop moderate-to-severe COVID symptoms. Those who followed a plant-based diet but included fish (pescatarian) had a 59 percent reduced risk of moderate-to-severe COVID symptoms. The healthcare workers who reported following a low-carb, high-protein (meat-centered) diet had nearly a 400 percent greater risk of suffering moderate-to-severe COVID symptoms. The authors concluded that a plant-based diet is significantly protective against developing moderate-to-severe COVID symptoms.[686] While both of these studies have limitations, their findings are consistent with past studies that show plant-based eating strengthens the immune system.[687]

POLITICS OVER SCIENCE

While progress has been made in the past several years to better inform the public of what truly healthful dietary choices look like, public health agencies in the USA still have much room for improvement in getting the word out.[688] The official dietary guidelines issued periodically by the USDA and Health and Human Services are influenced by the interests of food producers. Understandably, these folks take offense at reports that present their products unfavorably, and their strong lobbying efforts make that known to policymakers. According to some who have sat on the board of the USDA's dietary advisory panel, the result is that recommendations to the USDA and HHS get watered down and don't truly represent our current understanding of what constitutes healthful nutrition. Dr. Marion Nestle, a health policy expert and former chair of the Department of Nutrition, Food Studies, and Public Health at New York University was once a member of this dietary advisory panel. "I was told we could never say 'eat less meat' because [the] USDA would not allow it," she says.[689] The guidelines, Nestle adds, "have internalized food industry values."[690]

The other problem that has long skewed the dietary guidelines so that they favor industry over public health is the conflict of interest at the USDA. This federal agency was founded for the express purpose of promoting the products of the American agriculture and food industries. It was given the additional mandate of helping to formulate official dietary recommendations. Until the USDA is divested from this role it's unlikely that Americans will receive guidelines wholly reflective of what the scientific community believes.

THE FEAR FACTOR

If the idea of making sweeping dietary changes is worrisome to you, I understand. There was a time in my life when my dietary considerations were largely influenced by popular food myths and the advertising campaigns of food producers. I had yet to imagine how powerfully my choices could affect my health and I was confident that the choices I was making were sound. My breakfast typically consisted of four to five scrambled eggs, white bread slathered in butter, and several strips of bacon. Lunch was fried chicken or a tuna salad sandwich chock-full of mayonnaise, and dinner was a pork chop, burger, or steak often accompanied by fried tater-tots or some other nutritionally bankrupt accompaniment. Cheese was simply irresistible, and I found a way to work it into nearly every meal, and vegetables and leafy greens rarely made an appearance on my plate. Because I thought it afforded me athletic prowess, I was competitive about how much protein I consumed each day, and for good measure I prepared one or two protein powder shakes that further amplified the excess protein in my diet. I thought nothing of polishing off a pint of ice cream in one sitting, justifying it on the basis that it was rich in calcium.

It wasn't until I began to read the science about the long-term implications of eating this way that I began to change my diet. Yet I admit that I resisted and tried to rationalize my soon to be abandoned habits along the way. You may find this happening to you as well. Try not to let setbacks frustrate your progress. Keep forging ahead.

Change can be unsettling, but it can also be exciting. For many, making dietary changes that protect their health rather than staying with old patterns that are negatively affecting their health can be inspiring. A plant-based diet offers a multifaceted way to protect and optimize brain function and reduce the risk of neurological disease.

In late 2019 the results of a study that began in 1993 were published. The researchers looked at dietary patterns in 63,000 subjects aged 45 to 74. They followed up with them 26 years later to see who had become cognitively impaired. Those who had most strictly adhered to a plant-based diet had a substantially reduced risk of impairment.[691]

Currently, there are two diets that have received attention for their apparent ability to help reduce risk of dementia. They are the Mediterranean diet and the MIND diet. Both are improvements over the typical

Western diet, and both have been shown to lower the risk of key AD risk factors as well as dementia itself. Even here, though, there is evidence that both diets leave room for improvement.

For over a decade, researchers have gathered evidence indicating that a Mediterranean eating pattern is associated with a significant reduction in risk for cardiovascular disease, mental decline, and Alzheimer's.[692] The Mediterranean diet is centered upon vegetables, legumes, fruits, and whole grains. It includes a liberal intake of monounsaturated fats derived from olive oil and a relatively low intake of saturated fats. The diet recommends fish consumption twice weekly, and a moderate intake of poultry, cheese, and yogurt. Meat is to be eaten only rarely. Sweets are restricted.

The Mediterranean diet is a substantial improvement over the typical American diet, and the benefits are evident in research findings. A study of 2,258 people showed that for those who most closely adhered to this way of eating, risk of Alzheimer's was reduced by up to 40 percent.[693] Their brain structure and volume was also better preserved (less shrinkage).[694]

Building on the compelling findings from the Mediterranean diet research, scientists from Rush University Medical Center in Chicago reported they had devised a diet for which risk for AD was slashed even further. Called the MIND diet (Mediterranean-DASH Intervention for Neurodegenerative Delay) this eating pattern is a hybrid of the principles derived from the Mediterranean diet and a diet devised to lower blood pressure called the DASH (Dietary Approaches to Stop Hypertension).

While these two diets are similar in certain respects, the MIND diet encourages beans three times per week, leafy greens consumption every day, berries twice weekly, nuts most days per week, and, like the Mediterranean diet, permits moderate daily alcohol consumption. It suggests limiting butter and cheese consumption. The MIND diet also specifies that processed meats (sausages, hot dogs), fast foods, fried foods, sweets and pastries, and stick margarine be eliminated. Both diets discourage added salt.

A study of the MIND diet involved 960 participants aged 58 to 98 who were followed on average for 4.7 years. In people who followed the diet closely, risk for developing Alzheimer's was slashed by a remarkable 53 percent. In participants who followed the diet only moderately, risk was cut by 35 percent.[695] In this case, there's an important message: moderate dietary changes limit the degree to which you may be able to reduce your risk. Keep this in mind.

Another encouraging finding is that those who most closely adhered to the MIND diet's principles slowed their rate of mental decline and functioned cognitively *at a level 7.5 years younger than those who least adhered to the diet.*

The strength of both diets is that they promote a greater intake of protective plant foods. While both diets recommend cutting back or in some cases eliminating certain foods that are problematic, I believe their weakness is they both still permit problematic foods, even if in moderation.

The reduction in risk shown by the Mediterranean and MIND diets research is exciting because it demonstrates how powerfully our food choices can affect our health, positively or negatively. The risk reduction these diets confer comes from cutting back significantly on the foods that we have known for decades promote the primary risk factors for Alzheimer's: heart disease, stroke, high blood pressure, diabetes, and obesity, as well as inflammation and oxidative stress.

I want to drive home another point illustrated by the study of the MIND diet. The benefits that we gain from dietary and other lifestyle changes *are in proportion to the degree of change we are willing to make.* As noted above, subjects saw that their risk was reduced commensurate with how closely they followed the recommendations. Those who followed the diet moderately had a moderate risk reduction. Those who embrace the dietary recommendations fully saw a substantially greater reduction in risk. However, I'm not satisfied with a 35 percent to 53 percent reduction in risk. I have yet to meet anyone who is looking for a moderate reduction in their risk of dementia. Following the MIND or Mediterranean diet is like taking half the dose of your medicine.

I trust that you are reading this book because you are motivated to avoid becoming a victim of Alzheimer's disease. Therefore, I believe it is essential that we build upon the encouraging outcomes from these dietary patterns by no longer consuming chicken, fish, dairy, and, hopefully, alcohol.

To reiterate what I have stressed before, when tested, chicken is consistently found to be laden with neurodegenerative pesticides, dioxin, and other dangerous contaminants. Fish is simply the most contaminated food on any dinner plate. Chicken and fish both contain saturated fat and cholesterol, and recent research has found that when it comes to raising LDL (bad) cholesterol, chicken is just as problematic as red meat.[696] That's the stuff that promotes clogged-up blood vessels not only feeding the heart and brain but blood vessels within the brain itself. The most protective way of eating is to build your meals entirely from plants.

In this chapter, I will discuss all the foods within the Revolution Lifestyle. We will also take a closer look at so-called good fats and antioxidants and discuss the importance of choosing organics. You can enjoy the Revolution Lifestyle diet knowing that these foods are tasty, good for you, and protective of brain health.

We have so far covered some very compelling reasons *why* a plant-centered diet makes good sense as the centerpiece of the Revolution Lifestyle. Yet before you head out to the market to shop for your new list of dietary staples, I want to show you some of the *how* that makes plant-based eating so powerfully protective.

THE DIVIDENDS OF A PLANT-CENTERED DIET [697]	
Lowers body weight	Improves blood flow to brain
Lowers blood pressure	Improves arterial health
Reduces blood viscosity	Improves brain function
Lowers cholesterol levels	Decreases amyloid build up
Lowers blood glucose levels	Lowers homocysteine
Reduces insulin resistance	Protects against cognitive decline
Lowers saturated fat intake	Reduces oxidative stress
Lowers exposure to contaminants	Reduces inflammation
Improves sleep	Increases energy
Lowers healthcare costs	

PHYTOCHEMICALS AND ANTIOXIDANTS

Plants are truly remarkable. In addition to their diverse aesthetic beauty, they are packed with myriad compounds that offer health-protecting properties. In the developing world, an estimated 80 percent of people choose plants as their primary form of medicine,[698] and up to half of all pharmaceutical drugs sold by prescription today are derived from plants.[699]

One reason a plant-based diet decreases the risk of cognitive impairment and Alzheimer's disease is the presence of compounds called *phytochemicals*. Found in fruits, vegetables, whole grains, legumes, herbs, and spices, these compounds work in varied ways to lower risk for many diseases.[700]

Some phytochemicals are antioxidants that scavenge free radicals, while others help lower blood pressure, increase blood flow to the brain, support neurogenesis, and guard against neuroinflammation. Still others improve blood sugar levels and protect synapse function. Some phytochemicals may even turn on genes that protect neurons.[701]

I have been asked whether animal-based foods contain antioxidants. They do, in small amounts. They are derived from the animal's diet—many animals raised for consumption are, after all, vegetarians. Yet plant-derived foods have 64 times more antioxidants than foods made from animals.[702]

POLYPHENOLS

More than 8,000 different polyphenol compounds have been identified in a wide array of plant foods. They have been linked to a reduced risk of dementia, AD,[703] strokes, and Parkinson's disease,[704] as well as a reduction in the risk of hypertension, heart disease,[705] diabetes,[706] and cancer.[707]

Polyphenols use a variety of biological actions to reduce risk, including extinguishing free radicals, inhibiting the inflammatory response, modulating the action of certain enzymes, and increasing expression of brain-derived neurotrophic factor (BDNF), supporting neurogenesis.[708]

A polyphenol you have probably heard of is resveratrol, found in blueberries, cranberries, grapes, peanuts, and pistachios. This compound, which has both anti-inflammatory and antioxidant properties, is believed to facilitate the clearing out of amyloid protein, reduce neuron loss through combatting inflammation, help lower blood pressure, and protect neurons from oxidative stress.[709]

Another remarkable polyphenol is curcumin, found in the spice turmeric. Curcumin has shown great promise in helping to ward off neurodegenerative disease not only because it has very strong antioxidant and anti-inflammatory properties, but because it can reduce production of amyloid. Curcumin has also been shown to improve endothelial function and blood flow by increasing the availability of nitric oxide.

In a laboratory setting, the capacity for a food to combat free radicals is measured in a procedure called Oxygen Radical Absorbance Capacity (ORAC) and yields a total antioxidant capacity (TAC) rating. You may be surprised by some of the foods in the following list of the TAC Top 50.

RANK	FOOD ITEM	SERVING SIZE	TAC
1	Small red bean, cooked	½ cup 92 g	13,727
2	Blueberry, wild	1 cup 145 g	13,427
3	Red kidney bean, cooked	½ cup 92 g	13,259
4	Pinto bean, dry, cooked	½ cup 96 g	11,864
5	Blueberry, cultivated	1 cup 144 g	9,019
6	Cranberry	1 cup whole 95 g	8,983
7	Artichoke, cooked	1 cup hearts 84 g	7,904
8	Blackberry	1 cup 144 g	7,701
9	Prunes (8)	½ cup 85 g	7,291
10	Raspberry	1 cup 123 g	6,058
11	Strawberry	1 cup 166 g	5,938
12	Apple, Red Delicious	1 fruit 138 g	5,900
13	Apple, Granny Smith	1 fruit 138 g	5,381
14	Pecan	28.4 g (1 oz)	5,095
15	Potato, russet	1 potato 369 g	4,882
16	Cherry, sweet	1 cup 145 g	4,873
17	Plum, black	1 fruit 66 g	4,844
18	Potato, russet, cooked	1 potato 299 g	4,649

RANK	FOOD ITEM	SERVING SIZE	TAC
19	Black bean, cooked	½ cup 52 g	4,181
20	Plum, red	1 fruit 66 g	4,118
21	Apple, Gala	1 fruit 138 g	3,903
22	Walnut	28.4 g (1 oz)	3,846
23	Apple, Red Delicious	1 fruit 128 g	3,758
24	Apple, red	1 fruit 138 g	3,685
25	Apple, Fuji	1 fruit 138 g	3,578
26	Date, Deglet Noor	½ cup 89 g	3,467
27	Avocado, Haas	1 fruit 173 g	3,344
28	Pear, green	1 fruit 166 g	3,172
29	Pear, red Anjou	1 fruit 166 g	2,943
30	Apple, Gold Delicious, peeled	1 fruit 128 g	2,829
31	Hazelnut	28.4 g (1 oz)	2,739
32	Broccoli raab, raw	⅕ bunch 85 g	2,621
33	Navy bean, dry, cooked	½ cup 104 g	2,573
34	Orange, navel	1 fruit 140 g	2,540
35	Figs, dried	½ cup 75 g	2,537
36	Raisins	½ cup 82g	2,490
37	Cabbage, red, cooked	½ cup 75 g	2,359
38	Potato, red, raw	1 potato 213 g	2,339
39	Potato, red, cooked	1 potato 173 g	2,294
40	Pistachio	28.4 g (1 oz)	2,267
41	Pea, blackeye, dry, cooked	½ cup 52 g	2,258
42	Potato, white, raw	1 potato 213 g	2,257
43	Date, Medjool	½ cup 89 g	2,124
44	Asparagus, raw	½ cup 67 g	2,021
45	Grapes, red	1 cup 160 g	2,016
46	Pepper, yellow, raw	1 pepper 186 g	1,905
47	Grapefruit, red	half 123 g	1,904
48	Beets	½ cup 68 g	1,886
49	Potato, white, cooked	1 potato 173 g	1,870
50	Pepper, orange, sweet, raw	1 pepper 186 g	1,830
	Source: Journal of Agriculture and Food Chemistry		

FLAVONOIDS

Research has focused on the ability of flavonoids, a group of polyphenols, to protect neurons, boost neuron function, produce regenerative effects on compromised neurons, and to improve memory and learning.[710] These compounds have both antioxidant and anti-inflammatory properties, and some are believed to stimulate angiogenesis (the development of new blood vessels) and neurogenesis (the development of new neurons) in the hippocampus. Their consumption is strongly associated with a reduction in risk for Alzheimer's disease as well as an improvement in the symptoms of people already diagnosed with AD.[711]

A 5-year study involving more than 1,300 participants found that those who had the highest intake of flavonoids had half the risk for dementia compared to those with the lowest intake.[712] In another study 921 dementia-free men and women with an average age of 81 underwent a detailed assessment of their diet. They were then followed for six years. By the end of the study, the subjects who had the highest intake of dietary flavonoids were 48 percent less likely to have developed Alzheimer's disease.[713] Finally, a similar observational study was conducted with 2,800 people aged 50 and older who were then followed for up to 20 years. Approximately every four years a detailed report was taken of the foods they ate to determine the level of flavonoids in their diet. As an example, the low-flavonoid-consuming participants ate 1.5 apples, no berries, and no tea in a single month. The highest consumers of flavonoids reported eating 7.5 cups of berries, eight apples, and drinking about 19 cups of tea per month. The research team found that over the course of the study those who consumed the least apples, pears, and tea had double the risk of developing AD as compared to participants who consumed these foods. But if they were low consumers of blueberries and strawberries, their risk was four-fold higher.[714]

Apples, berries, and tea are not the only flavonoid-containing choices you can make. In fact, six different types of flavonoids are present in virtually all fruits and vegetables. Their absorption rate varies, however, so once again eating a variety of foods is the key.

CAROTENOIDS

The bright colors of fruits and vegetables are produced by carotenoids, which are pigments present in all plants. In green-leafed plants, colors are hidden by chlorophyll until autumn, when the pigments emerge. Carotenoids occur in red-, yellow-, and orange-colored foods, such as bell peppers, carrots, sweet potatoes, watermelon, pumpkin, and tomatoes, as well as in dark green vegetables like broccoli, asparagus, and spinach. These compounds protect plants from damage caused by oxygen and the sun's ultraviolet rays. When we consume the plants, their carotenoids protect our cells from oxidative damage caused by free radicals.

A carotenoid with both antioxidant and anti-inflammatory properties that is highly concentrated in the retina of the eye is called lutein. It is thought to protect against macular degeneration; and it is also highly concentrated in brain tissue and is associated with cognitive health.[715] Multiple studies have shown that people with higher concentrations of lutein have higher performance in executive function, language, learning, and memory.[716] In elderly subjects, lutein supplements were shown to improve learning efficiency and memory. While the richest dietary sources of lutein are spinach and kale, it is also found in broccoli, corn, bell peppers, romaine lettuce, parsley, peas, and pistachios.

Laboratory studies suggest that certain carotenoids, including beta carotene, lycopene, and retinoic acid may inhibit both the production and depositing of amyloid protein.[717]

VITAMIN K

Vitamin K does not have the status of vitamins C and D, but evidence suggests that this vitamin may play several roles in supporting cognition and helping protect against Alzheimer's, because it has both antioxidant and anti-inflammatory properties and is critical to the formation of a special type of fat (sphingolipids) found in brain cells.

Vitamin K is important to the health of brain cell membranes, is involved in preserving blood vessel elasticity, and maintaining insulin sensitivity and calcium balance in the brain. Calcium balance in neurons is essential to their function and survival.[718] Vitamin K also activates a protein that reduces the risk of calcium deposits on artery walls.

Studies have shown that vitamin K deficiency and insufficiency, especially in the elderly, is more widespread than previously thought. Older adults who eat a diet rich in vitamin K are less likely to report memory problems than those who have insufficient levels.[719] Further, deficiency is often diagnosed in people with Alzheimer's.[720] Although vitamin K is derived from both plants and animals, the healthiest sources of vitamin K are leafy greens and other vegetables, such as broccoli, kale, collards, turnip greens, Brussels sprouts, spinach, kiwi, avocado, and prunes.

Amount of Vitamin K in One Cup Cooked Vegetables

Broccoli: 220 mcg

Brussels sprouts: 218 mcg

Collard greens: 1,059 mcg

Kale: 1,062 mcg

Spinach: 889 mcg

Turnip greens: 529 mcg

WHAT ABOUT PROTEIN?

No other dietary nutrient is obsessed over like protein. People who follow a meat-and-dairy centered diet may be concerned about getting enough protein if they switch to a plant-centered diet. We are living at a time of protein mania fostered by high-protein diet books, lifestyle bloggers, and social media influencers singing the praises of protein for building muscle and more.

Many packaged food labels are emblazoned with "High Protein" or "Great Source of Protein" and there are aisles full of protein bars, powders, and mixes. Food manufacturers are now capitalizing on the trend by offering an increasing number of "protein-enhanced" products including pasta, bagels, chips, bread, peanut butter, brownies, pancake mix, and even bottled water. Nearly half of Americans now seek out such protein-enriched foods.

Collectively, companies that peddle protein supplements worldwide now generate $9 billion a year from these products. From the ubiquity of these products, one could infer that Americans have a problem getting sufficient dietary protein. Generally, they do not.

Protein propaganda is rich with unfounded beliefs, such as the one that says protein is only found in meat, or that to meet one's protein needs from plant foods one needs to eat them as combinations at particular times. Extra protein is credited with facilitating weight loss, increasing athletic prowess, and providing a great source of energy. These ideas have many adherents, but they lack supporting scientific evidence, and in many cases, have been robustly refuted.

The surprising fact is that most Americans consume twice (or more) of the recommended daily intake of protein with no benefit at all—and it can be argued that this amount is detrimental to their health.[721] Even more telling, a survey of more than 25,000 vegetarians—the largest ever undertaken—concluded that, on average, even those who eat no meat, fish, or dairy were exceeding their actual protein needs by 70 percent.[722] Yet over the last decade consumer desire for more protein has only grown. In a survey by the market research company NPD Group, 78 percent of respondents said they were seeking more protein in their diet, yet remarkably 71 percent had no idea what the recommended daily amount is.

There is a price to pay for protein excess. First, due to the myth that protein is only found in foods made from animals, the focus on protein tends to bring undesirable dietary additions—namely, saturated fat and cholesterol—while squeezing out the fiber-rich, antioxidant-rich, and anti-inflammatory foods our diets should be rich in.

Over the long term, ingesting too much protein is tied to dehydration, constipation, accelerated bone loss, and kidney disease, as the body works to process the excess nitrogen and waste products created during protein metabolism.

Think you are an exception because you live such an athletic lifestyle? Consider that Novak Djokovic, who won the 2019 Wimbledon championship, Scott Jurek, who won the Western States 100-mile Endurance Race, and Dotsie Bausch, a silver medal–winning Olympic cyclist all fueled their phenomenal athletic achievements on plant-based diets. Patrik Baboumian, who hails from Germany, is a strongman competitor with many records under his belt, including the record for the log-lift, lifting 400 pounds; and for the yoke walk, carrying 1,230 pounds for 33 feet. He too lives and trains on a plant-based diet.

PROTEIN CONTENT OF VARIOUS FOODS		
FOOD	SERVING SIZE	GRAMS OF PROTEIN
Quinoa	1 cup	8
Peanut butter	2 tbsp	8
Soybeans	1 cup	29
Lentils	1 cup	18
Black beans	1 cup	15
Chickpeas	1 cup	15
Tofu, firm	4 ounces	11
Green peas	1 cup	9
Soy milk	1 cup	7
Oatmeal	½ cup, dry	6
Wild rice	1 cup, cooked	7
Hemp seeds	1 tbsp	4
Chia seeds	1 tbsp	3
Pumpkin seeds	1 tbsp	4
Buckwheat	1 cup, cooked	5.7
Seitan	⅓ cup	21
Broccoli	1 cup, cooked	6
Nuts (all types)	1 ounce	7

Now that I have cautioned you about protein worship, let me add that there is growing evidence that the USDA's recommendation of 46 grams of protein a day for women and 56 grams a day for men may be lower than ideal and may not account for age-related muscle loss (sarcopenia). Loss of muscle—particularly in those who are physically inactive—starts as early as your forties. In the next two decades that loss accelerates and can lead to instability, risk of falling, and lower quality of life. To counter this, first we must keep active and exercise our muscles. Adequate protein is also important to slowing the rate of loss. A more prudent protein allowance would be a gram of protein for each kilogram of bodyweight. Later in the chapter I will illustrate what sufficient protein intake looks like.

CALCIUM

When you read or hear the word calcium, you probably imagine a glass of milk. We have been so conditioned to associate cow's milk with calcium that many people cannot name another source of the mineral, save for perhaps supplements. But dairy does not have a corner on the calcium market. In fact, we can get calcium from more than 50 different foods—sometimes more efficiently than we can from cow's milk.

While calcium is certainly important to health, there is a misperception that we cannot manage to get enough in our diet and therefore need to supplement with cow's milk and calcium pills. Where we really have trouble is not in *consumption* but in *retention*. This is because several features of the typical American lifestyle, including excess animal protein, high caffeine consumption, soft drinks, high sodium, high sugar, smoking, and sedentary living all cause the body to lose calcium.

When it comes to bone health specifically, the lifestyle proposed in this book, including a diet chock-full of all the nutrients required to build and sustain healthy bones (it takes more than calcium) coupled with regular bone-stimulating exercise, is ideal.

HOW MUCH CALCIUM IS IN MY FOOD?

FOOD SOURCES OF CALCIUM (MG OF CALCIUM PER 3.5 OUNCES)			
Amaranth	153 mg	Arugula	309 mg
Barley	57 mg	Black beans	47 mg
Blackstrap molasses	342 mg	Broccoli	177 mg
Brussels sprouts	56 mg	Butternut squash	84 mg
Chickpeas	80 mg	Collard greens	148 mg
Corn bread (one piece)	133 mg	Dandelion greens	147 mg
Figs, dried (10)	269 mg	Northern beans	121 mg
Green beans	58 mg	Kale	94 mg
Lima beans	55 mg	Lentils	37 mg
Mustard greens	104 mg	Navel orange	56 mg
Navy beans	128 mg	Okra	176 mg
Onion	57 mg	Orange juice (fortified)	350 mg
Peas	95 mg	Pinto beans	82 mg
Raisins	53 mg	Rhubarb	115 mg
Soy milk	100-500 mg	Soybeans	175 mg
Soy yogurt (6 oz)	250 ng	Sweet potato	70 mg
Swiss chard	102 mg	Tahini (2 tbsp)	128 mg
Turnip greens	197 mg	Watercress	120 mg
White beans	161 mg		
SEAWEEDS			
Agar	567 mg	Dulse	296 mg
Hiziki	1,400 mg	Kelp	1,093 mg
Kombu	800 mg	Wakame	1,300 mg
NUTS & SEEDS			
Almonds	254 mg	Brazil nuts	186 mg
Hazelnuts	209 mg	Peanuts	74 mg
Pistachios	131 mg	Sesame seeds	1,160 mg
Sunflower seeds	126 mg	Walnuts	83 mg

So far we have been looking at specific macronutrients, antioxidants, and vitamins in foods. Now let's look at the larger classes of foods that make up a healthful plant-based diet.

GRAINS

Grains have played an important role in many societies worldwide. In Central America corn is a dietary mainstay, while in the Middle East, millet is eaten regularly. In North Africa couscous is popular, and in Italy polenta is a favorite. Whole grains are a rich source of fiber, vitamins, and minerals, and if unrefined are an excellent source of complex carbohydrates. When whole grain foods are plentiful in the diet they help lower blood pressure, fight the buildup of arterial plaque, reduce colon cancer risk, and significantly cut risk of premature death.[723] Oddly, while the US is the largest producer of grains in the world, we do not favor them in our cuisine, exporting much of it and feeding the balance to livestock.

A drawback to a lot of the grain sold in the USA is that it has been refined. This is sometimes the case even when the packaging claims the product is a whole grain food. It is not uncommon for products to contain a small amount of whole grain added to a much more refined grain with added fat, sugar, and salt to make the claim of containing whole grain. This is most seen in packaged breads. The refinement process involves milling to make grains easier to eat and to enable them to cook faster, a process that also depletes their nutritional quality.

An important example is wheat. All wheat flour begins in its whole form. In refinement, the grain is ground, rolled, and sifted, separating the seed. What is retained is the powdered endosperm, which is then bleached with solvents, ultimately resulting in the white flour used for most of the pasta and bread and other baked goods. This flour has lost 25 percent of its fiber and 50 percent of its vitamins and minerals. Not only is refined white flour less nutritious, but due to the loss of fiber it is assimilated by our body more rapidly and causes a rapid rise in blood sugar.

It is healthiest to eat grains in their intact, whole form. Look for the Whole Grain Council seal on the package do be certain it is a genuine whole grain product.

THE FOLLOWING ARE GRAINS YOU MAY WISH TO INTEGRATE INTO YOUR NEW WAY OF EATING.

Amaranth

Amaranth's history dates to the Aztecs. Today, it is produced largely in China and Central America. This tiny, pale-yellow grain can be used like wheat. In baking, you can split a wheat-flour measurement, using half amaranth and half whole wheat. Amaranth has a high protein content and contains more calcium that any other grain.

Barley

Barley was first cultivated in China around 2000 B.C. Today, the most popular form is an ivory-colored form called pearl barley, which has had its bran removed. The most nutritious variety is called hulled barely. Its bran has been left intact and the fiber, calcium, and iron content are substantially greater. Barley is also a rich source of potassium. This versatile grain can be added to soups, broth, salads, or mixed with vegetables, and can even made into a hot breakfast cereal.

Buckwheat

Technically, buckwheat is not a grain because it is not part of the Gramineae grass family. However, it is used like a grain in a variety of dishes, including buckwheat pancakes. Buckwheat is rich in vitamin E, potassium, phosphorus, and B vitamins. It has a distinct nutty flavor and is gluten-free.

Cornmeal

A staple for Native Americans, cornmeal is made from ground corn. Like other grains, the best way to buy it is in its whole form with the germ and bran still present. While most people have had cornbread and corn muffins, this hearty grain can make terrific pancakes, hot breakfast cereal, and soft or formed polenta.

Kamut

Once known as "King Tut's wheat," this buttery-flavored grain is a relative of modern wheat. Kamut is higher in protein than many other grains and rich in minerals. You will find an increasing number of breads, cereals, and pastas made from kamut in stores today.

Millet

Considered a sacred food by the Chinese, millet is high in protein, B vitamins, copper, and iron. The grain is small and absorbs flavors well. Like barley, millet can be made into a tasty hot cereal. It can also be mixed into salads or casseroles or eaten in place of rice. Those who make their own granola at home may enjoy adding millet to the mix.

Oats

Oats contain calcium phosphorus, iron, vitamin E, thiamin, and B vitamins. Although oats were consumed by hunter-gatherer societies as far back as 32,000 years ago, and have always been a staple in the diet of the Scots, they did not reach America until the 1600s.[724] Most Americans eat oats as a hot cereal, in granola, snack bars, and, more recently, in oat milk. Oats can also be used to make muffins, pancakes, and bread.

Several publicized studies indicate that oats can help lower cholesterol levels. Fortunately, all oats retain their bran and germ, so the fiber content remains high. Oats are available in old-fashioned, quick cooking, and steel-cut varieties.

Quinoa

Pronounced keen-wah, this staple of the Incas has become quite popular in the past ten years. Known as the super-nutrient grain, quinoa is rich in protein, iron, riboflavin, manganese, zinc, potassium, and magnesium. It has a mild nutty flavor and comes in black, red, and white varieties. Quinoa is now used to make breads, pastas, baking flour, pancakes, and in place of couscous in salads.

Rice

There are numerous varieties of rice including long-grain, short-grain, wehani, black, wild, Arborio, and basmati. Although rice is the most popular grain food in the Americas, China consumes many times as much as the US. Like barley, however, the bulk of the rice consumed in the USA is the refined form of polished white rice. Brown rice is richer in fiber and nutrients such as magnesium and selenium, and it is easier on blood sugar levels.

Rye

One of the least used grains, rye is significantly higher in protein than whole wheat. It also contains B vitamins and iron. While consumed widely in Scandinavia, what little rye we eat in the US is in the form of rye bread, which is mostly refined wheat flour with added rye. Rye can be added to oatmeal, breads, muffins, rice, or, in its flake form, prepared as a hot cereal or mixed in with homemade granola.

Spelt

Cultivated for at least 5,000 years, this grain is becoming quite popular, particularly among people wishing to lower their intake of gluten. It has a nutty flavor and is rich in B vitamins. Spelt breads, bagels, and pastas have become increasingly more available in recent years.

WHAT ABOUT GLUTEN?

Gluten is a protein that occurs in wheat (including kamut and spelt), rye, and barley. Although oats are often mistakenly referred to as a gluten-containing grain, they are not. However, oats can become cross-contaminated with gluten if they are processed in a facility that also processes wheat, rye, and barley. So people with celiac disease are careful to only buy oats that are labeled "gluten-free." Gluten is also added to some processed foods as a binding or thickening agent. For those diagnosed with celiac disease, consuming gluten can be life-threatening because it causes damage to the small intestine. The intestine wall is lined with thread-like projections known as villi whose job it is to absorb nutrients from food and transport them to the bloodstream. The presence of gluten causes the immune system to mount an attack on the villi. In their damaged state, the villi can no longer perform their job well and serious nutritional deficiencies will follow.

In the past decade, concern over gluten has led to an explosion of gluten-free foods in markets. About three million Americans must avoid gluten due to their celiac condition, and an additional one percent of the population is allergic to wheat specifically. However, an estimated 30 percent of shoppers are now looking for gluten-free foods because they believe that they have a condition called non-celiac gluten sensitivity (NCGS). It is difficult to know how many people have this condition, but a study published in the journal *Digestion* made an interesting finding.

Researchers recruited 390 subjects who believed they were gluten-sensitive and reported various symptoms they suspected were caused by gluten. Each was placed on a gluten-free diet for six months and then had gluten reintroduced to their diet for one month. About 6.5 percent were diagnosed with celiac disease. Nearly seven percent were diagnosed with NCGS. Just 0.51 percent had a genuine wheat allergy. However, 85 percent of the subjects experienced no changes in symptoms while following a gluten-free diet.[725] An emerging theory is that there may be a third camp of individuals who have neither celiac disease nor a classic wheat allergy and yet experience symptoms when they consume gluten or wheat. This is referred to as non-celiac gluten sensitivity syndrome.[726] If you suspect you may fall into one of these camps, make an appointment with a gastroenterologist and or allergist and get tested.

LEGUMES

A legume is a plant that bears seeds enclosed in pods that split upon maturity. We eat these pods in the form of beans, peas, and lentils. Legumes are probably the oldest crop in the world, with evidence they were grown as far back as 10,000 years ago. Today, legumes make up a substantial part of the diets of people in Asia, Latin America, the Middle East, and India.

Perhaps due to their reputation as the poor man's protein, legumes were an ignored food in America until relatively recently. In fact, legumes are an inexpensive and highly versatile food that not only provides a significant amount of protein (12 to 20 grams per cup) and fiber, but also calcium, magnesium, iron, potassium, zinc, B vitamins, protective antioxidants, and omega-3 fats. Surprisingly, pinto beans and red beans contain a higher concentration of antioxidants than raspberries or cultivated blueberries. People who feast on legumes are well-served by the concentrated nutrition they provide. The most long-lived people in the world, who reside in the Blue Zones (more about them later), consume four times the number of legumes that Americans do. Another wonderful quality of legumes is that they are durable and store well for up to a year.

Most varieties of legumes are delicious eaten alone or as a side dish. They are also frequently added to soups, stews, salads, or chili, combined with a grain, or mixed in with a variety of vegetables. One of the reasons that legumes have not been popular in the past is the myth that they are difficult to cook. They are not.

FRUITS AND VEGETABLES

When one thinks of the distinction between fruits and vegetables, what usually comes to mind is sweetness. Botanically speaking, what distinguishes fruits from vegetables is that fruits are seed-bearing and emanate from a flowering plant. Vegetables are the other parts of plants including the roots, stems, leaves, and flowers. However, I am sure you can think of a couple of vegetables that you eat that contain seeds such as tomatoes, avocados, and cucumbers. Technically, these are indeed fruits.

According to the United Nations Food and Agriculture Office, there are more than 1,000 species of vegetables grown in the world, yet in the USA we only see about seven percent of that bounty. If you are like most Americans, your exposure to fruits and vegetables may be limited to a narrow band of favorites. The three most popular vegetables in the

USA are potatoes, tomatoes, and sweet corn, and Americans typically eat no more than three servings of vegetables a day. That paltry intake makes it impossible to acquire a sufficient level of antioxidants, fiber, phytochemicals, minerals, and vitamins that are requisite to sustaining good health.

Vegetables and fruits are a good source of dietary fiber, especially if they are eaten with their skin (with exceptions of course, such as bananas, pineapple, and melons!). They are also the chief source of protective antioxidants and phytochemicals. While many Americans rarely venture beyond than bananas and apples, at least 40 additional varieties of fruit are ours to explore, each with distinct colors, flavors, and protective properties.

As with legumes and grains, I encourage you to stretch beyond your zone of familiarity and see what else you may find appealing. Recall that the bulk of the protective phytochemicals, such as flavonoids, are concentrated in fruits and vegetables. Think of these foods as nutritional medicine.

NUTS AND SEEDS

Nuts and seeds are nutrient-dense and offer many protective compounds that support brain health and help ward off neurological disease. Eating nuts and seeds has been associated with lower cholesterol; a reduced risk for cardiovascular disease, high blood pressure, diabetes, cancer, and gallstones; improved immune function; and the safeguarding of arterial linings.[727] These benefits are attributed to antioxidant and anti-inflammatory compounds in the nuts and seeds, as well as other compounds that prevent blood platelet clumping. Nuts and seeds contain protein, vitamin E, calcium, magnesium, potassium, and fiber. A few (walnuts, flaxseeds, chia seeds, hemp seeds) are good sources of anti-inflammatory omega-3 fats. Nuts also contain folate, which is important for controlling homocysteine levels.

Numerous studies have shown better cognitive function in people who regularly consume nuts over their lifetimes.[728] In one study of 2,613 men and women aged 43 to 70, participants were given cognitive tests twice over a five-year period. Nut consumption was associated with better memory, information processing speed, cognitive flexibility, and global cognitive function. The subjects in the highest quintile for nut consumption had the cognitive function of people five to eight years younger.[729]

Almonds have been shown to increase levels of HDL, the form of cholesterol that is protective against heart disease[730] and that helps lower total cholesterol levels.[731] They may also help lower blood pressure, reduce inflammation, and raise levels of the "brain fertilizer," brain-derived neurotrophic factor (BDNF).

Hazelnuts are high in antioxidants, including vitamin E and selenium, and contain potassium, calcium, manganese, and B vitamins. Compared to healthy controls, patients with AD show a consistent deficiency in selenium.[732] Just ¼ cup of hazelnuts provides 50 percent of the recommended intake of the antioxidant vitamin E.

Pecans have the greatest concentration of antioxidants among nuts, including beta carotene, cryptoxanthin, lutein, and zeaxanthin, and are rich in magnesium, which lowers inflammation markers like c-reactive protein (CRP).[733] Pecans also contain a small amount of the omega-3 fat alpha-linolenic acid (ALA).

It's remarkable how a whole walnut appears to resemble the wrinkled texture of the two hemispheres of a brain. Maybe nature is telling us something. Several studies have shown that walnut consumption improves artery function.[734] Specifically, adding walnuts to the diet helps the endothelium (artery lining) by improving flexibility of the artery wall as well as dilation. These are qualities that enhance blood flow everywhere, including to the brain.

Walnuts are loaded with brain-supportive nutrients, including ALA.[735] Walnuts also contain the antioxidants vitamin E and melatonin, folate, polyphenols, and the neuroprotective substance gallic acid. Folate is often severely deficient in those suffering from cognitive problems, including Alzheimer's.[736]

In a study that looked at the dietary choices of 10,000 subjects, researchers found that cognitive function was consistently greater in those who consumed walnuts regularly, irrespective of whether they smoked, drank alcohol, exercised, or were overweight.[737] One only needs about seven or eight walnuts a day—about one-quarter cup—to do the trick. This amount provides nearly 100 percent of the suggested intake of ALA. I enjoy adding walnuts to my oatmeal, salads, or mixing them with sliced banana as a snack.

Some people avoid nuts because they find they gain weight easily when they consume them. Interestingly, although the mechanism is unclear, in some cases certain nuts may even assist in regulating body-weight. In a meta-analysis of 30 prior studies that looked at the influence of nut-eating on bodyweight, the authors concluded that nut eaters were no more likely to see an increase in body weight, waist circumference, or body mass index (BMI).[738] Having said that, my suggestion is that you limit portion size to no more than about the palm of your hand per day.

Whether enjoyed as a snack, mixed into a main dish, or sprinkled over a salad, nuts provide wonderful flavors as well as many protective elements.[739]

When nuts are roasted several undesirable things can occur. First, if nuts are roasted in oils, you now have the burden of heat damaged and refined oil. The higher the heat used and longer the duration the more oxidized they will become.[740] Roasting also may reduce levels of some antioxidants present in nuts.[741] After roasting, nuts are less shelf stable and will oxidize further at an accelerated rate compared to raw nuts. Also, roasting can produce small amounts of trans fats.[742] Fresh, whole, raw nuts should have little scent. If they smell like paint thinner, you can be certain they are not healthy to eat.

The best way to consume nuts and seeds is in their whole, raw form. Skip the roasting, skip the oil, and skip the salt. To sustain freshness, store nuts in an airtight package in the refrigerator.

Chia Seeds

These miniscule seeds contain boron, calcium, iodine, magnesium, zinc, and vitamins A, B, E and D. Like flaxseeds, chia seeds are a rich source of the omega-3 fat ALA. Including chia seeds in your diet has been shown to improve blood sugar levels and reduce blood pressure, which in turn protects cognitive function. Chia seeds have a high antioxidant capacity, and are fiber-rich, offering 11 grams per ounce of seed, and have been proven to be an effective means of providing sustained energy for endurance exercise.[743]

Flaxseeds

Legend tells us that in the eighth century the Emperor Charlemagne was so impressed with the health benefits of flaxseeds that his subjects were required by law to consume them. Although the king lacked the technology to study flaxseed as we do today, he had great instincts because flaxseeds offer many important health benefits.

Flaxseed meal is an excellent and inexpensive way to boost intake of the omega-3 fat ALA. Just two tablespoons of flaxseed meal provide almost 150 percent of our daily requirement for ALA. The lignans found in flaxseeds have antioxidant properties that can help to combat oxidative stress, as well as help lower bad (LDL) cholesterol, and reduce the likelihood of plaque depositing on arterial walls, thereby supporting blood flow to the brain and heart.[744] Flaxseed appears to be helpful in lowering blood pressure and improving insulin sensitivity as well. Compared to those taking a placebo, after just six months study participants who ate two tablespoons of flaxseed meal daily saw up to a 15-point reduction in systolic and 7-point reduction in diastolic blood pressure.[745] This improvement is superior to some commonly prescribed hypertensive medications.

Integrating flaxseed meal into the diet is simple. For example, add one to two tablespoons flaxseed meal to cold cereal, oatmeal, soups, or smoothies. It is also easy to add a tablespoon of flaxseed meal to salads and even pasta sauce, or to toss roasted vegetables in flaxseed meal.

To extract all the nutritional benefits, it is best to consume flaxseed in its ground form. Using a coffee bean grinder at home works fine, or simply purchase the pre-ground version. Refrigerated and sealed in an airtight container or zip lock bag, ground flaxseed will retain its freshness for about 12 weeks, after which it loses nutritional value and can become oxidized. Choose organically produced flaxseeds or flaxseed meal whenever possible.

Pumpkin Seeds

Pumpkin seeds, also known as pepitas, are rich in protein and magnesium, which support healthy blood vessels and blood pressure. They also have anti-inflammatory properties, and contain various antioxidants, calcium, vitamin K, iron, and omega-3 fats. Pumpkin seeds may improve blood sugar levels, as well as increase good (HDL) cholesterol levels. The seeds may also help reduce plaque formation and improve blood flow in arteries by elevating nitric oxide levels.

You can blend pumpkin seeds into a smoothie, sprinkle them on soups and salads, bake them into breads, or eat them alone as a snack.

An array of nut- and seed-based beverages are on the market today, including milks made from almonds, coconut, cashews, hazelnuts, hemp seeds, macadamias, pecans, and walnuts, as well as milks based on oats, peas, and soy. I encourage you to explore these options. Keep in mind that many, unfortunately, are sweetened with sugar in one of its various guises. However, nearly every brand offers an unsweetened option, which I recommend.

If you purchase almond or other nut milks in Europe, you will undoubtedly notice they are much creamier and richer in flavor. This is because the milks are made from a higher percentage of nuts overall. Most nut milks in the USA use 4 percent nuts. The European products regularly contain 6 to 8 percent. Because the beverages have been made this way, they have a richer and more satisfying flavor. A new brand that has yet to have national distribution but can currently be found in the eastern USA is the Elmhurst line of nut milks. To my knowledge, they use the highest concentration of nuts in their milks, which makes for an exceptionally good product. An alternative to buying ready-made nut and seed milks is to make your own at home. All that is required is nuts, water, a blender, and cheesecloth to separate the liquid from the nut/seed pulp.

25

SUPERFOODS FOR THE BRAIN

A s IMPORTANT AS it is to avoid foods that *damage* our brains, the Revolution Lifestyle promotes the consumption of foods that *protect* our brains. Not only does a plant-based diet substantially increase our intake of foods shown to be protective, among those foods are a few superstars. To qualify, a superfood must have a high concentration of protective nutrients such as vitamins, minerals, and antioxidants or phytochemicals. And its consumption must be widely associated with a lower risk of disease.

APPLES

You have heard the 150-year-old aphorism: *An apple a day keeps the doctor away*. Because daily apple consumption is associated with a markedly lower risk of four factors that increase the chance of Alzheimer's disease—cardiovascular disease, heart attack, stroke, and diabetes—I encourage you to follow this prescription. An apple contains just 60 calories on average but is a powerhouse of protective nutrition and fiber. Flavonoids, vitamin C, calcium, B-complex vitamins, potassium, and other compounds are packed into the skin. An apple eaten with its skin provides up to six times the antioxidants found in the flesh and will provide 30 percent of your recommended daily fiber intake, something in which Americans are almost invariably deficient. One flavonoid in apples, quercetin, has been found to protect neurons against oxidative stress, and daily apple consumption has been found to lower the risk of type 2 diabetes by 28 percent.[746]

Acting like "nature's statin," daily apple consumption has been shown to reduce LDL cholesterol levels by 23 percent in just six months, and to help prevent the oxidation of LDL cholesterol, making it less prone to clogging up arteries.[747] And there is more. Regular apple consumption is associated with reduced risk of inflammation and was associated with up to a 28 percent reduction in the risk of stroke.[748] These benefits, coupled with the ability for regular apple consumption to increase levels of the neurotransmitter acetylcholine are some of the reasons why apple eating protects cognitive health.

Fuji and red delicious have the highest concentration of antioxidants, but other varieties are just as important to include. The additional protective compounds in apples vary from one varietal to the next, so rotate the types you eat for the greatest benefits. Keep the skin intact as that's where the protective factors are concentrated.

Now the not-so-good news. When tested, apples are consistently among the top 12 most pesticide-laden foods when tested. Therefore, choose organic apples whenever you have the option.

AVOCADO

Yes, avocados are rich in fat, but their fat is the monounsaturated variety. Avocados also contain lutein, fiber, folate, manganese, magnesium, iron, potassium, and vitamins A, B, C, E, D, and K and are associated with a lower risk of cancer.

Avocados have also proven to help lower blood cholesterol and triglyceride levels,[749] as well as help lower inflammation.[750] The carotenoid lutein has been shown to improve cognitive function and is important to healthy vision. A study found that compared to those who avoided them, people who included avocados in their diet experience an increase in macular pigment concentration which is associated with better cognition. Why? Because when lutein concentrates in the macula it also gets incorporated into the brain. A team of researchers found that after six months of adding avocado to the diet of volunteers there were significant improvements in memory and spatial working memory (memory used to recall the location of an object).[751]

BEANS

Beans are not the first thing that comes to mind when people think of foods rich in antioxidants. Yet red, pinto, and black beans are among the most antioxidant-rich foods one can eat. In addition to being a great source of protein, beans also contain calcium, potassium, magnesium, iron, folate, zinc, and fiber. Studies have found bean consumers lower their risk of inflammation, cardiovascular disease, and fatty liver disease. Beans also help control blood sugar levels. A study that followed 3,300 participants over four years found that those who ate beans just over three times per week reduced their risk of developing diabetes by 35 percent.[752] Moreover, adding just a half-cup of beans a day to your diet can lower LDL cholesterol levels by about 10 percent. You may enjoy beans in vegetarian chili, a bean burrito, added to a green salad or soup, or in a bean-based veggie burger.

BERRIES

In addition to their wonderfully sweet flavors, fruits and berries are a rich source of many protective antioxidants and phytochemicals. These are the compounds in foods that combat inflammation and oxidative stress and offer other important benefits.

The scientific literature is replete with epidemiological studies showing that people who regularly consume berries are better protected against Alzheimer's disease, Parkinson's disease, cardiovascular disease, and the general effects of aging. The presence of both antioxidants and anti-inflammatory polyphenols and carotenoids, as well as vitamin C and folate that may activate antioxidant enzymes in the brain, are believed to be what make these foods neuroprotective.

Berry consumption has not only been associated with reduced risk of cognitive decline, but numerous double-blind, placebo-controlled (the gold standard) studies have found *improvements* in memory, learning, executive function, cerebral blood circulation, and general cognition after as little as 12 weeks of berry consumption.[753] Blackberries, black currants, boysenberries, raspberries, and strawberries should all be on your menu, but at the top of the super berry list are blueberries.

We have heard for years that blueberries are an antioxidant power-house, beating out 20 other fruits and vegetables for their antioxidant capacity, and ranking second only to red beans—if the berries are wild. Even the cultivated variety is close to the top of the list of the most antioxidant-rich foods. Yet there is so much more that this remarkable fruit can do to protect the brain.

Blueberries (and blackberries) pack a high level of the flavonoids called anthocyanins, which enter and accumulate in the brain. Anthocyanins have both antioxidant and anti-inflammatory properties, increase blood flow to the brain,[754] improve the health of blood vessels, and have been shown to improve memory in as little as 12 weeks in those who ate blueberries daily.[755] Another compound in blueberries, cyclic guanosine monophosphate, causes the smooth muscles that line arteries to relax, which allows for better blood flow. Daily blueberry consumption has also been shown to raise HDL (good) cholesterol.[756] Finally, blueberries are known to boost levels of BDNF.[757]

Be sure to seek out organic blueberries, as tests have identified over 47 different pesticides, including 14 neurotoxins, on the conventionally grown variety.[758] Although the season for US-grown fresh blueberries is short, one can find frozen organic blueberries in major supermarkets year-round.

Strawberries are rich in vitamins B6, C, E, K, and contain folate, calcium, and potassium. They are also a source of anthocyanins which have been shown to significantly boost short-term memory.

Strawberries also contain the flavanol fisetin,[759] which protects neurons and enhances their connectivity, particularly in the hippocampus.[760] Fisetin also seems effective at reducing inflammation[761] and may help reduce the depositing of amyloid protein as well as regulate blood sugar.[762]

Due to the very high level of pesticide residue found on conventionally grown strawberries (a single sample contained 20 different pesticides in one study), always seek out organically grown strawberries. They are highly perishable, so buy them as fresh as possible and eat them soon after you bring them home. If you wait to wash berries until just before you are going to consume them, they will last longer in your fridge.

CELERY

You probably never imagined unexciting celery would appear on a super-foods list. Surprisingly, this humble food has 15 different substances that can contribute to our pursuit of brain health. Celery is full of vitamin C and other antioxidants that protect against oxidative stress, and it also contains anti-inflammatory compounds that protect cells, blood vessels, and the heart. Celery may help reduce LDL (bad) cholesterol, and a substance called phthalide, found in celery, seems to lower blood pressure by relaxing the smooth muscle in artery walls. I add a stalk to my kale smoothie before breakfast every day. (It tastes better than it sounds.)

CHERRIES

Cherries contain the antioxidant and anti-inflammatory compounds quercitrin and isoqueritin, as well as melatonin, which is both a sleep-facilitating hormone and an antioxidant produced in the pineal gland of the brain.

Cherries are a potent ally in fighting inflammation and reducing levels of MCP-1, a molecule that promotes arterial-plaque formation. In a study published in the *Journal of Nutrition*, researchers found that after feeding subjects Bing cherries for 28 days, circulating levels of the inflammation marker C-reactive protein dropped 25 percent.[763] Everyone can benefit from reduced inflammation.

CHIA SEEDS

Purported to have been a favorite of the Aztecs and Mayans, chia seeds have become more popular in the past few years. There's good reason these ancient cultures would have favored these miniscule seeds, which look like oversized pepper grinds. They are rich in omega-3 fats, antioxidants, protein, calcium, magnesium, manganese, potassium, phosphorus, zinc, B vitamins, and fiber. Adding about three tablespoons of chia seeds to the diet daily shaved six points off systolic blood pressure and reduced a marker of inflammation (CRP) by 40 percent in just three months.[764] Chia seeds can easily be added to salads, dressings, applesauce, cereal, oatmeal, and smoothies.

CRUCIFEROUS VEGGIES

Bok choy, broccoli, Brussels sprouts, cabbage, cauliflower, and kale belong to the cruciferous group. These vegetables have been receiving high acclaim for their health protective qualities for decades, especially with regard to lowering the risk for cancer. This is thought to be because protective compounds including nitriles, indoles, isothiocyanates, and thiocyanates are created when these vegetables are digested.

In fact, these foods offer four levels of protection to support cognitive resilience, and therefore they should have a prominent place in your diet. First, one of the remarkable compounds they contain, sulforaphane, helps combat neuroinflammation and oxidative stress, and supports mitochondrial function in neurons. Second, sulforaphane supports the production of BDNF, and it's thought to enhance connectivity in the brain by enhancing synaptic function. Third, it appears that sulforaphane offers neuroprotection against a broad variety of toxic agents, including certain pesticides and heavy metals.[765]

Finally, researchers have found that the more cruciferous foods individuals ate, the lower the plaque levels in their carotid arteries.[766] Remember, plaque in the carotid artery is considered a reliable indicator of the presence of plaque blocking up blood vessels in the brain.

GRAPES

Grapes are packed with antioxidants, including vitamin C and beta carotene. They also contain resveratrol, which is believed to protect blood vessels from damage, facilitate the clearance of beta-amyloid, and possibly promote neurogenesis.[767] Darker grapes contain the class of flavonoids called anthocyanins which are antioxidants.

Because 56 different pesticide residues have been detected on conventionally grown grapes, including ten neurotoxins, I encourage you to seek out the organically grown variety.

POMEGRANATES

The pomegranate has had any number of medicinal properties ascribed to it since antiquity. So, it should be no surprise that the Royal College of Physicians in Great Britain features a pomegranate in its coat of arms. Although one rarely sees them in the fruit bowl, pomegranates offer an array of benefits that directly support brain health. They contain 21 different polyphenols, including one of particular interest called punicalagin, which stimulates neurogenesis, is an antioxidant, and combats neuroinflammation.[768]

In addition to combating oxidative stress and decreasing neuroinflammation, studies have found that drinking pomegranate juice reduces amyloid protein and improves synapse plasticity and improves memory. In one study, just one cup of pomegranate juice daily for 12 weeks resulted in a drop of inflammatory markers by 30 percent.[769] In another study, both memory and blood flow to the brain were enhanced with the consumption of eight ounces of pomegranate juice daily for four weeks.[770]

Pomegranate juice has also been used to prevent the postoperative memory loss that is commonly seen in patients who undergo heart surgery.[771]

Several studies have shown that because they are rich in potassium and reduce levels of angiotensin converting enzyme (ACE), which controls blood vessel diameter, pomegranates help in blood pressure regulation. In a study of adults with high blood pressure, five ounces of pomegranate juice daily for two weeks resulted in a significant drop in blood pressure.[772] Moreover, it appeared to improve the health of artery walls as well.

In another study, eight weeks of pomegranate juice supplementation resulted in a reduction of both total and LDL (bad) cholesterol.[773]

Additional elements in pomegranates that support brain health include vitamin C, vitamin K, folate, and potassium.

Clearly, pomegranates are a great addition to a healthy, brain-protecting diet. To avoid the tedium of trying to remove the seeds from the flesh, simply cut one pomegranate in half, then turn it over, seeded side down on a countertop or dish. Then use a wooden spoon to tap firmly and repeatedly on the fruit skin. The seeds will slip out easily. They can be eaten individually or added to soups, cooked rice, quinoa, and salads.

POWER GREENS

Leafy greens, such as spinach, kale, chard, collard greens, dandelion greens, bok choy, and turnip greens are nutritional powerhouses consistently linked to better cognitive function as well as many other positive outcomes. Greens like these are rich in antioxidants such as beta carotene, vitamin C and E, selenium, lutein, and zeaxanthin. They also are a good source of folate, which as we have seen is critical to keeping homocysteine levels in check. The vitamin K, omega-3 fats, lutein, potassium, and magnesium they contain are associated with improved cognitive function.[774] Also, a substance in spinach and arugula (along with broccoli and beets) increases cerebral blood flow and lowers blood pressure for hours after these foods are consumed.[775]

In a study of 960 participants in the Memory and Aging Project, subjects aged 55-99 were given two cognitive assessments over about 5 years. After adjusting for smoking, alcohol consumption and other factors, those who consumed at least 1.3 cups of leafy greens daily performed as well on cognitive tests as people 11 years younger than they were.[776]

In addition to protecting brain function, leafy greens protect bone integrity, reduce risk of macular degeneration, and lower risk of type 2 diabetes.

Make sure you consume leafy greens every day. They're that important. It's as easy as making a salad, adding fresh kale to a banana-mango smoothie in the morning, adding fresh spinach to your home-made lentil soup, or sautéing a blend of kale, spinach, and chard to enjoy with your dinner. Buy your greens as fresh as possible, such as at your local farmer's market, and wash them well before eating them. Kept in the crisper of your fridge, they are good for three to five days before they begin to spoil.

SWEET POTATOES

In Cleveland Heights, Ohio, lives supercentenarian Lessie Brown. As this book went to print, she was 113 years old and officially recognized by the Gerontology Research Group as the oldest living person in the US. She's often asked what her secret is.

Her daughter Bernie, who is 88 years old, shared that her mother had eaten a sweet potato every day until she reached age 110.[777] While we may think of sweet potatoes during the holidays, the long-lived Okinawans and the Papua New Guinea Highlanders have made sweet potatoes the centerpiece of their diets, and with great results.[778] Native to Central and South America, these superfoods have been consumed for thousands of years, and because they offer a remarkable lineup of important nutrients that support brain health, can be a wonderful addition to your diet year-round.

Sweet potatoes, which can be orange or purple, contain calcium and are rich in potassium, which supports healthy blood pressure but which many Americans are deficient in. They also contain antioxidants, including beta carotene, vitamin C, and vitamin E, and vitamins B1, B2, B3, B5, and B6.

One constituent of sweet potatoes is choline, which is important to neurotransmissions and reducing inflammation.[779] When selecting them at the market, look for potatoes free of splits and blemishes. Pay particularly close attention to the ends, where you may find signs of decay.

In addition to baking them, you can prepare sweet potatoes more quickly through steaming and boiling. To steam, simply cut the potato into quarter-inch slices and place in a steaming colander. For boiling, skin the potato and cut into quarter-inch cubes. Cover well with water and boil until tender. After baking or boiling, I enjoy mashing my sweet potatoes with a bit of cinnamon, nutmeg, and well-ripened banana or vanilla extract.

WATERCRESS: THE ORIGINAL SUPERFOOD

A couple of years ago I couldn't identify watercress on a plate before me. Further, I could not recall ever eating watercress. Yet I have discovered that this humble leafy green has serious bragging rights for its rich and unusual nutrient profile. Back in about 500 BC, Hippocrates, the father of medicine, said this: "Let food be thy medicine and medicine be thy food." He located his first hospital near a stream, because he wished to assure a good supply of watercress, which was core to the nutritional therapies he used with patients.

Watercress is part of the cruciferous vegetable family, so it's a relative of broccoli, Brussels sprouts, cabbage, and cauliflower. But I wanted to give it its own section because it's so extraordinary. Watercress is packed with protective antioxidants, including beta carotene, as well as several anti-inflammatory and anticancer phytochemicals, including glucosinolates, lutein, phenolic acids, and quercetin. It contains folate, calcium, vitamin C, vitamin E, vitamin K, vitamin B6, thiamin, potassium, iron and iodine, omega-3 fats, and some selenium. Watercress can be eaten alone or added to salads, pasta sauces, and smoothies or made into a soup.

CHOCOLATE IS NOT KALE

Many health writers like to promote chocolate as a superfood. The average American eats about 12 pounds of chocolate a year, and some believe they are protecting their health by doing so. While raw chocolate does contain antioxidants in the form of flavonoids, you will notice that I did not include it in the table listing the best sources of dietary antioxidants. There are several reasons. First, much of the chocolate research has been funded by the chocolate industry, which creates concern over how results are interpreted. Industry-funded studies are many times more likely to report results favorable to the funder than those not funded by a commercial interest.

Those flavonoids in chocolate? They make chocolate taste bitter, so in many instances, processors remove them. Flavonoids are not listed on the ingredient label so there is no way to know if they are present or have been removed from the chocolate you buy. Most chocolate is full of sugar which causes insulin spikes, promotes inflammation, and is problematic for the brain in other ways already mentioned. All too frequently chocolate is contaminated with lead, a neurotoxin, picked up from processing equipment, as well as with cadmium, which evidence suggests accelerates cognitive decline.[780] Cadmium can make its way into chocolate through the plant roots, especially if phosphate fertilizers have been used in cultivation. It also may be absorbed from the machinery used to process chocolate.

In 2014, an analysis of some of the most popular chocolates was commissioned by the organization As You Sow. Out of 127 chocolate products, 96 had lead and/or cadmium at levels that exceeded California's legal limit, yet there was no disclosure made to consumers on the packaging. The companies put on notice included some of the biggest names in chocolate: Chocolove, Equal Exchange, Ghirardelli, Godiva, Hershey's, Kroger, Lindt, Mars, Mondelēz, See's Candies, Theo Chocolate, Trader Joe's, and the Whole Foods 365 brand. [781]

If you love chocolate, I suggest that you limit your consumption. Alternatively, you can seek out raw cacao (not cocoa). Cacao is the natural and unrefined form of the cocoa plant that has been fermented and dried. You have probably come across cacao nibs, which are cacao beans that have been chopped up. Used to make all of the chocolate products you are familiar with; cocoa powder is made by processing cacao with very high heat. This process destroys a significant amount of the nutritional properties of the raw bean. Raw cacao is free of sugar, retains nutritional value, can be used in baking and added to smoothies, oatmeal, granola, fruit salad, hot drinks, and snack mixes. A brand you may wish to look into is Terrasoul. This company reports that their cacao powder is third-party lab tested for heavy metals, including lead and cadmium.

PROTECTING YOURSELF WITH ORGANICS

In previous chapters, we have seen how important it is to free your body (and brain) of the burden of synthetic chemical pesticides. Meat and dairy typically have 5 times the level of pesticide contamination as plant foods. So when your diet is centered upon plants, you are sharply reducing your exposure to pesticide residues. An additional important step we can take to lower our exposure to them is to choose, when available, organically farmed foods—that is, foods certified as being raised without the use of toxic chemicals. Foods that are produced without harmful chemicals are truly superior to conventional foods. First, they are safer. Second, organically produced foods may offer greater nutrition with more vitamins and antioxidants.[782]

Scientists who study pesticide exposure through diet by measuring chemical breakdown products (metabolites) in urine have shown that after just one week of eating organic food, traces of these chemicals can be slashed by nearly 90 percent.[783] The table that follows draws upon the USDA's most current data produced in its pesticide monitoring program. Although the pesticides detected vary in their effects (e.g., neurotoxins, carcinogens, developmental toxins, hormone disrupters, reproductive toxins), because my focus is Alzheimer's, I'm noting only the number of neurotoxins. For the entire inventory of foods and chemical types detected, see www.whatsonmyfood.org.

THE DANGEROUS DOZEN: CONVENTIONAL FOODS WITH THE HIGHEST PESTICIDE RESIDUES		
FOOD	**# OF PESTICIDES**	**NEUROTOXINS DETECTED**
Apples	47	5 neurotoxins
Blueberries	47	14 neurotoxins
Celery	42	12 neurotoxins
Cherries	42	7 neurotoxins
Grapes	56	10 neurotoxins
Nectarines	33	9 neurotoxins
Peaches	62	12 neurotoxins

THE DANGEROUS DOZEN: CONVENTIONAL FOODS WITH THE HIGHEST PESTICIDE RESIDUES		
FOOD	**# OF PESTICIDES**	**NEUROTOXINS DETECTED**
Pears	35	7 neurotoxins
Spinach	54	11 neurotoxins
Strawberries	45	7 neurotoxins
Sweet Bell Peppers	53	10 neurotoxins
Tomatoes	35	6 neurotoxins

Pesticide residue data derived from the United Stated Department of Agriculture (USDA) Pesticide Data Program (PDP); Punzi, JS, et al., "USDA Pesticide Data Program: Pesticide Residues on Fresh and Processed Fruit and Vegetables, Grains, Meats, Milk, and Drinking Water," *Outlooks on Pesticide Management,* June, 2005. Updated 2015.

The second most effective step to lower our exposure to pesticide residues is to eat low on the food chain and avoid meat, dairy, and fish products, where the highest concentration of pesticide residue is consistently found.

As a third step, we need to avoid purchasing and using pesticide products in our homes or yards, and not hire others to do so unless they can guarantee they are using the latest generation of alternative nontoxic substances, such as orange oil. Following these three steps will slash the level of pesticides to which we are currently exposed.

What can we expect from going organic? The Swedish Environmental Research Institute engaged a family that was eating conventionally produced foods and performed a baseline assessment, through urine samples, of the types and levels of pesticides each family member was exposed to. In the second phase of the study, the family ate only organic food. By going organic, the family's pesticide load, as determined by urinalysis, virtually disappeared.

Keep in mind that this is Sweden: the USA has more lax regulations about the types of chemicals allowed in agriculture and the tolerance levels permitted on food. The full report is available online, but the table reproduced here shows the dramatic difference that can be made in our pesticide exposure when we choose organic foods.[784]

In a US study, four families who were put on a diet of only organic foods saw up to a 97 percent reduction in the level of four dangerous pesticides detected in their urine after only one week. It was encouraging to note that glyphosate, the activate agent in Roundup that seems to have found its way into a vast number of foods, was reduced by 70 percent in the test period.[785]

The following 15 foods have been identified by the Environmental Working Group as the "Clean 15." When tested by the USDA and the FDA, these foods are consistently found to have the lowest residues of pesticides on them.[786] If you find yourself without organic produce as an option, these are the foods you can purchase with confidence. Either their skin or other feature makes them more impervious to insects, so they tend not to be treated heavily with pesticides.

THE CLEAN 15: FOODS WITH VERY LOW PESTICIDE RESIDUES			
Avocados	Asparagus	Cabbage	Cantaloupe
Cauliflower	Eggplant	Grapefruit	Honeydew melon
Kiwis	Mangos	Onions	Papaya
Pineapple	Sweet corn	Sweet peas	

A FINAL WORD ON HEALTHFUL FOODS

A brain-healthy diet is one that is brimming with fresh flavors and lively textures and colors. If you have been eating a more typical American diet heavy on animal foods and high in fat, you may be surprised by how much better you feel eating according to the Revolution Lifestyle. Choosing organic foods and eating lower on the food chain protects you from environmental contaminants, including neurotoxins, clears out plaque in blood vessels, improves blood flow to the brain, helps balance blood sugar, and reduces inflammation and oxidative stress. By centering your diet on plant foods—and especially those high in antioxidants and phytochemicals—you are taking the most powerful step possible to reduce your risk of Alzheimer's disease.

26

BRAIN-SUPPORTING SUPPLEMENTS AND SEASONINGS

IDEALLY, WE WOULD get all the nutrients we need from our food, because the benefits of many micronutrients are to some degree dependent upon the presence of other compounds in food. Some micronutrients occur in a variety of forms in food but not in supplements. Research with individual supplements has not always shown positive outcomes compared to the consumption of foods that contain a variety of nutrients. This is likely due to the synergistic nature of nutrients in the foods we eat. In other words, the nutrients support or facilitate one another and possibly offer additional benefits when they work together.

Having said this, there is a valid concern that as we age, our bodies' ability to absorb certain nutrients from foods declines. Moreover, various prescription medications can reduce nutrient absorption, as can Crohn's disease and celiac disease.

Surveys have also shown that a condition called atrophic gastritis, a chronic inflammation of the stomach lining, occurs in about 4 percent of people aged 60 to 69, 32 percent of those 70 to 79, and up to 40 percent of those 80-years and older.[787] Nutrients that are poorly absorbed when this condition is present include folate, vitamin B12, calcium, iron, and beta carotene. In surveys of people suffering from cognitive decline, deficiencies are consistently seen with vitamins B1, B2, B6, B12, C, and folate.[788]

In summary, although food is always the preferred source of nutrients, when it comes to protecting the brain, evidence suggests that it's a good idea to add certain supplements our diet.

TOP 12 BRAIN-PROTECTING SUPPLEMENTS

Based on the available evidence, I believe there are a dozen supplements worth considering to help support cognitive resilience and reduce your risk of Alzheimer's disease.

B Vitamins

More than 100 studies show an association between dementia and suboptimal levels of B vitamins. A deficiency of vitamin B1, also called thiamine, is common in AD patients.[789] B vitamins are essential to brain health for several reasons. They are involved in the production of energy and are essential to the formation of the myelin sheaths that cover and protect neurons and assure effective communication between neurons. They are also critical to the production of neurotransmitters, serotonin, dopamine, acetylcholine, and norepinephrine, which carry signals between neurons. B vitamins also help produce the hormone melatonin, which is involved in the regulation of the sleep cycle. Sufficient restful sleep is required to clear waste and toxins (including amyloid protein) from the brain that might otherwise build up and lead to neuron damage.

Vitamins B6, B12 and folic acid keep homocysteine levels in check. As we have already seen, elevated homocysteine levels are an independent risk factor for AD. When given to subjects with elevated homocysteine levels, B vitamins slowed the advance of mild cognitive impairment and reduced the rate of brain shrinkage by up to sevenfold.[790]

Several common prescription medications, including Metformin, a popular diabetes medication, have been associated with vitamin B12 deficiency.[791]

In people with MCI and elevated homocysteine levels, cognitive decline has been slowed with supplementation of vitamins B12, B6, and folic acid,[792] and cognitive function has been improved in Alzheimer's patients who were given B12 supplementation.[793]

Rather than taking several different B vitamin supplements, look for a B-complex formula that includes the following B vitamins and doses:

B1 (50 mg)

B3 (50 mg)

B6 (50 mg)

Folic acid (400 mcg)

B12 (250–500mcg)

On a strictly plant-based diet it is essential to take a B12 supplement. However, because surveys now show widespread B12 insufficiency and deficiency I recommend that even omnivores take this supplement.

Vitamin C, 500 mg

Vitamin C might be the most celebrated vitamin of all, due to its role in immunity and as an antioxidant. Studies show vitamin C is strongly linked to cognitive function as well. When tested, those with the poorest performance on memory tests fell into the bottom 10 percent of vitamin C intake.[794] Further, a study of 3,385 men aged 71 to 93 found that, when taken with vitamin E, vitamin C reduced their risk of dementia by up to 88 percent compared to those who did not take the supplements.[795] As a reminder, top food sources of vitamin C include kiwifruit, bell peppers, strawberries, oranges, papaya, broccoli, and tomatoes.

FOOD	QUANTITY	VITAMIN C
Strawberries	1 cup	89 mg
Papaya	1 cup	87 mg
Pineapple	1 cup	79 mg
Kiwi	1 med	71 mg
Orange	1 med	70 mg
Cantaloupe	1 cup	57 mg
Kale	1 cup, cooked	53 mg
Broccoli	½ cup	51 mg
Brussels Sprouts	½ cup	49 mg

Vitamin D, 1,000–2,000 IU

You have probably heard someone say, "Go out in the sunshine and get yourself some vitamin D!" Called the sunshine vitamin, vitamin

D is a hormone that's synthesized in the body as a result of sun exposure. While our yesteryear exposure to the sun may have worked historically to keep the vitamin at sufficient levels, today that's not the case. Surveys consistently show widespread deficiency in the USA and elsewhere.[796] Recent surveys indicate 24 percent of Americans and 37 percent of Canadians are deficient in vitamin D.[797] This may be due to several factors, including the rise in sedentary living, which means some people are simply not getting outside to move their bodies with exercise and as a result are not exposed to UV light required to generate sufficient vitamin D. The heightened use of sunscreen and general sunlight avoidance due to a growing concern over skin cancer are also possible factors. In the elderly, the process of producing vitamin D from sunlight becomes less efficient. Whatever the reason for the decline in vitamin D sufficiency, there is ample evidence to warrant supplementation.[798]

Over the last decade, there has been an explosion of research into the protective effects of vitamin D. No longer can we think of the vitamin as related to just bone integrity. It is also an important antioxidant, plays a role in the production of glutathione (a critical brain antioxidant itself), enhances immune function, and helps control inflammation. There is also emerging evidence indicating severe vitamin D deficiency may as much as double risk for cardiovascular disease.[799]

Vitamin D receptors are found throughout the brain and are particularly concentrated in the hippocampus. Vitamin D plays a neuroprotective role, including helping to clear amyloid plaques,[800] helping to regulate neuroinflammation, and supporting calcium homeostasis.[801] It should be no surprise that studies repeatedly finding low vitamin D levels are associated with not only cognitive impairment in adults in their thirties,[802] but AD pathology and a substantially increased risk of MCI and AD in adults in their sixties and older.[803] The risk of cognitive impairment is up to fourfold higher in those who are most deficient.

During the initial COVID-19 outbreak, hospitals noticed a trend in patients related to their vitamin D status. Those who entered the hospital with insufficient blood levels of the vitamin had up to an eightfold greater risk of severe respiratory illness compared to those who arrived with sufficient levels.[804] The advantage afforded by sufficient vitamin D was attributed to its ability to help minimize the dramatic inflammation commonly seen in the lungs of COVID-19 patients.

When looking for a supplement, be sure to choose the D3 version, which is better at sustaining blood levels of vitamin D.

Vitamin E, 400 IU

Vitamin E is a critical antioxidant that protects the brain cells, and a diet rich in vitamin E–containing foods is associated with a decreased risk for AD. Research has suggested that vitamin E deficiency may lead to an increase in amyloid deposits by hampering the clearance of amyloid from the blood and brain.[805] While studies of the value of vitamin E supplementation have been inconsistent, a few impressive studies have shown that vitamin E supplementation alone significantly delayed mild cognitive impairment and reduced the risk of AD.

In a double-blind, placebo-controlled, parallel-group, randomized clinical trial, 613 participants with mild to moderate AD were given either 1,000 IUs of vitamin E or a placebo and followed for five years. Compared to people taking a placebo, subjects who received the vitamin E saw a 19 percent reduction in the annual rate of decline in their condition.[806]

In another study, patients with AD who took a vitamin E supplement had reduced damage to neurons as well as a slowed progression of the disease.[807]

Again, the greatest protection comes from dietary sources of vitamin E, and this is due to the variety of distinct compounds (there are eight naturally occurring forms) that collectively constitute the vitamin. At least eight different tocopherols found in food have vitamin E activity. If you choose to take a vitamin E supplement, seek out the mixed form that includes alpha, delta, and gamma tocopherol. As a reminder, top food sources of vitamin E include almonds, sunflower seeds, avocado, spinach, butternut squash, peanuts/peanut butter, and broccoli.

Choline, 500 mg

Choline is critical to produce the neurotransmitter acetylcholine, which is essential to cognition and memory, among other roles. Choline has also been shown in lab studies to reduce development of amyloid plaques. Although the liver produces small amounts of choline, we get the bulk from our diet. As with vitamin D, a survey found broad choline insufficiency in the USA.[808] Since choline is concentrated in foods like beef and eggs, which are at the core of the standard American diet, it's unclear why this insufficiency exists. Plant-based foods rich in choline include navy beans, green peas, quinoa, soy beans, tofu, chickpeas, wheat germ, broccoli, shiitake mushrooms, and peanuts.

Coenzyme Q10, 200 mg

Coenzyme Q10 (CQ10) is a vitamin-like element involved in the production of energy and preservation of the membrane of every cell. In the absence of adequate CQ10 levels, brain cells are unable to produce sufficient energy. In addition, CQ10 is an antioxidant that protects brain cells from oxidative stress.[809] Healthy foods sources include broccoli, cauliflower, lentils, oranges, peanuts, soybeans, spinach, and strawberries.

Reports on this compound's use in preventing mental decline have been mixed, but we know that natural bodily production of CQ10 declines with age. About 35 percent of Americans are deficient in CQ10. Furthermore, levels can be reduced sharply by several widely used prescription medications including statins and antidepressants.[810] Even if you do not use either of these medications, supplementation may be wise.

Note that there are two forms of CQ10, ubiquinone and ubiquinol. Either is acceptable, but ubiquinol is utilized more efficiently by the body.

DHA/EPA, 125 mg / 250 mg

The best supplement source of DHA/EPA, which is derived from lab-grown (golden) microalgae, has been shown to be nutritionally equivalent to what would otherwise be derived from fish.[811] After all, algae is the source from which fish obtain the long-chain omega-3 fatty acids found in their flesh.

The strain of algae used in microalgae supplements, crypthecodinium cohnii, is synthesized in an FDA-certified lab and certified free of the environmental contaminants invariably found in fish and fish-oil supplements.

Iodine, 140 mcg

Iodine is required to produce thyroid hormone. Our bodies cannot make iodine, so it must be derived from foods or supplements. Lack of iodine is a leading cause of reversible mental decline worldwide and an estimated one billion people worldwide are at risk of deficiency. Severe iodine deficiency can result in a drop of 10–15 IQ points.

While it isn't entirely clear why, over the last 40 years there has been a fourfold increase in iodine deficiency worldwide. Some have suggested that since iodized salt historically has been a primary source of the trace element for many, the increase in deficiency may be attributable to public-health message encouraging a reduction of dietary salt intake.[812] However, given the degree to which restaurant food, and particularly fast food, is spiked with salt, this seems questionable. As we have seen, those following a typical Western diet are already exposed to far too much salt, which can elevate blood pressure. Add to this the contamination of table salt with microplastics and there is good reason to steer clear of added salt and obtain iodine from healthier sources.

Plant-food sources rich in iodine include quinoa, soy milk, tofu, sea kelp, navy beans, sea vegetables, broccoli, pinto beans, oats, wheat germ, strawberries, and potatoes.

A WORD ABOUT CALCIUM

You may be wondering why calcium is not included in this list of suggested supplements, and especially since I strongly suggest you eliminate all dairy from your diet. After all, postmenopausal women, and many elderly men, are typically told to consume calcium supplements in addition to consuming dairy because of a widespread belief that doing so protects one from bone fracture. The fact is that the evidence supporting calcium supplementation to prevent bone fracture is thin. So unconvincing is the evidence that after reviewing 135 studies on the subject the United States Preventive Services Task Force recommended against taking calcium supplements.[813] It is not just that the body of research is inconclusive. The use of calcium pills has been repeatedly linked to an elevated risk of kidney stones.[814] They are contaminated with lead,[815] and even more seriously, taking them appears to present an increase in risk for heart attack and stroke.[816] It is believed that unlike calcium from plants which is absorbed more gradually, the calcium from supplements may enter the bloodstream too quickly and end up depositing on artery walls, thereby increasing the risk of atherosclerosis. The best source of calcium is leafy green vegetables and other plant foods. The best way to build and keep bones strong and fracture resistant is to stimulate them through daily physical activity.

SUPPORTIVE SPICES AND HERBS

When one thinks of foods rich in antioxidants, fruits and vegetables typically come to mind, not herbs and spices. Yet many of these flavor enhancers are a terrific source of protective compounds and are an easy way to boost antioxidant intake.

GOTU KOLA

The gotu kola herb has been used in both Chinese and ancient Indian Ayurvedic medicine for at least 2,000 years to speed wound healing, serve as a sedative, and enhance cognitive function. More recent interest in its potential neuroprotective properties stems from a study in which certain constituents of the plant effectively blocked the damage that would be caused to neurons by amyloid protein.[817]

A randomized, placebo-controlled study found both mood and cognitive improvements after just two months of taking a 750 mg extract.[818] In another study of subjects aged 65 and older who were suffering from mild cognitive impairment, a daily dose of 1,000 mg for six months provided significant improvement in the subjects' condition.[819] Improvements in hypertension, a risk factor for AD itself, were also noted in this study. These benefits may come from gotu kola's antioxidant properties.

As a dried herb, gotu kola can be taken by adding one-quarter to one-half teaspoon to a cup of boiling water, twice daily. As a powdered herb, 1,000 mg can be taken in capsule form, one to two times per day. *Note: There is currently insufficient evidence about the safety of this herbal supplement for pregnant or breastfeeding women.*

SAFFRON

Derived from the crocus flower, saffron has been used medicinally for at least 4,000 years. Today it is most used as a seasoning in Spanish cuisine. Known as the world's most expensive spice, its production is very labor-intensive, as the fine threads must be delicately extracted from the stigma of the saffron flower. There is evidence that saffron has mood-enhancing properties that can have a positive effect on mild to moderate depression, possibly through helping balance neurotransmitters.[820] It has also been shown to enhance cognitive function, including memory and concentration, and to inhibit the clumping of proteins (both amyloid and tau) and the formation of brain plaques and tangles. Saffron extract may also reduce the impact of chemically induced damage to the dopamine-producing cells of the brain.[821] Its benefits may come in part from three antioxidant compounds that it contains and from its ability to fight inflammation.[822]

Saffron supplementation in several clinical studies involving individuals with mild to moderate AD has shown positive results.[823] In a double-blind, randomized, placebo-controlled study, patients with mild to moderate AD were given baseline assessments using a dementia-rating scale. Then they were randomly assigned to receive either 15 mg of saffron or a placebo pill twice daily. After a 16-week period, the subjects were reassessed and researchers reported a significantly better outcome on cognitive function tests in those who received the saffron compared to the subjects who received the placebo.[824] Saffron was also used in a head-to-head double-blind placebo study where those with moderate to severe AD were given either 30 mg of saffron extract or 20 mg of the leading AD drug, memantine. Each subject was then tested monthly using a severe cognitive impairment rating scale (SCIRS) and other assessment protocols over the course of a year. Those who received the saffron extract benefitted equally with those receiving the drug as regards slowing the rate of cognitive decline.[825] Yet unlike memantine which carries the risk of headache, constipation, sleepiness, dizziness, blood clots, psychosis, and even heart failure, saffron appears to be free of any serious side effects.

In capsule form, 15 mg of saffron can be taken twice daily. Pregnant women should consult their healthcare provider before taking saffron, as it has a uterine stimulant effect.

TURMERIC

Used in curries and traditional Asian, Indian, and Middle Eastern dishes possibly going as far back as 2,500 years, the ancient Indian herb turmeric has truly remarkable medicinal qualities. Curcumin, a component of turmeric, has anti-inflammatory, antioxidant, antiseptic, and pain-relieving properties.

More than 1,000 studies to date have looked at the medicinal qualities of curcumin. In one of the most compelling findings, curcumin was shown to improve the cognitive function in patients diagnosed with AD, leading researchers to believe curcumin may have a role to play in AD prevention as well as treatment. In addition to its anti-inflammatory properties, curcumin promotes neurogenesis, enhances synaptic plasticity, and promotes the synthesis of DHA.[826]

In an astonishing report, three AD patients were given 764 mg turmeric each day for 12 weeks. All three patients suffered from anxiety, apathy, agitation, depression, irritability, and wandering, and two suffered from urinary incontinence. After treatment began, all their symptoms markedly improved. In case #1, the patient's delusion, depression, agitation, anxiety, and irritability were all resolved. She regained her ability to dress herself and was no longer incontinent. She even began to laugh, sing, and knit again, and regained recognition of her family members. After a year on the spice, she exhibited no symptoms of dementia. In case #2, the patient had suffered from hallucinations, which were also resolved. In case #3, there were similar improvements in psychological symptoms as well as improvements in cognitive skills, including the ability to perform calculations, strength of concentration, and ability to write. In all cases the burden on the caregivers was significantly improved, and the patients have been described as living peacefully and serenely at home with family.[827]

In a double-blind study, researchers at UCLA gave 40 participants aged 51 to 84 PET scans to check for the presence of plaques and tangles in their brains. Then they randomly put participants on 90 mgs of curcumin or a placebo two times daily and followed their condition for 18 months with reassessments performed every six months. At the end of the study, those who had received the curcumin showed a 28 percent improvement in memory function as well as less accumulation of both tau and amyloid.[828]

In another study from UCLA, researchers showed that curcumin may enable immune cells, called macrophages, to ingest and clear away amyloid more effectively.[829] This, along with the ability to reduce inflammation, may be why AD patients who have been treated with curcumin have had improvements in memory and cognitive function, and in other symptoms.[830]

Curcumin has also been shown in animal studies to inhibit the formation of both amyloid protein and tau tangles. In one study, mice with AD that were given small doses of curcumin experienced a 40 percent drop in levels of amyloid compared to untreated mice.[831]

As a powerful antioxidant, curcumin also inhibits the formation of dangerous free radicals, which damage neurons.[832] It also boosts the activity of superoxide dismutase, which is considered the most important antioxidant in the body. This benefit alone may improve cognitive function. Finally, when clinically tested against the drug Voltaren (Diclofenac Sodium), used to treat rheumatoid arthritis (a disease characterized by joint inflammation and swelling), curcumin performed significantly better than the drug did.[833]

Collectively, these findings and the qualities of curcumin might partially explain why the populations that consume the most turmeric have the lowest incidence of AD.[834]

With all the positive reports about curcumin, a wide variety of turmeric products have reached the marketplace, and not all can be expected to yield the results research has indicated. In particular, proprietary formulas that isolate curcumin often do not produce the expected results. This may be because the curcumin in turmeric works synergistically with coexisting compounds. The positive outcomes that have been seen in those who have been treated with it clinically have involved the whole spice (turmeric), and not isolates or proprietary formulas.

The advisable amount of turmeric supplementation is one-half to one teaspoon per day as a dried powdered root (the type bought in grocery stores); 400–600 mg in capsule form twice a day; or 15–30 drops of a tincture two times per day.

Ideally, seek out organic turmeric that has been tested for the presence of heavy metals. The percentage of turmeric that is curcumin varies from product to product due to processing methods and source species. Products with 2.5 percent curcumin are typical. Sources that are four percent or higher are desirable. Also, Stanford researchers recently discovered that turmeric products produced in Bangladesh are contaminated with lead, a neurotoxin, because local processors have been using lead chromate, an industrial yellow pigment normally used for coloring toys and furniture, in their processing of turmeric.[835] *Note: Avoid turmeric/curcumin supplements if you take blood thinners such as warfarin (Coumadin), are about to have surgery, are pregnant, or have gallbladder disease.*

ANTIOXIDANT-RICH HERBS & SPICES	
Allspice	Basil
Cayenne	Cilantro
Cinnamon	Clove (ground)
Cumin	Ginger
Oregano	Peppermint
Marjoram	Parsley
Rosemary	Saffron
Sage	Turmeric
Thyme	

TOP 17 HERBS & SPICES

The table shown above highlights the top herbs and spices that are rich in antioxidants and anti-inflammatory agents. Try to add between one-half to one teaspoon of dried herbs and spices to your foods daily. An easy way to quickly season any dish with a variety of antioxidant-rich herbs and spices is to try the seasoning called Sprinkle by Bragg. This salt-free product contains 24 organic herbs and spices that make a wonderful addition to soups, salads, and main courses.

27

MAKING THE TRANSITION WHILE EATING OUT ... AND AT HOME

ARE YOU READY to take all your newfound wisdom about diet, supplementation, and herbs and put it into action? Once you know what's best for protecting your brain, it's exciting to implement it.

A key challenge to changing the way you eat is how to follow your new plan while eating out. This is important because, prior to COVID-19, surveys suggested the average American was eating out about four times a week. If you are not accustomed to eating plant-based dishes, your first foray to a restaurant might be worrisome. Will there be enough meat-free choices? Rest assured many restaurants are ready and eager to accommodate their health-conscious guests. Research firm Global Data found that between 2014 and 2017 the number of people who said they eat exclusively plant-based meals rose by 600 percent. The hospitality industry is responding to this burgeoning interest accordingly. There are now 24,000 restaurants in the US that focus their offerings on plant-based cuisine 1,470 of which are entirely vegan. New ones are opening all the time.

ROOM AT THE TOP

A few years ago I was invited to dinner at an exclusive restaurant in San Francisco called Atelier Crenn. The chef, Dominique Crenn, is among the elite chefs who have won three Michelin stars. Before we visited the restaurant, I asked if they could accommodate my need to have a totally plant-based dinner. Chef Crenn created a culinary experience unlike anything I had ever before encountered. That night I was served ten courses of the most delicious, innovatively prepared, and beautifully presented food entirely composed of plants. The chef shared with me that requests for completely plant-based options have grown exponentially since she opened her restaurant, and in 2019 she eliminated meat from her menu. And Chef Crenn is not alone.

In 2021, Eleven Madison Park's chef, Daniel Humm, announced that going forward the world-famous Manhattan restaurant would be serving only plant-based foods. Having garnered every prestigious award sought by restauranteurs around the world, Humm decided that a menu of meat and dairy was no longer sustainable. Within three months the chef announced he had a waiting list of 50,000 hoping to enjoy his new cuisine.

Crossroads, in Los Angeles, is another great option. This discreet venue in West Hollywood is packed every night with guests looking for exciting new culinary experiences. Its chef and bestselling cookbook author, Tal Ronnen, has completely raised the bar for what can be expected of a vegan restaurant.

Then there's Vedge in Philadelphia. What the chefs of this bustling eatery accomplish! As with Crossroads, many people are vying for a seat at a table there.

Would you believe that many of the world's 50 best restaurants now offer an entirely vegan menu option? At L'Arpege in Paris, celebrated chef Alain Passard reportedly became bored with typical offerings and decided to branch out and provide customers plant-based options.

Also, a few dollar notches down, check out Sutra in Seattle, Plant in Asheville, North Carolina, Candle 79 in Manhattan, Shizen in San Francisco, and Cafe Sunflower in Atlanta, just to name a few.

Of course, most of us don't regularly visit award-winning restaurants, and it's certainly not necessary in order to enjoy great vegan food. I share these with you because I want you to know that plant-based eating is going both mainstream and upscale.

A popular and growing chain that offers exclusively vegan fast food, Veggie Grill is now the largest vegan restaurant company in the USA.

Presently, Veggie Grill restaurants are in California, Massachusetts, New York, Oregon and Washington.

If an exclusively plant-based restaurant has yet to arrive in your town, there are plenty of other options already available, many easy on the wallet.

CHINESE

Chinese restaurants are a haven for vegan diners. In addition to soups, many dishes are centered upon vegetables and either rice or noodles. You will also find soy dishes, such as edamame, cold sesame noodles, rice paper rolls (the healthy alternative to fried spring rolls), and steamed vegetarian dumplings, among other tasty dishes. One caveat: The salt-shaker tends to be used liberally in Chinese dishes. Ask if the kitchen will prepare low sodium versions of your selections.

ITALIAN

Italian restaurants have an abundance of pasta dishes from which to choose. Many are now offering whole-grain and gluten-free pasta options. A classic, pasta primavera, is pasta mixed with a variety of vegetables. Although cheese is popular in Italian dishes, many classic dishes can be made vegan. A great starter is bruschetta, generally chopped tomato and garlic on toasted bread. A classic vegetable risotto dish can be made without cheese. Polenta with vegetables and marinara is often on the menu and can be made dairy-free.

MEXICAN

At Mexican restaurants, many dishes contain beans, rice, salsa, and vegetables. You can ask for vegetarian enchiladas, a tostada, or a burrito. Just be sure to ask them to hold the cheese.

MIDDLE EASTERN

Middle Eastern restaurants are an excellent option for vegan diners. You can choose from a variety of vegetable, grain, and legume dishes. A popular meal is Yalanji Yaprak—baked eggplant stuffed with vegetables. Another option is couscous, which is steamed bulgur wheat, served over vegetables and hummus. Mujadara, a classic choice, is made from lentils, rice, caramelized onions, and aromatic spices.

GOT NON-MEAT?

For people who crave the taste and texture of meat, a growing number of meat replacement products on the market seem to pass the test. The most popular line is called Beyond Meat, which has captured the attention of investors like Microsoft founder Bill Gates (who has also invested in synthetic-meat producer Impossible Foods, maker of the Impossible Burger), and even conventional meat processor Tyson Foods. Made from pea protein isolates, yeast, potato starch, and other ingredients, the meat replacement comes in a variety of forms including the Beyond Burger, Beyond sausage links, Beyond chicken strips, and Beyond beef crumbles.

Other major brands offering mainstream meat replacement options include Gardein, Field Roast, and Amy's. Even Omaha Steaks has gotten in on the action, offering dairy-free veggie burgers that contain organic ingredients and can be delivered to your doorstep.

Although I'm personally not a fan of meat substitutes, they can be very attractive to people who miss eating meat or are struggling with their transition. They have a familiar mouth feel, are convenient, and have an appealing taste. However, keep in mind that they should not be considered health food. Some contain ingredients that truly should not make up a significant part of your diet. Be sure not to allow convenience foods like meat replacements to displace truly healthful foods—whole grains, legumes, fruits, vegetables, nuts, and seeds. Those are the foods that contain all the truly protective and life-enhancing elements. It's quite easy to use healthful ingredients to make your own plant-based burgers at home. You will find countless recipes online.

Another meat substitute is jackfruit, which grows on the jack tree and was first cultivated 3,000 years ago in India.[836] Each jackfruit can weigh as much as 100 pounds. Recently it has become a popular replacement for meat in the USA, because it can be prepared in various ways that resemble meat. Eaten on its own, jackfruit is soft (when ripe) and has a sweetness like mango or banana. As a young fruit (less ripe), jackfruit absorbs other flavors well, which enables it to masquerade as many different familiar dishes. Although it is traditionally used in curries and in a popular breakfast dish made with rice, I am seeing it show up on menus in mock "pulled pork" sandwiches, burritos, fajitas, and in vegetable hash. The fruit is rich in fiber, potassium, magnesium, carotenoids (including lutein and zeaxanthin), and vitamins C and B6. A popular brand of prepared jackfruit sold in supermarkets is Upton's Naturals, which offers flavors such as chili-lime, Thai, bar-b-q, curry, and original. I encourage you to experiment with this versatile newcomer.

WHAT ABOUT SOY?

Soybeans are a legume that was first cultivated in China in the 11th century BC.[837] Soybeans are free of cholesterol, low in saturated fat, high in protein, fiber, and vitamin E, and can be a healthy, versatile addition to your diet. Having said that, some people are allergic to soy and must avoid it.

When I speak of soy foods, I am referring to a range of preparations: natto, miso, edamame, soymilk, tofu, and tempeh. I suggest avoiding soy protein isolates because this chemically processed product may contain aluminum and solvent residues.

Be aware that most soy products sold in the USA today are the genetically modified versions treated with the glyphosate-based herbicide Roundup. Glyphosate residues are likely to be in the food. Unless you select soy foods that carry the USDA Organic certification seal, that is what you are consuming. Avoid chemically treated GMO soy at all costs.

Natto

Used as a topping for rice, vegetables, and miso soup, natto is made from fermented whole soybeans.

Miso

Miso is a smooth paste made from fermented soybeans, usually combined with rice and a bacterial culture. It is often added to various stocks to make the traditional Japanese miso soup, which in its plant-based recipe contains mushrooms, tofu, green onions, and seasoning.

Soy Milk

Soy milk is made by soaking, boiling, and then blending soybeans with water and removing the pulp. It is a rich source of protein and B vitamins. As with other plant milks, there are many varieties of soy milk on the market, some with a good amount of sugar and additives. Westsoy brand offers an organic soy milk with zero sweeteners or additives of any kind—water and soybeans are the only ingredients.

Tofu

Sometimes referred to as soybean curd, tofu has a cheese-like consistency and effectively absorbs flavors in any dish. The firm variety can be cut into cubes and added to soups, vegetables, casseroles, or even grilled. The soft version, known as silken tofu, blends nicely into sauces, soups, and smoothies.

Tempeh

An Indonesian tradition, traditional tempeh is made by fermenting soy with either rice or millet, which forms a chunky cake. Although it is not yet as popular as tofu, it's very versatile. With its nutty flavor, it works well in dishes like chili, stews, soups, and salads, and as thin slabs in sandwiches. Like tofu, tempeh can be marinated and absorbs other flavors well. Because it holds its shape well, it can be skewered and grilled.

REPLACING CHEESE

As with plant-based meats, options for dairy-free cheeses have expanded tremendously in recent years. Beyond the more common soy-based cheeses, there are now products made from seeds, nuts, and tapioca root. Perhaps the most compelling are the nut-based innovations from Miyoko's and Follow Your Heart brands. Whether it's cheese to spread on a cracker or cheese to melt on your pizza, there are sufficient options to help you make the transition away from dairy-based cheese without leaving you feeling deprived.

REPLACING EGGS IN RECIPES

When it comes to cooking and baking without eggs, you have several easy (and tasteful) options. Depending on the recipe, applesauce, bananas, and ground flaxseeds all work well in place of eggs.

One tablespoon of ground flaxseeds mixed with three tablespoons of water replaces a single egg. Half a banana (one-quarter cup) also works well in place of one egg in recipes. The sweeter and riper the banana, the more flavor will be imparted to the dish. One-quarter cup of unsweetened applesauce will do the trick as well. There are also egg substitute powders made by Bob's Red Mill and Ener-G.

If it's scrambled eggs that you'll miss, consider scrambled tofu with antioxidant-rich spices and vegetables. Another option is to use ackee, a fruit from West Africa. Because ackee is yellow, has a creamy consistency, and absorbs flavors well, it makes for a delicious and healthful alternative to scrambled eggs. In my travels to London, I always enjoy stopping in at the Wulf & Lamb café in Chelsea, where they offer a delicious scrambled ackee along with other innovative plant-based dishes.

ALZHEIMER'S REVOLUTION DIETARY GUIDELINES		
FOOD GROUP	**SERVINGS PER DAY**	**SERVING SIZE**
GRAINS	3 or more	½ cup oats ½ cup brown rice ½ cup quinoa 1 cup whole wheat pasta 1 slice bread
VEGETABLES	4 or more	½ cup cooked broccoli ½ cup sweet potato 1 cup spinach or kale
FRUITS	3 or more	1 medium apple ½ cup chopped fruit ½ cup berries ¼ cup dried fruit
LEGUMES	2–3	½ cup lentils ½ cup black beans 1 cup tofu 1 cup fortified soy milk
NUTS & SEEDS	1–2	1-ounce walnuts 1 tablespoon peanut butter 1 Tablespoon chia seeds
WATER	6–8	8-ounce glass

FOOD GROUP	FOODS FROM WHICH TO BUILD YOUR MEALS
WHOLE GRAINS	Amaranth, barley, buckwheat, bulgur, quinoa, millet, rye, triticale, pasta, cereals (oatmeal, shredded wheat, quinoa), breads, tortillas, corn, popcorn, cornmeal, corn flour, brown rice, oats, spelt, kamut
VEGETABLES	Artichokes, asparagus, bamboo shoots, beets, broccoli, Brussels sprouts, cabbage, carrots, cauliflower, chard, cucumber, garlic, eggplant, jicama, kale, leeks, parsley, sprouts, lettuce, peas, peppers, pumpkin, onions, tomatoes, mushrooms, potatoes, spinach, squash, yams
LEGUMES	Adzuki beans, black beans cranberry beans, fava beans, flageolets, Great Northern beans, kidney beans, lima beans, mung beans, navy beans, pinto beans, red beans, soybeans, black-eyed peas, chickpeas, red lentils, green split peas, yellow split peas, brown lentils, green lentils, tofu, soy milk

FOOD GROUP	FOODS FROM WHICH TO BUILD YOUR MEALS
FRUITS	Apples, blackberries, cranberries, guavas, mangoes, peaches, pineapple, apricots, blueberries, figs, kiwis, melons, pears, raisins, bananas, boysenberries, grapefruit, lemons, oranges, plums, raspberries, dates, cherries, limes, papayas, prunes, strawberries, pomegranate
NUTS & SEEDS	Almonds, Brazil nuts, cashews, chestnuts, coconut, hazelnuts, macadamia nuts, pecans, pine nuts, pistachio nuts, peanuts, walnuts, pumpkin seeds, sunflower seeds, chia seeds, sesame seeds, flaxseeds

The first table provides you with guidelines for the suggested number of servings and serving sizes of the five food groups the Revolution Diet is built on. The second table is a reference for the foods around which to build your meals. Many of us get into food jags where we eat pretty much the same thing day after day. We are fortunate to have such a broad array of foods to draw upon in formulating meals. I encourage you to branch out and explore the many options available.

IMPORTANT INSIGHTS FROM FASTING

Fasting—abstaining from food for a period ranging from 12 hours to a few days to as long as weeks, is rooted in many religious traditions. Of course, long-term fasters are drinking water and usually having vitamins, broth, lemon juice, or other things that offer minimal sustenance. Only very recently has the scientific community begun to consider how fasting may offer benefits for brain health.

Fasting results in comprehensive changes that suggest potential protection for the brain. So what happens when we restrict or forgo food entirely, and how might we acquire these benefits without practicing a conventional fast?

It turns out that during a "pure fast," when one abstains from eating entirely, a remarkable number of responses occur in the body and brain that favorably change some AD risk factors and may support long-term cognitive health.

Fasting induces an altered metabolic state that sources back to a long-ago adaptation in times of food scarcity. Nature favored those who could survive during times when nutrition could not be readily sourced, and that survival advantage was passed on to subsequent generations. The adaptive response is referred to as metabolic switching. In this response, the body has depleted its liver store of glucose (blood sugar), the body's preferred source of fuel, and begins to convert fat into fuel.[838] An array of changes follow that preserve health and extend the period before one starves. The question yet to be fully answered is whether regular intermittent fasting, which triggers this metabolic switching, could confer lasting benefits in terms of a reduction in the risk for AD and other diseases.

Anyone who has fasted for even 24 hours has likely noticed how their senses become more acute (this is called hyperesthesia). Taste, smell, hearing, and even vision all become heightened during a fast. When fasting, people also are more alert, experience improved memory, and learn new information more rapidly. Some report greater clarity of thought as well and, counterintuitively, feel more productive.

One process that is activated during a fast is called autophagy. In simple terms this is a process whereby the brain clears out damaged molecules and dysfunctional mitochondria and thereby helps preserve synapses and neurons and improve cognitive function.

Remember our friend brain-derived neurotrophic factor (BDNF), which supports synapse health, boosts the production of new neurons, and protects them from assaults? Fasting elevates levels of this desirable substance.

By now you understand that a key player in advancing AD is inflammation. It turns out that fasting sends certain proinflammatory cells (monocytes) to sleep and cuts production of other ones, lowering overall levels of inflammation, including in the brain.[839]

As you will recall from Chapter 8, type 2 diabetes develops as one become insulin resistant. When feeding is restricted to within a span of eight hours in a day or less, insulin sensitivity increases.[840]

Reductions of up to 11 points and even normalization of blood pressure have been noted during fasting states.[841]

There are presently studies in process that seek to determine whether or not repetitious, intermittent fasting leads to improved cognitive health and whether the positive changes mentioned may carry over and be lasting. We should see results in the next two to three years.

Changes Induced by Metabolic Switching

Lowered blood pressure

Lowered resting heart rate

Reduced blood cholesterol levels

Reduced oxidative stress

Improved blood sugar regulation

Reduced inflammation

Reduction in neurologic symptoms

Increase in BDNF

Reduced free-radical production

ALIGNING MEALS WITH YOUR CIRCADIAN RHYTHM

These kinds of changes are certainly positive, but to date there simply is not enough research to say that when triggered intermittently they will lower risk of cognitive decline in the long term. However, it's clear that limiting the time period in which we eat can help align us with our body's natural circadian rhythm and that by conforming more closely to that rhythm we can acquire many of the important benefits noted above.

The circadian rhythm is dictated by both a "master clock" in the brain's hypothalamus, which is influenced by light, as well as other mechanisms in various organs. Essentially, this regulating system tells us when to wake, eat, and sleep, and dictates the rise and fall of certain hormones and of body temperature. For example, when our eyes detect daylight, the brain triggers the release of cortisol to arouse the body and mind, making us more alert and energized. As the sun sets, cortisol levels wind down and melatonin levels ramp up, preparing us for sleep. Early in the day our body has greater insulin sensitivity and cells use glucose more efficiently. That's not the case at night. In the early evening, when many people are eating their biggest meal of the day (many people eat as much as 40 percent of their daily calories at dinner), our caloric needs are greatly reduced, and insulin sensitivity is lower. Eating at night is counter to our natural rhythm for digestion and the body's natural sleep-wake cycle.

The pure fast that requires not eating at all can be challenging for some and may also, initially, be accompanied by headache and fatigue. The good news is that this type of fast isn't necessary to gain the benefits mentioned above and to realign your body with its natural circadian rhythm. We can gain some of the same benefits derived from a pure fast simply by shortening the window of time within which we consume meals, thereby extending our fast period. While some individuals choose to limit their mealtimes to an eight-hour window on a daily basis, you may wish to try it out two days per week. Your food intake could occur between 8 a.m. and 4 p.m., after which you consume only water until 8 a.m. the next day. If you are an earlier riser, the window could be 7 a.m. to 3 p.m. This provides you with a 16-hour fasting period. Of course, the shorter the window for consuming meals, the longer the fasting period will be. The result is that you may see improved digestion, better control of blood sugar, weight loss, reduced blood pressure, enhanced sleep quality, improved mood—you may just generally feel better.

28
PURE WATER IS ESSENTIAL

WHEN IT COMES to water, think about quantity and quality. We must get enough of it, and it must be free of contaminants.

Adequate hydration is essential not just to metabolism, maintaining electrolyte balance, blood circulation, production of saliva, and regulation of body temperature, but also to healthy cognitive function.[842] Water accounts for 75 percent of brain mass. As you become dehydrated, attention, concentration, coordination, memory, and problem solving are all compromised measurably.[843] It takes just 1 to 2 percent of body water loss to impair cognitive function. This may be in part because with inadequate hydration blood vessels will constrict and pressure rises.[844]

Yet not all of us pay attention to our thirst. Moreover, elderly people often have an impaired sense of thirst which puts them at higher risk for dehydration.

WATER IS A PURIFIER WE LOSE CONTINUALLY

One of water's critical roles in the body is facilitating the excretion of wastes and toxins from cells by way of perspiration, urination, and defecation. Through these processes, as well as evaporation through the skin and by simply breathing, we are losing water all the time.

DEHYDRATION OCCURS BEFORE THIRST

By the time we experience thirst, we are already dehydrated (that is, we have lost 1 to 2 percent of the water in our body) to such a degree that cognitive function is likely to be affected.[845] Even mild dehydration has been shown to cause short-term memory problems, poor concentration, increased reaction time, moodiness, and anxiety. For the highest level of brain function, it's important to be adequately hydrated throughout the day.

WATER FILTRATION IS ESSENTIAL

Investing in a reliable water filtration system has never been more important. In 2021, the EPA prepared a report that noted 66 different chemicals are "known or anticipated to occur" in US public drinking water systems and presently are not subject to any regulation.[846] In an investigative piece, the *Los Angeles Times* reported that 86 drinking water systems serving nine million Californians are contaminated with two extremely toxic substances, perfluoroalkyl and polyfluoroalkyl compounds. Linked to developmental problems, thyroid disease, cancer, and elevated cholesterol, these were the key ingredients in Teflon cookware, Scotchgard waterproofing, and flame-retardant foam.[847] The Natural Resources Defense Council estimates 77 million Americans rely upon municipal water systems that regularly violate drinking water contaminant standards.

Both chlorine and chloramine (chlorine combined with ammonia) are used to disinfect municipal drinking water. They do a great job eliminating the risk of waterborne diseases like typhoid and cholera, but they eliminate healthful bacteria as well. Also, chlorine tends to react with organic matter in water to produce trihalomethanes (THMs) that with long term exposure present a risk for bladder cancer.[848]

PRESCRIPTION DRUGS

Disturbingly, and due largely to hospitals, but also consumers, throwing unused drugs into drains and toilets, we have created yet another water contamination problem. Water tests reveal that 80 percent of streams and municipal water supplies[853] now contain a lengthy list of pharmaceuticals including hormones, painkillers, antidepressants, antipsychotics, antibiotics, heart medications, and tranquilizers—all compounds that public water systems are not designed to filter.[854]

LEAD & COPPER

As we saw in Chapter 16, drinking water can, sadly, also be a major source of lead. In 2016, the world learned about the threat of lead in municipal water when the Flint, Michigan, water crisis exploded in the media. Lead from aging pipes was leaching into the community's drinking water after officials failed to add certain corrosion inhibitors to the water. Authorities repeatedly assured residents the water was safe to drink and posed no risk. Yet lead levels were in some cases hundreds of times over the EPA's prior safety limit. In the end 12,000 children and adults were adversely affected by the exposure in Flint. Today, the World Health Organization, the CDC, and the EPA all agree that no level of lead exposure is safe, and the EPA has set a goal for the maximum contaminant level for lead in drinking water as zero.

Unfortunately, exposure to lead is not limited to Flint. Children and adults in at least four million households in the US are currently exposed to unsafe levels of lead, according to the CDC. Further, in 3,000 "hot spots," lead poisoning exceeds that which occurred in Flint.[855] The EPA's own survey revealed 130 US municipal water systems exceeded the level previously considered safe and 10 systems had levels four times higher. In 1986 the US federal government mandated that solder used for connecting copper drinking water pipes in homes must be lead-free. Therefore, if you live in a home built before 1986, chances are you're being exposed to lead through your drinking water.

Earlier we looked at the problem of excess copper depositing in the brain where it promotes free radicals and advances problems with concentration and memory. Both activated carbon and reverse osmosis filtration systems will remove lead and copper from your drinking water.

Although carafe-style water filters are inexpensive, they often provide what amounts to a taste filter rather than effectively removing many contaminants.

As a further way of avoiding exposure to contaminants, choose non-leaching, reusable beverage containers, such as those made from glass or stainless steel. These are the ideal materials for water bottles, beverage dispensers, pitchers, and travel mugs.

A FINAL DROP OF ADVICE

Hydrate adequately each day. Although actual needs vary according to one's age, health status, climate, and amount of physical activity, recommendations are that we consume between 72 and 104 ounces (9 to 13 eight-ounce cups a day). Please do. And be sure to hydrate both before and after exercise or sports.

Lastly, if you drink alcohol, try to drink water alongside your alcoholic drinks, or at least rehydrate before bed; alcohol leads to dehydration.

29
HOW TO GET THE LEAD
AND ALUMINUM OUT

The REVOLUTION LIFESTYLE plan for reducing the risk of Alzheimer's calls on us to reduce our exposure to toxic substances to the greatest degree possible. By eliminating fish and shellfish from your diet, you have already taken an important step to protect yourself from exposure to mercury, a potent neurotoxin. In this chapter, we focus on minimizing your exposure to two other neurotoxins: lead and aluminum.

GETTING RID OF LEAD

As we saw earlier, lead presents many dangers to the brain and may be a contributing factor in cognitive decline. Lead is present in more places than we might imagine, but there are many opportunities for us to minimize our exposure to this brain toxin. In the last chapter we saw that lead in drinking water is a common problem that can be eliminated through proper filtration. However, water is not the only beverage with hidden dangers.

APPLE JUICE, GRAPE JUICE, AND WINE

Apple and grape juices have a surprising amount of lead in them, due to the 100-year history of fruit growers using lead-containing pesticides in farming. In a *Consumers Union* test of more than 80 samples of apple and grape juices, not only was a significant amount of lead present, but 25 percent exceeded the FDA guideline for maximum exposure in bottled drinking water. Always choose organic juices and fruits to minimize such exposure.

Considerable lead (and other heavy metals) has been detected in wine as well. Federal authorities found lead levels that exceed the EPA's drinking water limit in more than 600 domestic and imported wines.[856] As you'll recall, the Revolution Lifestyle program recommends avoiding alcohol; cutting lead exposure is just one of many reasons to do so.

LIPSTICK

Lipstick is a source of lead that millions of makeup-wearers expose themselves to daily, if not multiple times a day. Because it's applied on the lips, ingestion of the lead content is likely. This risk factor can be eliminated either by foregoing the product entirely or by choosing lipsticks that have been tested and are free of lead.

PRODUCE

Even if grown organically, produce may be a source of lead because of the long history of lead-containing pesticides as well as atmospheric lead resulting from lead-containing gasoline. The good news is that by soaking and washing your produce well, you can remove a substantial amount of the lead dust it may contain.

FISH AND SHELLFISH

Due to the discharge of lead-containing industrial waste into waterways and the ocean, fish and shellfish are another source of lead.[857] Avoiding unnecessary lead exposure is another reason to avoid fish and shellfish.

CHOCOLATE

As previously noted, chocolate can be another source of both lead and cadmium. A recent sampling of 42 products from the biggest names in chocolate found that just a single serving of 26 of their chocolate products exceeded the California state limit for reproductive harm.[858] At this time it appears there is no way to reduce exposure other than to avoid chocolate. Chapter 24 discusses healthier alternatives for those who love chocolate but wish to avoid the contaminants.

PROTEIN POWDERS

Even in the absence of protein deficiency, millions of Americans consume protein powder supplements daily. This is not only stressful to the kidneys, as *Consumer Reports* revealed, but consuming protein powders also exposes one to hazardous levels of lead, mercury, arsenic, and other neurotoxic contaminants.[859] A single serving of several of the top-selling products exposes a consumer to so much lead that if the state of California were paying attention, the products would need to be labeled under Proposition 65 as a toxic hazard. Protect yourself from exposure to heavy metals and give your kidneys a break by passing up unnecessary protein powder supplements.

TEA

It was crushing to me to learn that in an analysis of 30 green, black, white, and oolong teas, researchers found that they all contained lead. After a three-minute steep, 73 percent of the teas had lead levels that exceeded the guidelines for consumption during pregnancy and lactation. After a 15-minute steep, 83 percent of the teas exceeded that guideline.[860] The lead in tea comes from the soil it's grown in. Much of the tea consumed is sourced from China, where leaded fuel was permitted until 2000. The soils used for farming there still contain substantial levels of lead.

FINALLY, OLD PAINT

Another common source of lead is old paint that's flaking or forming a fine dust that is nearly imperceptible to the naked eye. If you live in a dwelling with old paint, consider a fresh coat of no-VOC paint over it to seal in the toxin rather than risk creating lead dust through a removal process. And of course, do not let curious children anywhere near it.

GETTING THE ALUMINUM OUT

In previous chapters we saw that aluminum is another brain toxin that should be avoided. In addition to drinking water, sources of aluminum include certain teas, some processed foods, and some personal-care products. Tea plants are generally efficient at absorbing aluminum from soils, particularly acidic soils.[861]

According to the US Agency for Toxic Substances and Disease Registry, the following foods and beverages have been found to contain significant levels of aluminum.[862]

SOURCES OF ALUMINUM		
American cheese	Antacids	Baking powder
Cinnamon	Clams	Cocoa
Garlic	Oysters	Muffin mix
Mustard (prepared)	Nutmeg	Pickles
Processed cheese	Salt (w/aluminum additives)	Spinach (non-organic)
Tap water (unfiltered)	Tea (non-herbal)	

The amount of aluminum that we absorb from a particular food depends on how much it contains, other foods and drinks consumed with the contaminated food, and the condition of our gut, as well as the bioavailability of the aluminum—that is, whether it's bound to other elements in the food that prevent or reduce its absorption. Both alcohol and coffee enhance aluminum absorption from foods.

Beware that the following foods, medications, and personal care products contain varying levels of aluminum:

Products Containing Aluminum

Antacids (as aluminum hydroxide)

Antiperspirant (as aluminum chloride or aluminum zirconium)

Buffered aspirin (as aluminum hydroxide)

Non-dairy creamers (very high)

Frozen cheese pizza (very high)

Nonsteroidal anti-inflammatory drugs (NSAID) (as aluminum hydroxide)

Calcium supplements (as a contaminant)[863]

Iron supplements

Intravenous (IV) feeding solutions

Many pancake mixes (as "sodium aluminum phosphate)

Conventional toothpaste (as aluminum oxyhydroxide)

More tips include:

- Avoid using aluminum foil to wrap and store foods. Choose glass food storage containers or the newly popular waxed fabrics for storage.

- Avoid taking antacid medications that contain aluminum, as many popular brands do. Read the ingredient labels of all over-the-counter medications to be sure they are free of aluminum.

- Avoid antiperspirants. Unlike regular deodorant, antiperspirants use aluminum as the active ingredient. You will absorb the aluminum through your skin, especially if you have a small cut from shaving.

- To reduce exposure to aluminum, be sure to avoid using aluminum-surfaced pots and pans. Safer alternatives are pans composed of an aluminum core (for heat conductivity) and have a stainless-steel finish that prevents food coming into contact with the aluminum. Some cookware does not have the protective stainless outer layer.

- Avoid purchasing water, teas, sodas, beer, and other beverages sold in aluminum cans; the aluminum may migrate into the liquid and is higher in dented cans.[864]

When it comes to the things we ingest—foods, beverages, herbs, spices, water—there is a lot to be aware of. You have powerful new insights about what foods best support your brain health, where to seek them out when you are on the road or at restaurants, and how to prepare them for yourself and your loved ones at home. There is an almost over-whelming number of vegan websites, blogs, and cookbooks available with a wide variety of recipes to try. Keep expanding your repertoire and invite family and friends to join you. In this way you can build a supportive community around this new and powerfully protective way of nourishing yourself.

30
HOW TO SLEEP LIKE A BABY

As noted earlier, many of us simply do not prioritize getting enough rest, and millions struggle with a sleep disorder. We now know that getting a full eight hours of deep, restful sleep is critical for creating and preserving memories and clearing metabolic waste that otherwise may hinder optimal brain function and accelerate neurodegeneration. A foundational approach is required—we must arrange our lives in a way that assures we can achieve regular, quality sleep. Here are some strategies for giving yourself the very best chance of consistently achieving quality sleep.

EAT WELL

An overlooked yet influential factor in whether we obtain restful sleep is the food we choose to eat. You now understand how critical it is to brain health that you choose a plant-based diet that is low in saturated fat and full of antioxidants and fiber. Sleep researchers have recently come to understand that a diet rich in saturated fat and refined sugars and low in fiber works against quality sleep. Individuals who follow such a diet are not only more likely to wake up repeatedly in the night, but they are also less likely to achieve what's called slow-wave sleep.[865] This is the most restorative phase of sleep, when we consolidate memories and dream.

REMOVE SOURCES OF AMBIENT LIGHT

Ambient light has a negative impact on sleep and increases insulin resistance. Light sources in a bedroom—things like clocks, phones, computer chargers—can give your brain the wrong message, because sensors in the eye can detect light even when the eyelid is closed. The sensing of artificial light may alter the production and release of melatonin, known as the "sleep hormone," which may in turn deprive you of the deep restful sleep essential to brain health.[866] Melatonin triggers the lowering of cortisol, blood pressure, glucose, and body temperature, and we do not want to disrupt its regular cycle.

Surveys show that up to 40 percent of individuals sleep with a bedside lamp, T.V., or bedroom light source on. Make every effort to sleep in a dark room. Remove extraneous light from clocks, cell phones, computer chargers, radios, tablets, security system keypads, and any other technology that emits light, however dull. Use blackout curtains for intrusive streetlights and wear an eye mask, if necessary, to create a truly dark sleep environment, and you will wake more rested and refreshed.

EAT EARLIER

Our natural circadian rhythm causes levels of the sleep hormone melatonin to rise a few hours before we go to bed. Eating late disrupts melatonin production and signals your body that you are fueling up for activity. Try eating your last meal closer to between 5:00 and 6:00 p.m.— and avoid after-dinner snacking.

DON'T SLEEP NEAR YOUR CELL PHONE

Cell phones can do more than interfere with melatonin. The radio frequency they emit has in some cases been associated with a reduced production of a sleep-promoting neurohormone called Lipocalin type prostaglandin D. A study found that people who sleep with a cell phone in close proximity had lower levels of this substance and required more than twice as much time to fall asleep.[867]

DE-STRESS

Stress can interfere with sleep, so practicing your favorite stress-management technique can be an important first step in getting a good night's sleep. Likewise, a period of meditation before bed can help clear your mind and get you to the state most receptive to sleep. (More about meditation coming up.)

CONTROL NOISE

If noise is a factor, consider the use of earplugs or masking the sounds with a white noise device. Or visit simplynoise.com for access to a free app that offers wonderful soundscapes of running water, ocean, and rainfall that can effectively mask other environmental sounds.

AVOID CAFFEINE LATE IN THE DAY

Avoid drinking caffeinated drinks, such as coffee, tea, and sodas, as well as chocolate, late in the day, or entirely. The caffeine in these foods and drinks can interfere with the process of going to sleep and may also contribute to premature awakening. Also, be aware that some over-the-counter pain relievers contain caffeine.

AVOID ALCOHOL

Avoid alcohol before bed. Some people believe a nightcap will help them sleep. But alcohol interferes with the brain's sleep-regulating mechanism, diminishing quality of sleep. Also, its diuretic effect may cause you to wake up in the middle of the night to urinate.

COMMIT TO A SCHEDULE

Because the body thrives on regularity, commit to a regular sleep schedule if possible, retiring at the same time each evening and waking at the same time each morning—even on the weekend.

AVOID BLUE LIGHT FROM SCREENS

Avoid television, computers, cellphones, tablets, e-readers, and the use of other screen technology just before bed. All stimulate the brain and reduce levels of melatonin, making it more difficult to settle into a sleep state. On Apple computers and iPhones, you can set the screen to Night Shift mode which cuts blue light substantially. There are also several brands of blue-light-blocking glasses you may wish to try.

WARM BATHS HELP TO RELAX

Take a warm bath just before bed and and/or consider a simple stretch routine to help you relax.

KEEP THE ROOM COOL

Keep the temperature of your bedroom cool in the evening. About 65 degrees is best.

INVEST IN A GOOD BED

Sleep is critical to your brain health as well as your overall health.[868] Since you will spend about one-third of your life in bed, don't compromise on the quality or comfort of your mattress. Bed technology has improved greatly in the last decade, bringing memory foam, modifiable latex, and ergonomically adjustable bed systems to the market. Be sure you have a comfortable and supportive mattress and pillows.

CLEAR YOUR MIND

Clear your mind of troubling thoughts that may keep you awake. If that sounds impossible, try this time-tested aid: Write your concerns on a pad of paper or in a journal. This act can help you let go for the night and attend to your concerns once you wake up.

USE AUDIO RECORDINGS OR RELAXATION APPS

Consider using a guided relaxation audio recording. There are also several story-telling apps designed to help the mind relax and thus invite sleep.

AVOID MEDICATIONS FOR SLEEP IF POSSIBLE

Be aware that if you use sleeping medications such as Ambien, there is some risk of reversible cognitive impairment, as well as many other reported side effects.[869] It's worth putting all the above strategies to work for you before resorting to prescription sleeping aids.

If you have tried the above suggestions for improving sleep and still find yourself unable to experience a solid night's rest, consider getting a medical evaluation to determine if you have a sleep disorder, such as parasomnia, sleep apnea, or restless leg syndrome. Some conditions can be treated through cognitive behavioral therapy. To find a sleep professional, visit the National Sleep Foundation website at sleepfoundation.org.

31

INOCULATING YOURSELF AGAINST STRESS

FOR DECADES WE have known that chronic psychological distress is unhealthy, that it can wear us down and make us more susceptible to illness. As it turns out, stress is as bad for our brains as it is for our bodies. Stress increases the risk of cognitive decline and AD.[870]

To investigate the link between stress and Alzheimer's some 500 adults aged 70 and older were enrolled in the Einstein Aging Study in the Bronx, New York. The researchers developed a Perceived Stress Scale (PSS) to quantify the degree to which participants felt stressed. For those who were in the highest quintile of the five PSS tiers, the risk of developing cognitive impairment was 2.5 times higher than those in the lowest tier. Participants who describe their work environment as stressful, had experienced trauma or physical or psychological abuse in the past, had lost a spouse or endured a divorce, or who had a "stress-prone personality," were found to be at higher risk for Alzheimer's.[871]

In another study, researchers found that for each major life stressor people endured their risk of developing AD later in life increased by 20 percent.[872] We will all face stressors in our lives. The more we can work to manage our responses to them, the better our chances at reducing our risk of AD. Let's look at some techniques for doing that.

FIGHT OR FLIGHT

Psychological stress probably influences the risk of dementia because of the release of stress-related hormones like epinephrine, adrenocorticotropin, and cortisol. These compounds elicit a state of arousal in the body, raising your heart rate, blood pressure, breathing rate, and blood sugar. This primal response is meant to save your life in an authentic emergency, preparing you to spring to action and defend yourself (fight) or run away from a threat (flight). The hormonal and physical changes brought about by such an instance of acute episodic stress subside after 20 to 60 minutes. Yet many of us may trigger these same powerful changes in response to circumstances that are not life-threatening but are chronic in nature: traffic, an argument with a loved one, conflicts at work, or financial strain. The result is that the body's physical stress response is chronically retriggered, with little opportunity provided for recovery.

PERCEIVED STRESS AND THE IMPORTANCE OF COPING

The degree to which stressful events affect us negatively depends largely upon our perception: When we *believe* that challenges exceed our ability to adapt and cope, we experience stress. Our confidence in our own capacity to manage a situation matters quite a bit. So does our assessment of the importance of a situation. And, of course, temperament matters as well.

For these reasons, different people will experience the same situation differently. One person could find throwing a party for 50 guests to be an exhilarating and rewarding experience, while for someone else the same event could elicit feelings of great stress. Moving to a new home can for many people produce feelings of stress, while for others it may be exciting.

We often assume that stressful situations are inherently negative. The word *stress* tends to evoke visions of looming deadlines, angry bosses, or worse. But positive life events can be challenging, too. Getting married, planning a vacation, having a child, or starting a new job can all cause feelings of stress.

Managing how we respond to stress is critically important to the Alzheimer's prevention lifestyle. A negative response to stress—that is, feeling overwhelmed by stressors—triggers biochemical and physical changes in the body that promote established risk factors for AD. Clinical studies have shown that those who are exposed to chronic stress demonstrate cognitive impairments and an acceleration of cognitive decline.[873] A negative response to stress disrupts neurotransmitter function. Over an extended period, this has a particularly negative effect on the hippocampus region of the brain.[874]

Repeatedly activating the fight-or-flight response can have a deleterious effect on the brain.[875]

It impairs learning and memory, inhibits neurogenesis, decreases levels of nerve growth factor and changes the physical structure of the hippocampus.[876] And chronic stress leads to inflammation of the brain.[877]

One of the ways chronic stress may contribute to risk is through causing the dysfunction of synapses. The steady release of cortisol and other stress hormones can lead to changes that detach synaptic connections and shrink dendrites (the projections on neurons that receive electrochemical transmissions from other neurons), degrade communications between neurons, chip away at memory, and damage and ultimately kill cells in the hippocampus.[878]

Those who live in a persistent state of stress have been shown to have elevated levels of inflammation-promoting molecules in the brain.[879] Chronic stress also causes changes in the size of the region of the brain called the amygdala by binding to cortisol receptors inside neurons. This causes the neurons to allow more calcium to cross their membrane. Excessive calcium in turn excites the neurons, which end up firing too frequently, ultimately hastening their death.

Even more interesting is that researchers at the UC Irvine Institute for Memory Impairments and Neurological Disorders have shown that cortisol significantly promotes the production of amyloid precursor protein, the precursor to beta amyloid, which constitutes the brain plaques found in AD, and tau protein, which constitutes the hallmark tangles seen in AD.[880]

SAVE THE TELOMERES

Telomeres are the protective caps on the ends of DNA strands that shield our chromosomes and the genetic information they contain.

They have been likened to the plastic tips (aglets) found on the ends of shoelaces, because telomeres prevent the fraying of chromosomes, which could lead to damaging the genetic material and is also considered a biomarker of age.

All cells in our body are constantly renewing themselves through a replication process called mitosis. The process is essential to keeping hair and skin youthful and the liver, heart, pancreas, bones, and immune system functioning in top form. However, the number of times a cell can divide is limited by the length of its telomeres. So, your telomeres dictate the life span of all your cells.

High levels of stress, among other factors, can hasten the shortening of telomeres, and literally the shortening of one's life.

In younger cells, an enzyme named telomerase keeps telomeres from shortening too quickly. However, over time and with continued cell division, less of this enzyme occurs and the length of the telomeres decreases. Some cells stop replicating. Moreover, as more cells enter this dormant phase, they begin to secrete immune cells called cytokines that promote inflammation. People with short telomeres also happen to be at greater risk of Alzheimer's.[881]

Chronic stress and the elevated cortisol levels it generates, insulin resistance, depression, and oxidative stress all reduce the availability of telomerase. When that occurs, it can accelerate the shortening of telomeres, which in return accelerates aging, promotes illness, and ultimately leads to the early death of cells.

OTHER PHYSIOLOGICAL EFFECTS

An unhealthful response to stress also causes a rise in immune system cells called leukocytes and neutrophils. These cells increase inflammation in the walls of blood vessels, restricting blood flow to the brain and elsewhere, and can contribute to the risk of hypertension. This process may also encourage existing plaques to dislodge from the blood vessel wall, raising the risk of a stroke or heart attack.[882]

MANAGING STRESS

The good news is that there are powerful ways to inoculate ourselves against chronic stress. Life will always throw us challenges, but the choice is ours as to how we react to and deal with them. By integrating one or more of the following strategies, we can avoid succumbing to the primitive stress response that can be so toxic and damaging to the body and brain.

Stress-reduction strategies have the most powerful and healthy effect when practiced on a regular basis. One of the most attractive ways that we can dial down the stress response in our body is to engage with nature. It is no secret that most of us feel mentally better after we spend time at a beach or in the woods, and now scientists have begun to gain a better understanding of why. It turns out that when we enter natural surroundings, we undergo physiological changes. Most important, levels of the primary stress hormone, cortisol, begin to plummet after just ten minutes of entering calming areas where we feel close to nature. Researchers who wanted to quantify changes in physiological stress chose to measure both cortisol and alpha amylase levels in the saliva of 36 urban residents over the course of an eight-week study. The participants were encouraged to have three experiences a week lasting ten minutes or more that made them feel close to nature. Like cortisol, the digestive enzyme alpha-amylase tends to rise with physical and psychological stress. The researchers reported that levels of cortisol dropped 21.3 percent on average per hour. The greatest drop in levels of alpha-amylase (28 percent per hour) occurred in those who stayed still instead of walking during the nature experience. Cortisol levels were not affected by movement.

The "sweet spot" for these benefits seemed to be in the first 20 to 30 minutes, after which the reduction in alpha amylase and cortisol continued but at a reduced rate.[883] Other studies have found a similar response to brief retreats to nature.[884] With expanding urbanization it's increasingly difficult for many people to access nature. Is there a place nearby, such as a park, that you could visit for half an hour a day a few days a week or more to gain this benefit?

MEDITATION

One of the most important skills we can develop as part of the Revolution Lifestyle plan to build cognitive resilience and reduce the risk of AD is meditation. In the past decade, interest in meditation has grown substantially, and today we hear some of the most successful corporate executives, scientists, actors, and athletes have turned to meditation to help them stay at the top of their game. Shown to literally build more brain volume, meditation enhances memory, reduces feelings of stress, improves sleep, and offers a host of additional benefits that have been documented through extensive research. Although it's not yet entirely clear how meditation leads to all these positive outcomes, the evidence that it does is highly compelling.

There are dozens of types of meditation, including Vipassana, Zen, kundalini, guided meditation, and mindfulness techniques. Many people believe that one of the easiest methods of meditation, and certainly the one with the greatest amount of research backing its positive impact, is transcendental meditation, or TM.

Generally speaking, meditation is about sitting still, quieting the mind, and focusing attention inward. The effect may be achieved through focus on breathing, visualizing imagery by way of a guided audio recording, or through the repetition of a word or sound called a mantra, which aids in concentration. While many forms of meditation emanated from religious or spiritual practices, meditation today is largely a secular practice.

After a couple of false starts with other types of meditation, nine years ago I was introduced to TM by the bestselling book *Transcendence* by Norman Rosenthal, MD. The book inspired me to enroll in a four-day course, and I have been a regular practitioner since. It would be impossible to overstate the benefits that I feel I have gained from TM. After a month of regular practice, close friends almost invariably told me things like, "You seem calmer" or "I notice that you are more relaxed in stressful situations." Seeing the benefits that I was enjoying, my now 90-year-old mother and three of my siblings enrolled in their own meditation training. They too have found that meditation has great rewards.

Some 340 peer-reviewed studies and more than $26 million in National Institutes of Health funding have revealed the remarkably positive impact meditation can have on a variety of health conditions, including hypertension, anxiety, post-traumatic stress disorder (PTSD), depression, metabolic syndrome, cardiovascular disease, and stroke. Regular practice of TM has been shown to help in reducing cortisol, ending insomnia, and improving brain function and memory.[885] In many cases TM resulted in outcomes comparable to or better than those derived from prescription medications, without any of the side effects that sometimes come with medications. Meditation alone may be helpful in enhancing and preserving cognitive function and reserve.[886]

In studies focusing on TM, benefits relevant to helping reduce the risk of AD include:

- 47 percent reduction in death from cardiovascular disease[887]
- 40 to 55 percent reduction in depression and PTSD[888]
- 42 percent reduction in insomnia[889]
- 40 percent reduction in psychological distress[890]
- 25 percent reduction in cortisol levels[891]
- Reduced reactivity to stressors[892]
- Lowering blood pressure as effectively as medications[893]
- Increased telomerase activity levels[894]
- Increased brain glucose metabolism[895]

We have examined the importance of unimpeded blood flow to the brain. Meditation can help here as well. To examine the influence of meditation on cerebral blood flow, researchers performed brain scans on subjects before introducing them to an eight-week meditation program. The subjects were injected with a contrast solution that helped researchers see how effectively blood flowed to their brains. Then they gave the subjects tests that focused on verbal fluency and memory. After eight weeks of the meditation program, brain scans and the neuropsychological evaluations were repeated. Not only was blood flow to the brain shown to have improved significantly, but the subjects also showed marked improvements in memory.

In another study, researchers evaluated unemployed men and women who were seeking a job and were under elevated stress due to their circumstances. The participants were taught to meditate and given baseline brain scans and had blood drawn to look for markers of inflammation. After four months of regular meditation, the researchers took new scans and blood samples from the participants. The blood samples showed much lower levels of markers for inflammation and the scans showed improved communication between regions of the brain that manage stress and facilitate states of calm.[896]

MEDITATION BUILDS BRAIN VOLUME & COGNITIVE RESERVE

The benefits of meditation may be even greater over the long term. Evidence shows that with meditation practice brain structure not only changes but brain volume is increased. Just think about that—your brain literally gets larger when you meditate.

Using functional MRI and PET scans, Sara Lazar, a neuroscientist at Harvard Medical School, and her research colleagues have shown that long-term meditators develop a thicker cerebral cortex and a higher concentration of gray matter in the temporal lobe, frontal lobe, and hippocampus, and experience significantly less loss of brain volume with aging, as compared to non-meditators. Like physical exercise, meditation can be helpful in developing greater cognitive reserve to forestall age-related brain atrophy. Lazar's team found that long-term meditators 50 years old have brain matter in the frontal cortex at levels similar to 25-year-olds. [897]

You need not meditate for decades before realizing positive change in your brain. Apparently, it only takes a couple of months. Lazar and her colleagues showed for the first time that meditation changes the physical structure of the brain in as little as eight weeks.[898] Along with the physical changes came improved memory. Participants were told to meditate 40 minutes a day, yet the average duration was only 27 minutes. Physical changes took place in areas associated with anxiety and stress as well as in the hippocampus. In these regions, brain matter became thicker and denser. Moreover, researchers found that meditation reduced the concentration of gray matter in the amygdala, a region of the brain associated with fear, anxiety, and stress. It's likely that the benefits would have been even greater if all the participants had meditated for the suggested 40 minutes a day.

To repeat, studies have consistently shown that when practiced regularly, meditation reduces not just stress, anxiety, depression, and anger; it also lowers blood pressure and reduces the risk of stroke and heart attack.

MEDITATION AND AGING

In a study published in the *Journal of Neuroscience*, scientists studying the benefits of transcendental meditation reported a remarkable finding. They measured blood pressure (which rises with age), near-point vision (which diminishes with age), and auditory discrimination of higher pitches (which diminishes with age). Long-term TM practitioners (meditating five years or longer) have a biological age, on average, 12 years younger than their chronological age. Even short-term meditators (less than five years of meditation), were biologically five years younger than their chronological age.[899]

MEDITATORS NEED LESS HEALTH CARE

The most impressive study that I have seen regarding the positive influence of meditation practice on overall health was a 14-year study using governmental health insurance records in Quebec. The study showed that for patients 65 years or older who learned TM, health expenditures dropped at a rate of 14 percent a year. In five years, when compared to those not practicing TM, there was a 70 percent reduction in healthcare expenditures in the trained subjects.[900] It's difficult to imagine any other single factor that could produce such an outcome. However, if there were something such as a pill that produced no dangerous side effects and led to a 70 percent reduction in healthcare costs within five years, you can bet any national healthcare system would be handing out prescriptions for free.

Meditation Improves Brainwave Coherence

Over time, meditation practice leads to what scientists refer to as greater brainwave coherence and integration. Each part of the brain produces brainwaves, faint electrical impulses, of varying frequencies. During the day most of us have a brainwave pattern that appears disorderly. When brain waves of a particular frequency from different parts of the brain become synchronized they are said to be in coherence, which results in more harmonious brain function. Using an electroencephalograph or EEG, a device that uses electrodes placed around the scalp to measure brain wave activity, researchers find that in meditation slow alpha waves become the dominant type and brainwaves assume a more orderly and rhythmic pattern. This is the same brainwave state that we wake up in after a restful night of sleep and when many people feel they are most creative.

Greater brainwave coherence results in improvements in every aspect of cognition. Not only is memory enhanced, but creativity, comprehension, and focus improve, as well. An additional benefit for those we live or interact with is that meditation tends to develop parts of the brain that foster greater patience, empathy, moral reasoning, and understanding.

Greater brainwave coherence can be evident in new meditators after just a few weeks of practicing meditation, and with regular practice greater coherence extends into periods when one is not meditating.

It's worthwhile to add meditation to your daily routine, if for no other reason than that it has been shown to have a positive effect on multiple risk factors for Alzheimer's. Any form of meditation that works for you (and that you practice regularly) offers benefits simply too great to miss out on. I encourage you to explore the various options available in your community. To locate a meditation instructor near you, see Resources.

YOGA

Yoga involves performing a series of physical poses or postures that stretch the muscles, encourage controlled breathing, concentration, visualization, and relaxation, and produce greater flexibility. Like meditation, yoga has been shown to reduce feelings of stress and anxiety, improve mood, and reduce risk factors for chronic illnesses such as heart disease and high blood pressure. Yoga can increase cerebral blood flow, improve neuron connectivity, and help retain cognitive reserve. Almost any town now has one or more yoga studios. Many health clubs also offer regular yoga classes, and there are also countless free YouTube yoga classes and yoga apps available.

People of all ages do yoga, and there is no flexibility prerequisite! UCLA researchers recruited a group of middle-aged Americans with mild cognitive impairment for a study on the effects of different activities on cognition.[901] Participants first underwent brain scans to see how different regions of their brains were communicating with each other. Half the group then participated in a memory enhancement training class for one hour per week and practiced training games at home for 15 minutes each day. The other half of the group participated in one hour of yoga and meditation instruction weekly. After three months, both groups underwent brain scans again and took cognitive performance tests. While both groups showed improved cognitive performance, the group that used yoga and meditation showed much greater improvement in cognitive function as well as greater connectivity in parts of their brains that were scanned.

Not only do we see greater brain connectivity in people who do yoga, they also experience positive changes in the physical structure of the brain. Research from the Hospital Israelita Albert Einstein in São Paulo, Brazil, showed that elderly yoga practitioners had greater cortical thickness than did healthy non-practitioners. This finding suggests that yoga may help develop cognitive reserve that will in turn help protect against cognitive decline.[902]

TAI CHI

Tai chi has been likened to meditation with movement. It involves performing a series of gentle movements in a slow and focused manner, accompanied by deep breathing. Like yoga, it helps strengthen muscles while reducing feelings of stress and anxiety; it also helps practitioners develop greater balance and coordination as weight is regularly shifted from one foot to the other.

In an eight-month study, researchers from the University of South Florida and Fudan University in Shanghai studied 120 adults in their sixties and seventies who practiced tai chi for 30 minutes three times a week; they found significant increases in brain volume (as measured by MRI before and after the study), improved memory, and improved cognitive function when compared to people who did not practice tai chi.[903]

Another study of 389 subjects with MCI or dementia found improved cognitive function after five months of practicing tai chi three times a week. The improvements were still present one year later.[904]

In a 2017 meta-analysis that reviewed 39 prior studies of the cognitive improvements seen from various types of exercise, tai chi consistently showed improved cognitive function in people aged 50 or older.[905] Two results that may explain the cognitive improvements experienced by those who practice tai chi are that it lowered blood pressure 9.12 mmHg systolic and 5 mmHg diastolic on average, and that both LDL (bad) cholesterol and triglycerides were reduced in practitioners.[906]

Ongoing study of tai chi in those who already have dementia has shown one additional benefit is a sharp reduction in their risk of falling brought about by the improved sense of balance tai chi affords. The chance of a fall and suffering serious injury, such as a hip fracture, is doubled in those with dementia.[907]

The great thing about tai chi is that, like yoga and meditation, once you know the sequence of movements or techniques you can practice it anywhere, whether at home or on the road, and you don't need special equipment or a special facility to do so.

QIGONG

Qigong (pronounced *chee-gong*) is an exercise similar to tai chi in that it involves a series of physical movements that benefit balance and coordination. It also lowers blood pressure, reduces inflammation, improves circulation, and enhances immune function.[908] Both cortisol and adrenaline levels are reduced and blood circulation to the brain is increased during qigong practice.[909]

Studies have also reported that practitioners of qigong experience a reduction in both anxiety and depression, and these benefits are seen in those who practice it for as little as seven minutes a day. While tai chi requires adequate space to make broad sweeping movements with the body, qigong can be practiced standing, lying down, or sitting in a chair. When practiced together with tai chi, qigong has been shown to increase brain plasticity and lower risk of cognitive decline.[910]

TAKE A BREAK FROM YOUR CELLPHONE

Cellphones can be a significant contributor to feelings of stress. Today, the average cellphone user looks at their screen 221 times a day. That's more than 1,400 hours a year; time lost that could be used for more healthful activities with family and friends and in the world around us. There is a growing body of evidence that, as convenient as these devices are, they bring an unconsidered cost to many people's lives. For many people, just hearing the continuous notification chimes of their phone triggers a stress response. These devices may generate a chronic sense of obligation to reply to emails, texts, and social media posts for fear that one is otherwise missing out on important developments.[911] In turn, this fear elevates cortisol levels, which, in turn, can raise blood pressure.

I encourage you to become more aware of your cellphone use. How often are you on the device? When do you use it and why? How do you feel when you are using it, and when you aren't? Would you be willing to reduce the time you spend on the device each day or even shut the phone off for 24 hours? Simply becoming more conscious of your usage and how it makes you feel may be helpful in regulating your usage and the subsequent impact on your health.

A FINAL WORD ON STRESS

As you have seen, stress doesn't just make you miserable; it also has the potential to affect your cognitive health adversely. Incorporating just one of the stress-reducing strategies described in this chapter within your personal Revolution Lifestyle program has the potential to yield tremendous benefits.

32
YOUR BRAIN WANTS YOU TO MOVE

I KNOW THAT FOR some, exercise is a dreaded word. But if you are really committed to protecting your brain and enhancing cognitive function, this is one of the most effective tools available. I suspect that once you see how powerfully protective it can be your relationship with physical activity will change. Next to brain-supporting nutrition, nothing is as critical to preserving brain volume, memory, and general brain function than regular vigorous exercise. Exercise literally changes the size, structure, and function of your brain.

The list of known benefits offered by exercise is lengthy, and it keeps growing. For decades we have known that those who are committed to keeping their bodies as fit as they can be are rewarded with minds that stay fit as well—and now we know why. Aerobic exercise is a powerful Alzheimer's preventative—a one-stop-shop that can prevent, if not reverse, more than ten known risk factors including cardiovascular disease, elevated cholesterol, inflammation, being overweight or obese, high blood pressure, insulin resistance, diabetes, stroke and ministrokes, depression, and insomnia.

The largest long-term studies have shown that those who remain the most fit reduce their risk of Alzheimer's by about 50 percent. So it's unfortunate that today only 18 percent of medical schools in the USA even broach the subject, with a single course in exercise science, for their students.[912]

The research findings related to exercise and cognitive health are truly remarkable. We know that regular exercise enhances the brain's ability to maintain old network connections and to develop new ones. Exercise counteracts mental decline,[913] reduces oxidative stress,[914] builds brain volume, helps maintain synapses, is believed to promote neurogenesis,[915] increases blood vessel elasticity,[916] promotes the growth of new blood vessels in the brain, increases brain glucose metabolism,[917] and reduces inflammation.[918] In fact, scientists have shown that brain function is enhanced after just one 30-minute session of aerobic exercise![919] If there were a prescription drug that offered such benefits, it would be a multi-billion-dollar bestseller.

Living in the age of COVID-19, it would be remiss of me if I did not point out that, due to its immune system strengthening effect, regular exercise is strongly associated with a decreased risk of COVID infection, reduced severity of symptoms, and lower risk of death.[920]

What is especially inspiring is that you don't need to be "athletic" or have started exercising in your youth to reap great benefits now, no matter where you are starting from. For someone who has been leading a sedentary life, significant improvements in memory and cognitive function can be experienced from as little as 12 weeks of regular, vigorous aerobic exercise.[921]

Researchers from Rush University Medical Center placed actigraphs (small devices that record movement) on 716 dementia-free adults to measure their level of daily activity over 3.5 years. Participants in the bottom 10 percent for physical activity were 2.3 times more likely to develop Alzheimer's disease as those in the top 10 percent.[922]

Australian researchers went farther and followed subjects aged 45 to 55 for 20 years to see how exercise would affect risk. At the end of the study, the researchers concluded that exercise was the number-one defense against cognitive decline.[923]

Other researchers created a meta-analysis where they pooled the findings of 15 prospective studies that involved more than 33,000 subjects who were followed for up to 12 years. Those who were most physically active were 38 percent less likely to experience cognitive decline.[924]

In an exciting study of adults aged 20 to 67, aerobic exercise performed four times weekly at 75 percent of one's maximum heart rate (MHR) for six months resulted in significant improvement in cognitive function as well as an increase in brain volume.[925] Researchers divided participants into two groups: the control group who would perform a simple stretching program and those who would perform aerobic exercise. The exercisers could choose any form of exercise they wished if they maintained their prescribed heart rate. All the participants were given a battery of cognitive exams before they embarked upon their training programs. Six months later they were tested once again. *The 40-year-old exercisers performed in their second round of tests with the mental acuity of people ten years younger. The 60-year-olds performed similar to people 20 years younger.* No cognitive improvements were seen in the group that did stretching only.

At the University of Texas Southwestern Medical Center, a similar study was performed. A research team took a group of individuals aged 60 and older who were experiencing memory loss and divided them into two groups. For 12 months half did stretches, and the other half aerobic exercise. At the beginning and end of the test period, the subjects were given memory tests and blood flow in their brains was measured. At the end of the study, the stretchers had virtually no benefit to their cognitive function. However, the exercisers experienced a 47 percent improvement in their memory and measurable increases in blood flow to the hippocampus. There is no drug that can produce that outcome![926]

The most comprehensive study of exercise and risk of Alzheimer's came from Trondheim, Norway. There researchers looked at 30,000 individuals over the course of two decades. Those who remained the most physically fit cut their risk of AD by 50 percent. Moreover, the protection exercise affords was acquired even by those who did not become physically active until midlife.[927]

TYPE OF EXERCISE COUNTS

There are three types of exercises: aerobic, flexibility, and resistance. While a complete exercise program should include all three, aerobic exercise, which increases your breathing and heart rate, is the most important for preserving cognitive function, because it triggers the powerful changes that I describe below. Aerobic exercise is rhythmic and sustained. Examples are brisk walking, jogging, running, cycling, swimming, and group aerobics classes. To achieve the benefits that are described below, aerobic exercise is essential.

HOW AEROBIC EXERCISE PROTECTS THE BRAIN & MEMORY

Exercise results in a host of favorable changes that are critical to maintaining brain function and protecting memory, including increased brain blood flow through dilation of existing blood vessels, the creation of new blood vessels (angiogenesis), the production of new nerve cells (neurogenesis), and enhanced connectivity between neurons through the production of new synapses (synaptogenesis) and protection of existing ones.[928]

When we are sedentary, we impede the brain waste removal process discussed in the sleep section. A number of processes and enzymes that are critical to degrading and transporting waste (including amyloid protein) out of the brain are hampered by inactivity.[929] Not only are these processes restored to their proper function, but regular exercise is an aid to quality sleep, which is when the most substantial brain waste removal takes place.

Exercise appears to be a key factor in promoting the cognitive reserve that permits some people to maintain a high level of cognitive function late in life even though their brains may already have pathological changes associated with AD.[930]

All of the positive exercise-induced changes that enhance and protect cognition come about because exercise activates various agents in the body. Let's take a look at some of them.

VEGF

A compound that is elevated by aerobic exercise is vascular endothelial growth factor (VEGF). Evidence suggests it protects against cognitive decline.[931] In addition to supporting the development of neurons, one of the chief jobs of this fascinating substance is to promote vascular health, and in particular, to promote the creation of new blood vessels (angiogenesis).[932] Some degree of its protection may come from assuring that adequate blood supply reaches neurons. Those who maintain higher levels of VEGF retain better cognitive function with age and experience significantly less shrinkage of the hippocampus. Alzheimer's patients have low levels of VEGF.

IRISIN

Another protective compound that is boosted with regular exercise is the hormone irisin. Levels of this hormone are depleted in those who have Alzheimer's as well as those who are sedentary, but high in people who exercise regularly and are cognitively healthy.

During exercise, muscles secrete irisin and send it out to various tissues in the body, including the hippocampus, where it works in a variety of ways to protect memory. Irisin promotes neurogenesis, supports synapse plasticity, improves insulin sensitivity, protects against neuronal damage caused by oxidative stress, and blocks the harmful effects of amyloid protein.[933] Researchers are already postulating that irisin might be useful as a drug for the prevention or treatment of Alzheimer's. But why wait for the drug when you can already stimulate production of irisin simply by performing regular exercise?

BDNF

Physical activity causes an increase in production of our old friend brain-derived neurotrophic factor (BDNF).[934] I want you to develop a healthy obsession with BDNF. This amazing chemical, likened to "Miracle-Gro for the brain," is believed to support neurogenesis in the hippocampus, build new synapses and attach to receptors at synapses protecting brain cells from injury and death.[935] BDNF is also critical to the regulation of calcium within neurons. Calcium dysregulation in neurons is a common and early symptom in many neurodegenerative diseases, including Alzheimer's and Parkinson's.[936] Remember, BDNF levels tend to be very low in people diagnosed with AD.[937]

In a study of 2,130 dementia-free subjects aged 60 and older, blood BDNF levels were measured and then the group was followed for ten years to see who developed dementia and Alzheimer's. Over the next decade, those who maintained the highest levels of BDNF were less than half as likely to develop dementia and AD compared to those who had the lowest BDNF levels.[938]

Researchers at Rush University's Alzheimer's Disease Center showed that people who maintain higher BDNF levels are able to retain more of their cognitive capacity, even if amyloid plaques begin to form.

Effects of BDNF

- Supports neurogenesis
- Prevents death of nerve cells
- Promotes growth of synapses
- Promotes memory consolidation

CATHEPSIN B

When we exercise aerobically a protein called cathepsin B becomes elevated in the blood. This protein is positively associated with both greater fitness and better memory. It's produced in and secreted by muscles and is involved in their recovery after strenuous exercise. Cathepsin B also crosses the blood–brain barrier and supports the production of new neurons and greater connectivity in the hippocampus. As blood levels of the protein rise, people perform better on tests of memory and thought process. When tested, those who exercise consistently maintain the highest levels of the protein in their blood and show the greatest improvement in memory function.[939]

KLOTHO

Named after a Greek goddess, Klotho is a protein that is associated with cognitive resilience. Levels naturally decline in humans with age, and lower levels are associated with higher levels of inflammation, memory impairment and general cognitive decline.[940] Higher levels of klothos are associated with great cognitive reserve, enhanced synaptic function, and greater cognitive health as well as longevity. So compelling is the research on Klothos that some scientists are exploring the viability of synthesizing the protein and administering it to people therapeutically. But you can simply perform robust aerobic exercise to keep your klotho levels elevated.

IMPROVING BLOOD FLOW TO THE BRAIN

In the short term, by increasing the diameter of blood vessels, exercise increases blood flow to the brain, which carries oxygen, glucose, and other factors to neurons.[941] Neurons therefore become better nourished. In the long term, exercise reduces the stiffness of carotid arteries that feed the brain, leading to lower pressure and a sustained increase in blood flow. Further, exercise increases the number of small blood vessels that supply blood to the brain, a process called angiogenesis.[942] One literally grows more blood vessels, which further improves blood irrigation in brain tissue. A study led by neurologist Scott Small at Columbia University showed that after a three-month exercise program, capillary volume in the hippocampus of study subjects increased by 30 percent.[943] This means more blood, more oxygen, and more nutrients reaching the brain cells.

Even after exercise, when one is at rest, blood flow will be greater in a person who exercises compared to one who does not.[944] New blood vessels can compensate for (work around) damaged blood vessels. Exercise reduces the risk of blood-vessel disease (which deprives brain cells of oxygen and nutrients).

PRESERVING & INCREASING BRAIN VOLUME

As previously discussed, just as the muscles of our limbs shrink with age and disuse, the brain shrinks over time. From about age 30, we lose an estimated one percent of our brain volume every two to three years. Mind you, this estimate is based upon average people who unfortunately make many lifestyle choices that accelerate brain shrinkage. Exercise can help us resist this trend by stimulating neurogenesis and boosting blood flow to the brain.[945]

Dr. J. Carson Smith and colleagues at the University of Maryland School of Public Health showed for the first time that physical exercise can reduce the risk of brain shrinkage, a sign of neurodegeneration, in individuals at heightened risk for developing AD.[946] The subjects of his study were individuals aged 65 to 89 who carried the APOE4 gene, yet who had normal cognitive abilities. Each had a family history in which a first-degree relative had received a clinical diagnosis of AD or had a history of memory loss and loss of other cognitive functions, confusion, or judgment problems, but did not receive a formal diagnosis of AD before death. All subjects underwent structural MRIs at the start of the study and at its completion. During the 18-month period of the study, subjects who didn't exercise lost three percent of their brain volume in the hippocampus. Yet all the participants who exercised several times a week preserved their brain volume.

In another study, sedentary participants were randomly assigned to either an aerobic exercise group or a stretching group.[947] At the start of the study, there was no difference between hippocampus volume in the two groups. MRIs were taken of the participants' brains at six months and then again at 12 months. At the completion of the study, not only did the brains of the aerobic-exercise participants increase by over two percent (hippocampus region), but the brains of the control group members who only stretched shrank by about 1.5 percent in that same period. Improved memory function was also found in those who experienced an increase in brain volume. The participants exercised at 50 to 60 percent of their maximum heart rate for the first seven weeks and then 60 to 75 percent of their maximum heart rate for 40-minute sessions for the remainder of the study.

Dr. Scott McGinnis, a neurologist at Brigham and Women's Hospital and an instructor in neurology at Harvard Medical School notes that even if you have been living a sedentary life and as a result have experienced more rapid shrinkage of your brain, you can reverse that loss of brain volume in as little as 6-12 months by beginning an exercise program today.[948]

Agnieszka Burzynska, a professor of neuroscience at Colorado State University and her colleagues studied a group of 250 sedentary but otherwise healthy adults over aged 60. The researchers divided the group into those who would only perform stretching, those who would learn and practice line dancing, and those who would walk briskly for 40 minutes three times weekly. The participants were selected because of their age and the fact that they were generally inactive. Before beginning the program, the men and women had their aerobic fitness level accessed, were given memory tests, and had images taken of their brains to quantify volume. The participants followed their routines for six months and then returned to the lab to be reevaluated. Both walkers and dancers had developed greater aerobic fitness, both had an increase in brain volume, there were improvements in both structure and function improvements, and even lesions had shrunk. Yet improvements on memory tests were seen only in the walkers. No positive changes in brain volume, structure or memory were noted in the control group that only stretched.[949]

INCREASING NEUROPLASTICITY

It is one thing to stimulate production of new neurons (neurogenesis), but if they aren't integrated into the existing neuronal network, they will eventually die off. Exercise recruits new neurons into the network.[950] Exercise also increases neuroplasticity, which increases brain cells' ability to recover from injury and assaults and to redirect pathways between neurons, thereby forming new neuronal pathways.[951]

REDUCING INFLAMMATION

A critical benefit from exercise is its systemic anti-inflammatory effect. Researchers recently discovered that regular exercise increases the number of microbes in the gut that produce anti-inflammatory substances that suppress levels of proinflammatory cells.[952] Stephen Rao PhD, a neuropsychologist at the Cleveland Clinic's Lou Ruvo Center for Brain Health who has studied the effects of exercise on brain health and reducing the risk of dementia, has reported that vigorous exercise specifically reduces brain inflammation.[953] It's believed that the reduction in inflammation comes in part as a result of suppressing the activation of microglial cells.[954]

INCREASING INSULIN SENSITIVITY

Insulin resistance, a precursor to diabetes, is a risk factor for cognitive impairment and AD. Exercise is effective at improving insulin sensitivity and protecting against diabetes.[955] Specifically, researchers have found that the reduction in glucose use by the brain that is seen in MCI and AD can be countered by performing at least three 50-minute aerobic exercise sessions per week at an intensity level of 70 to 80 percent of one's maximum heart rate.[956]

REDUCING HYPERTENSION

Regular exercise has been shown to be effective at both reducing the risk of and helping to reverse hypertension.[957] One of its effects is to reduce blood vessel stiffness. Various studies have shown a risk reduction between 34 and 65 percent among people who regularly engage in the most vigorous physical activity.[958] For those who have hypertension, exercising aerobically for at least 30 minutes daily has been shown to lower blood pressure 5 to 8 mm Hg. A meta-analysis of 300 studies that looked at the use of either exercise or medications to lower blood pressure found that overall, a structured exercise program was as effective as most blood pressure medications.[959]

EXERCISE PROTECTS EVEN ULTRA-HIGH-RISK INDIVIDUALS

Looking at individuals with a rare gene mutation that places them at high risk for early onset Alzheimer's disease, researchers found that those who exercised five times per week performed significantly better on cognitive performance tests, had lower levels of markers such as tau in their spinal fluid, and delayed their diagnosis of dementia by 15 years compared to those who carried the gene but did not exercise.[960]

CAN EXERCISE REVERSE MCI?

Even when mild cognitive impairment, a precursor to AD, is present, aerobic exercise has been shown to slow the advancement of the disease[961] and, in one study, to reverse MCI.[962] Improvements in cognitive function have been seen from as little as six months of regular exercise.[963] Even in people who have had ministrokes that have damaged brain tissue and impaired their memory and ability to think, significant improvements in memory and attention were gained through following a regular high-intensity aerobic exercise program.[964]

IS EXERCISE HELPFUL AFTER AN ALZHEIMER'S DIAGNOSIS?

For many of the reasons listed above, exercise can play an important part in slowing the progression of Alzheimer's disease and even improving cognition, as well as improving mobility and the performance of activities of daily living – including in patients in later stages of the disease.[965] In 2013, Stratford Commons Memory Care Community, an Alzheimer's support facility in Kansas, began to explore the effect of exercise on brain function.[966] In an experiment, researchers compared the status of Alzheimer's patients at 12- and 24-week intervals.[967] Half were encouraged to exercise, and half remained sedentary. Sedentary individuals continued to worsen during this period, whereas those who exercised remained cognitively stable, and in some respects improved. Positive changes were seen in executive function and word fluency, reaction time, hand-eye quickness, and attention. Elsewhere, researchers studied patients in five nursing homes who had mild to severe AD. By following an exercise program that involved just one hour of moderate exercise twice a week, they slowed the progression of the disease by one-third.[968]

In the ADEX Study at the Danish Dementia Research Center, patients diagnosed with AD who performed aerobic exercise at 70 to

80 percent of their max heart rate four times a week for just 16 weeks reduced common side effects that accompany AD, including mood problems, anxiety, irritability, and depression.[969]

Other research shows that vigorous exercise can reduce the amount of tau protein in one's cerebrospinal fluid.[970] To date, nothing else has been shown to be effective at lowering tau protein levels. Since high levels of tau protein in the brain are predictive of how rapidly one will move from MCI to Alzheimer's, exercise may be a powerful means to slow the otherwise inevitable decline.

In a fascinating and serendipitous occurrence, Dr. Jay L. Alberts, a neuroscientist at the Cleveland Clinic Lerner Research Institute, agreed to join a charity bike ride with one of his patients. The purpose of the ride was to raise contributions and awareness for Parkinson's disease research. However, Dr. Alberts and his patient, Cathy Frazier, did much more to benefit those who suffer from PD. Due to the physical limitations of his patient, the doctor suggested the two of them ride together on a tandem bicycle. During a rest stop, Alberts noticed that Cathy's hand tremor had improved markedly—in fact, it was absent, and his hunch was that her improvement was somehow related to the cycling they were doing. With no other reasonable explanation, Dr. Alberts set up a clinical study in which he and colleagues used functional MRI to evaluate how cycling might affect symptoms in PD patients. They learned that while pedaling a bike for exercise results in greater connectivity in brain regions associated with movement, the greatest benefits are seen in those who exercise between 60 to 80 percent of their maximum heart rate.[971] Participants enjoyed a 35 percent reduction in symptoms and a 51 percent improvement in motor functioning.

Where doctors once prescribed rest to PD patients, as with Alzheimer's disease they now understand that the best approach to slowing the progression of the disease is to encourage patients to get regular vigorous exercise. The chance observation made on the charity bike ride and the clinical research that followed inspired a worldwide movement called Pedaling for Parkinson's, where PD patients come together in organized classes to reap the benefits of stationary cycling.

ARE THERE ADDITIONAL BENEFITS TO EXERCISE?

It's clear that when it comes to protecting your cognitive health, vigorous exercise is a potent ally. Yet there are other very important benefits from exercise that we should not overlook. Committing to regular aerobic exercise will significantly reduce your risk of the number-one killer in the USA, cardiovascular disease (CVD). Those who adhere to a vigorous exercise program over the long-term enjoy about a 40 percent reduction in the risk that they will succumb to CVD. Regular exercise can also help you attain deep, restful sleep. Aerobic and resistance exercise also help increase insulin sensitivity. Finally, exercise is a reliable way to improve one's mood and has an impressive outcome for those contending with depression. Although physicians are much more likely to prescribe medication over exercise, studies have repeatedly found that for some patients, regular aerobic exercise can lead to improvements that are comparable to prescription medications, yet without the side effects that drugs may bring.[972]

THE IMPORTANCE OF REGULARITY

The amazing array of protective elements that exercise offers is found in no other single action we can take. However, it's important to note that, for the greatest benefits, we must exercise consistently and stick with it for the long term. An important study that involved seasoned athletes found that after just ten days of forced inactivity they began to develop a degree of insulin resistance, and the increase in both volume and distribution of blood to the hippocampus was diminished.[973] This is to say nothing of their BDNF, irisin, and cathepsin B levels. This study affirms how important it is to remain committed to a consistent exercise routine.

RESISTANCE EXERCISE

As I have already noted, when it comes to brain health, aerobic exercise is where we derive the greatest benefit. However, there is much to be gained from resistance exercise, not just in terms of its role in helping protect brain health but also in maintaining strength, stability, muscle tone, and bone integrity. Resistance exercise can be as simple as performing calisthenics, such as push-ups, that employ your own bodyweight. However, many more exercises can be performed using free weights (barbells and dumbbells) as well as the wide array of fitness machinery that permits you to make incremental adjustments in the amount of resistance your muscles contract against and to train your muscles in a highly focused manner.

Whether you use free weights or machines, a general guideline is to perform one to two exercises per body part (e.g., chest, shoulders, back, legs). For each exercise, strive to complete three sets of 10 to 12 repetitions. It's important to select a resistance level that challenges you to complete the number of repetitions but does not overwhelm you. As a rule, repetition numbers 8 through 10 should not be a cinch. But the resistance level should also not cause you to perform physical contortions to complete the repetitions, something which can lead to injury.

STAY FLEXIBLE

Stretching is also a form of exercise that is critical to maintaining joint range of motion and preventing injury. It is also relaxing and can be supportive of quality sleep when performed right before bed.

HOW MUCH EXERCISE IS REQUIRED?

While it is clear there are many important benefits to be gained from moderate exercise, clinical studies have consistently shown that the greatest benefit, both as a preventive as well as in improving early cognitive impairment, is gained at a specific intensity, duration, and frequency.

For general health, the WHO and other public health organizations now recommend 150-300 minutes of moderate-intensity aerobic exercise weekly. At the minimum, this equates to exercising 30 minutes five times a week. Much of the science related to exercise and neurological health underscores the value of striving for 300 minutes per week, particularly if one is already experiencing cognitive decline.[974] It's clear that exercise protects against cognitive decline in a dose-response manner. In other words, the more we do, the better off we are.[975]

HOW TO CALCULATE YOUR TARGET HEART RATE

Calculate your target heart rate using the following formula: 220 - age = maximum heart rate (MHR) x 60 percent (for the low end of the target range) and 70 percent (for the higher end). Your maximum heart rate is the rate you shouldn't exceed.

As an example, I am 56 years old. Here's how I would calculate my rates:

220 - 56 = 164 (maximum heart rate, or MHR)

164 x 60 percent = 98 (lower target heat rate)

164 x 70 percent = 114 (upper target heart rate)

For women, use 226 minus your age.

This equation shows the recommended heart-rate range for someone my age. If you have not exercised much in the past, you will want to stay closer to 50 percent or 60 percent of your MHR. Those with more conditioning will exercise at a higher heart rate. As you become more conditioned, you can gradually raise the intensity toward the upper range.

MEASURING HEART RATE

Many of today's aerobic exercise machines in health clubs have heart-rate monitors integrated into handle grips that provide a reading of one's heart rate on the machine's screen. Based on whether exercisers are above or below their target heart rate, the machine will adjust the operating speed or grade to keep the exerciser within their target range. I have experimented with a variety of these built-in monitors and find them to be less than accurate.

An alternative is to wear a heart rate monitor on your wrist. They are inexpensive and easy to use. Alternatively, devices such as the FitBit or Apple Watch will track your heart rate along with activity levels as well as provide daily reminders to keep you involved in your fitness program. I use the Apple Watch to track my heart rate on both stationary bike and treadmill workouts and appreciate the ability to look back at the cumulative data and see my progression over time.

IS A TRAINER REQUIRED?

Although a trainer is not required to have a successful workout, some people enjoy having an expert guide them through their program and monitor their progress. I do suggest that if you are new to the world of fitness training, you hire a trainer for at least an initial session. A trainer can orient you to the array of equipment available, show you how to use the equipment properly, ensure you are employing good form, and design a routine that assures you are getting the most from your efforts. And the encouragement of someone who is invested in your success is always helpful. Although I have been exercising consistently for 40 years, on occasion I will hire a trainer for a few sessions to gain new insights. Exercise science is continuously evolving and there are new understandings as well as increasingly better equipment to employ. An occasional session with a trainer helps me stay on the cutting edge of efficiency and effectiveness.

Of course, no one needs a trainer or a gym to start an exercise program. Download a tracking app, head out for a walk or a run, and when you are done you can see the distance you've gone along with your average pace. There are also apps and websites that can help you find local hikes so you can combine your exercise with some nature time—another stress reducer, as we have seen.

IT'S NEVER TOO LATE

It is never too late to begin to exercise and enjoy its benefits; even start-ing a program at age 80 affords some protection against AD, according to researchers from Rush University Medical Center.[976] Eight out of 11 studies of elderly individuals who followed an aerobic exercise pro-gram have shown that with improved cardiorespiratory fitness comes improved cognitive performance.[977] I have a good friend who is in his 80s and didn't take to exercise until late in life. He enjoys using the elliptical machine and gets a lot of attention at the gym because he exercises daily for one hour at 85 percent of his MHR, undoubtedly inspiring those decades his junior.

GET CHECKED OUT FIRST

Please be sure to see a doctor before you begin any exercise regimen. It's important that any physical limitations you may have are taken into consideration.

PROTECT THE NEXT GENERATION: START THEM SOON

Researchers have reported that women who exercise when pregnant may induce epigenetic alterations (alterations in gene and protein expression) in their offspring that will protect them from developing AD later in life by improving brain plasticity and possibly other fac-tors.[978] Unfortunately, kids have become increasingly sedentary and are carrying their inactivity into adulthood. We must do everything we can to encourage and reward physical activity as well as instill an appreciation and understanding for the many health benefits that regular, lifelong exercise provides.

JUST BEGIN WALKING

If you are new to exercise, a simple, safe, and effective way to ease into aerobic activity is by walking briskly. Walking is a particularly good choice for people who are overweight, who have been sedentary, or who may have an orthopedic or other condition that limits activity. When performed at a brisk rate, walking can have a beneficial aerobic effect. Even at a slow pace, when we walk and our feet come in contact with the ground, small pressure waves travel through the arteries and increase blood supply to the brain, and this improves cognitive function. With time, you will be conditioned enough to try out other forms of aerobic exercise, if these are appropriate for you. As a beginner, you can begin with a 10-minute walk a day for the first two weeks. In subsequent weeks, extend your daily walks by 5 minutes until you have reached 30 minutes, six days per week. If you are already somewhat active, then begin with 30-minute walks. At first choose a pace that you are comfortable with. Your goal should be to reach a pace that accelerates your breathing but still permits you to carry on a conversation comfortably.

The best way to begin a walking program is to start out on flat surfaces such as a community bike or walking path or residential streets in your neighborhood. As your body becomes more conditioned you can increase the intensity of your walks by walking on surfaces with a moderate grade.

Be sure you have good, stable shoes to walk in. You need not purchase expensive athletic shoes to walk. But you do need to be sure your shoes are appropriate for walking (crocs, sandals, or fashion boots will not suffice). They should be comfortable, have a well-padded and even sole, and sufficient lateral support at the ankles. If you are shopping for walking shoes, look for ones with a flared heel, as this provides greater stability.

Sedentary living is strongly associated with an increased risk of Alzheimer's disease. It's also a major risk factor for early death. A long-term study of 13,000 people showed that the amount of exercise they got correlated with how long they lived. The quantity of exercise we get is also a reliable predictor of how well we will function as we age.[979] The more exercise we get the better!

Some researchers believe that women who exercise when pregnant may induce epigenetic alterations (alterations in gene and protein expression) in their offspring that will protect them from neurodegeneration later in life by improving brain plasticity and possibly reducing amyloid deposits.[980] So they may impart greater cognitive resilience in their unborn child. Unfortunately, kids have become increasingly sedentary and are carrying their inactivity into adulthood. We must do everything we can to encourage and reward physical activity as well as instill an appreciation and understanding for the many health benefits that regular, lifelong exercise provides.

The good news is that your own physical activity level is another risk factor you are in control of and can change starting today. By making exercise a regular part of your lifestyle you will both protect your brain and increase your longevity. In the next chapter we'll look at strategies for exercising the mind.

33
KEEPING THE MIND ACTIVE

O UR MINDS RESPOND to a lack of stimulation the way our muscles respond to a lack of exercise—they degenerate. Cognitive fitness is partly sustained through continual cognitive challenges, the classic "use it or lose it" scenario. Without adequate mental stimulation and social engagement, our synapses become dysfunctional, neurons may be lost, and the brain atrophies, setting us up for cognitive impairment.[980] Individuals who remain engaged with meaningful and intellectually stimulating activities, keep socially active, or even pursue higher levels of education enjoy extended protection against brain atrophy, slow cognitive decline, and reduce the risk of dementia. As was noted in Chapter 3, collectively these factors are believed to help build cognitive reserve.

COGNITIVE INACTIVITY AND RISK OF AD

Researchers at the Rush Alzheimer's Disease Center and Rush-Pres-byterian-St. Luke's Medical Center in Chicago enrolled Catholic clergy, including 700 priests, nuns, and brothers, all 65 years of age or older, in a five-year study. Baseline assessments were conducted, then every year participants were reevaluated using 21 cognitive tests that measured aspects of memory, language, and attention. Daily activities, including reading books, newspapers, and magazines; taking museum trips; or engaging in card games, checkers, or crossword puzzles, were rated with a 1-5 point value system. The frequency with which participants engaged in a particular activity determined the points they were assigned. The most cognitively active were 47 percent less likely to develop Alzheimer's.[981]

In another study, called the Advanced Cognitive Training for Independent and Vital Elderly trial, adults aged 65 and older with no cognitive impairment were given ten sessions of memory training, reasoning training, or processing-speed training.[982] The participants' cognitive skills were significantly improved in all these areas. What is even more impressive is that their improvement persisted a decade after they stopped the training sessions.

At the Carrick Brain Center in Dallas, Texas, what appears to be some degree of brain restoration in Alzheimer's patients has been demonstrated recently by Dr. Andre Fredieu and colleagues.[983] Using a program of specific brain exercises or mental challenges designed to revive both memory and personality, patients have resumed driving and cooking. Some even recognized their grandchildren for the first time in years. The exercises are aimed at improving connectivity between regions of the brain that have deteriorated. In one exercise, called axis rotation, patients are subjected to a variety of full body movements while they sit in a motion-controlled apparatus. The particular movement stimulates the vestibular region of the brain (which relates to our sense of balance and spatial orientation) and seems to reawaken memories in the patients. Another exercise, where the patient focuses attention on a dot while moving his or her head, improved connectivity in regions of the brain that had already deteriorated.

TV does not count as mental stimulation. Researchers followed 3,200 adults aged 18 to 30 for 25 years and recorded their daily television viewing time. After 25 years, the participants were tested for cognitive performance, including memory, processing speed, and executive function. Those who watched four or more hours of TV a day showed significantly poorer cognitive function at midlife.[984] According to the Nielsen organization, the average American watches more than five hours of TV every day.[985] And the more time we spend sitting in front of a TV, the less time we have to exercise.

Quite the opposite of passively watching television, continual mental stimulation through learning increases brain volume. In one study, randomly chosen college students were taught how to juggle. Their brains were scanned before the juggling lessons, three months into the training, and three months after the training ended. Researchers found that several regions of their brains increased in volume three months after they learned this new skill.[986]

Learning new skills seems to increase the number of synapses. Using an electron microscope, a team of scientists at the University of Illinois Beckman Institute for Advanced Science and Technology looked at post-mortem brain tissue samples. The samples were divided into groups according to the amount of education and the professional skills needed for the subject's occupation. Those who had greater levels of education and jobs that required more skills had 17 percent more synapses for each neuron compared to those with the least amount of education and occupations that did not require a high level of skills.[987]

On a recent trip to London, I took a taxi from Heathrow airport. As we approached the city, we encountered substantial traffic. My driver turned off the main route and began taking a dizzying selection of back streets. I asked him if he was using a navigation app that had suggested an alternative route. "Navi ain't my way, mate. I'd rather keep growing the ol' hippocampus than rely on them programs," he explained. I was delighted to hear my driver use the word hippocampus and to learn that he knew its purpose. Although he was not previously aware, I shared with him that in a study conducted prior to the widespread adoption of electronic navigation devices, researchers used functional MRI and PET scans to compare the brains of taxi and bus drivers in London. It turned out that taxi drivers had a significantly larger hippocampus compared to the bus drivers.[988] In addition to its critical role in learning and memory, the hippocampus is also involved in the use of complex spatial information used to navigate. While bus drivers were relegated to a fixed route, learning virtually nothing new about how to navigate their way each day, taxi drivers were constantly driving to new destinations at the direction of their passengers. They also needed to make navigation decisions on the fly based on traffic patterns, time of day, and routes that could change randomly because of construction.

When we learn new things, we set BDNF signaling into action at sites where synapses will develop. This triggers neuron firing in what are called theta rhythms. These rhythms, essential to forming memories, involve numerous neurons firing synchronously up to eight times per second in the hippocampus. Brain researchers believe that theta rhythms weaken as we age. Yet regular stimulation through ongoing learning, as well as the other lifestyle strategies we have discussed, may be able to keep the BDNF signaling and theta rhythms strong and more consistent.

In one study, researchers found that in subjects who engaged in the most frequent mental activity late in life the rate of mental decline was 32 percent lower compared to those who engaged in mental activity only on occasion.[989] After they died, the participants' brains were autopsied. Striking was that even with the presence of Lewy bodies, plaques, and tangles, people who were most mentally active maintained greater protection of their mental prowess, suggesting that the benefit of mental activity was independent of the pathologic features.

Researchers at UC Berkeley have also reported that people who get a high level of mental stimulation produce lower levels of amyloid protein. Using PET scans, the research team looked at the brains of subjects who had no symptoms of dementia. The more mentally active the subjects were over their lifetime, the fewer amyloid plaques were present in their brain scans, suggesting that cognitive activity may help reduce a hallmark pathologic feature of AD.[990]

Lastly, we have known for years that people who retire early are more prone to mental decline and dementia, presumably due to a lack of mental stimulation and social engagement. In 2013, a massive study of 429,000 subjects conducted by Carol Defouil and colleagues at the Bourdeaux School of Public Health was published. The team found that for each year participants put off their retirement, their risk of developing AD was further delayed. For people who waited until age 65, the risk of developing AD was lowered by 14 percent compared to those who retired at age 60, suggesting a 2.8-year delay in cognitive decline for each year we remain engaged with our work.[991]

The general observation is that greater cognitive stimulation is associated with greater brain volume, less plaque deposition, greater glucose metabolism, and lower rates of cognitive decline and dementia.

HOW COGNITIVE STIMULATION IMPROVES BRAIN HEALTH

A prevailing theory about why education, and social and mental activity in general, may provide protection against AD is that the mental stimulation may build cognitive reserve, so that there's more to spare over time. The theory of cognitive reserve has been underscored in a study showing that people who died cognitively intact, with no signs of dementia, often showed AD pathology at the time of brain autopsy. Yet they exhibited no outward symptoms of it.[992] These individuals had greater brain volume and a greater number of large neurons.

Education and mental stimulation also create more elaborate connectivity in the brain. It is not just that the brain may have greater volume, but that there are more synaptic connections between neurons—what's called synaptic density. More neurons to spare and more connectivity promotes greater plasticity, neural reserve, and neural compensation. In the end, this happens because of lifestyle choices.

STRATEGIES FOR COGNITIVE STIMULATION

Cognitive stimulation is clearly valuable in warding off cognitive decline and dementia. For that reason, it's an important part of the Revolution Lifestyle. There are many enjoyable ways to stimulate your brain. Number one on most lists is reading.

I suggest you commit to reading for at least 30 minutes each day. It doesn't matter when or what you read—"just do it."

While reading alone is fine, the experience of reading can take on an added dimension of mental stimulation and provide companionship as well if we join a book club. This gives us the opportunity to meet with others and enjoy social interactions around our reading—even if circumstances require that we do so by way of Zoom! It can be a wonderfully affirming experience to learn that others found books as rewarding or enriching (or annoying) to read as we have, or to gain insights we may have missed that others gleaned from their reading.

If you don't want to engage in discussions about the books you're reading, there's a new movement called Slow Reading Clubs. Folks come together at cafés, bookstores, and other places where there's space to congregate comfortably, then spend an hour sitting quietly together reading their own books. The intention is to have a regularly scheduled weekly gathering where people can read in the company of others. If there is not a Slow Reading Club near you, you can start your own. See Resources for more information.

Another option to encourage and support regular reading is the online reading community found at Goodreads.com. This free website allows users to browse through other users' libraries, see what these readers are currently enjoying (or not) and read their reviews. The site also allows participation in discussion groups and online book clubs.

BILINGUALISM PROVIDES PROTECTION

Neurocognitive studies have shown that people who are bilingual or multilingual have an added advantage when it comes to warding off mental decline. Using functional MRI, which measures brain activity by recording changes in blood flow while subjects perform tasks, we have learned that people who speak two or more languages need to activate less of the brain to accomplish a comparable task performed by a monolingual person.[993] Bilinguals also develop a broader neural network which is more resistant to degeneration; once again they have greater cognitive reserve to resist decline. The result is people who speak two or more languages have been found to delay the onset of Alzheimer's by an average of five years.[994]

Although the exact mechanism by which protection is conferred is unclear, some believe that the action of suppressing one language in order to invoke the other, known as switching, may be a protective mental maneuver. Compared to monolinguals, bilinguals develop a larger inferior parietal cortex region of the brain.[995]

Today there are many ways to learn a new language, including classes at community colleges and free online language instruction websites, such as Duolingo.com. Babbel.com is another popular site, although it does require payment of a fee.

MUSICIANS GROW BIGGER BRAINS

Studying music is a highly stimulating and mentally challenging activity that promotes structural brain changes that appear to contribute to cognitive reserve. There is a significant difference in volume in motor, auditory, and visual-spatial regions of the brain in those who play music professionally (for at least one hour daily) compared with amateur musicians and non-musicians.[996] Brain volume tends to be greatest in professional musicians, intermediate in amateur musicians, and lowest in non-musicians. Studying a musical instrument creates not just more neurons and synapses but greater connectivity as well.

While the greatest benefits may be derived by those who begin studying a musical instrument early in life, there's good reason to believe it's never too late to become a musician and reap the cognitive benefits of doing so. Two years ago I became determined to add music study to my repertoire of strategies to support cognitive health. I couldn't decide whether to learn to play piano or guitar, so I found a professional who could teach me both. In addition to feeling good about the reported structural and cognitive changes in the brain this may afford me, I cannot overstate the degree to which music practice has enriched my life. I highly encourage you to find a way to become musically engaged.

DO ONLINE MEMORY GAMES REALLY WORK?

A growing number of online mental exercise services claim they offer a way to work toward greater brain fitness. Companies such as Lumosity and Neuronation offer online brain-training exercises intended to improve attention, increase brain speed, improve memory, reduce response time, and increase productivity. So far, however, there is insufficient evidence to confirm such outcomes, and some in the scientific community have expressed skepticism that there is much to gain from the exercises other than entertainment value. However, this doesn't mean the claims of brain exercise game manufacturers are without any merit. If some products and services are effective, the challenge is figuring out just which ones are.

One study conducted at the University of California San Francisco showed particularly encouraging outcomes. The study involved participants aged 20 to 85 who trained on a video game called Neuro Racer created by scientists at UCSF.[997] Prior to participants embarking on the training, scientists measured the subjects' degree of cognitive decline. After participants had completed the training, the scientists found an increase in brain-wave activity, which in some senior participants reached levels equivalent to that of untrained 20-year-olds. When given memory and attention tests before and after the training, participants showed they had significantly enhanced cognitive function. Compared with the control group, participants who trained using the game improved in multitasking skills and memory function after 12 hours of training over a one-month period. Even when tested six months after the study had been completed, seniors who had participated in the training retained their improvements in cognitive function, suggesting that the game training led to a reversal in their decline. Neuro Racer is now available in app stores. If you choose to use this program note that the improvements noted above were seen after three one-hour play sessions per week over four weeks.

In the Advanced Training in Vital Elderly study, the largest cognitive training study conducted to date by the National Institutes of Health, participants saw a remarkable benefit. With a focus on what is referred to as speed-of-processing, 2,802 dementia-free individuals with an average age of 74 played a video game called Double Decision. They were presented with a screen that had a central object as well as an object that they would see in their peripheral vision. For example, they might see a car in the center of the screen and a road sign in the periphery. As the game advanced, less time was provided to identify both objects and distracting elements were also introduced. Over the course of the initial six weeks, some participants received up to ten training sessions lasting 75 minutes each. Controls received no training. Each participant was followed for ten years, with four training "booster" sessions at 11 months and again at 35 months, with cognitive testing and functional assessments performed at years 1, 2, 3, 5, and 10. The researchers found a significant dose-response benefit. The more training sessions one completed, the better their cognitive health when tested. Those who completed the most sessions had a 29 percent reduction in risk of developing dementia over a ten-year period.[998] A similar type of training is available by subscription on the internet at BrainHQ.com

HOW TO BECOME A MEMORY OLYMPIAD

For the past 20 years, competitors known as "mental athletes"—some in their 70s—have gathered for the USA Memory Championship, a memory Olympics event for those with exceptional recall skills. Some events include reciting a list of 300 words in a particular order or recounting 40 pieces of biographical information from four people introduced to the athletes on stage. While some observers have explained these individuals' abilities as resulting from photographic memories and the like, it turns out that these athletes are no different than most of us. Virtually anyone can train their own mind to do the same "tricks."

The secret these mental Olympians use is an ancient mnemonic technique called *method of loci training*. *Loci* is the plural of *locus*, or location. Used by the ancient Romans and Greeks, the strategy involves linking things you wish to learn or remember with places you know well, such as your home or another location.

In a study with subjects who were trained to use this technique, remarkable improvements in memory were achieved and sustained four months after the training stopped. The subjects spent 30 minutes a day practicing over a six-week period. At the beginning of the study, they could recall an average 26 of 72 words presented to them. By the end of the study, the subjects recalled 62 of 72 words.[999]

Many mnemonic training devices are available on the Internet, including the popular Memoriad.com. Or check out the online Boot Camp for the Brain curriculum, seven two-hour modules developed by the administrators of the USA Memory Championship.

BREAKING THE MONOTONY

It's easy to slip into an autopilot lifestyle in which our daily activities become repetitive. We drive the same routes, socialize with the same people, eat the same foods, and hold the same general perspective. This may feel comfortable, but the lack of novel experiences and the brain stimulation those kinds of experiences bring may lead to a degree of brain laziness. There's evidence that novelty is helpful to maintaining cognitive function.[1000]

Simply changing the route that we drive home (without the assistance of GPS) can shake things up, because it requires more engagement and exposes us to different stimuli. We have all had the experience of suddenly being unable to account for a stretch of time during a drive. Most often this happens when we are traveling a familiar route—perhaps one by which we commute each day. This activity is so familiar, it has entered the domain called semantic memory, where we store general facts about our environment and the world. When we take a different route through an unfamiliar area, we activate the hippocampus in ways that enable us to reorient ourselves to a new spatial layout and to form new topographical memories.[1001] We become like the cab drivers mentioned above, figuring out our place and direction in the world anew. We do this by noting new landmarks and spatial relations between those landmarks. This may develop new synapse connections in our brains and enhance the overall communication between brain cells. New experiences also trigger the release of the neurotransmitter dopamine, which is involved in focus and attention, securing memories in the brain, and motivation.

If we rely on GPS navigation devices to lead us through unfamiliar territory, we may be less conscious of these landmarks and spatial relations, and thus forego some degree of important brain stimulation. Consider turning GPS off and plotting a new route the old-fashioned way.

ART APPRECIATION AND CREATION

Visiting a museum at least once a month and signing up for docent-led tours can expose us to new facts and historical insights, stimulate our minds, and even inspire us. A welcome benefit is that after just 30 minutes of exposure to art one finds pleasant, cortisol levels are lowered markedly.[1002] We have seen earlier that this "stress hormone" promotes inflammatory agents, impairs memory, and shrinks dendrites. Keeping cortisol levels lower is critical to brain health.

While viewing paintings and other forms of art stimulates multiple regions of the brain, creating our own works of art can be of even greater benefit. In a study in which half the participants viewed and were engaged in discussions about it and the other half produced their own artwork, those who produced art enjoyed even greater cognitive enhancement.[1003] Using MRI technology, the brains of both groups were scanned at the beginning and end of a ten-week program. Those who created art developed greater connectivity in their brains, probably since they employed both cognitive and motor processing in their creative process.

LISTENING TO LECTURES

Another way to engage our minds actively is by attending lectures, either in person or online. Attending a talk can be mentally stimulating in multiple ways, while having the added benefit of social interaction. TED talks offer a vast and continually growing archive of stimulating lectures accessible by TV, computer, or tablet. Topics range from science to politics, social change to religion, inventions to foreign policy. Each month new lectures from leading thinkers of all cultures around the world are added to the video library. TED talks are a regular part of my own ongoing education effort, and not just for the purpose of keeping my cortisol level down.

There are so many wonderful ways that we can stimulate the mind, strengthen neurological connections, and develop protective cognitive reserve. Doing so not only helps protect us from dementia, but at the same time enriches our life experience with pleasure, new insights, and knowledge. What new strategies will you adopt to keep your mind active?

34

BUILDING COMMUNITY

Building and maintaining robust social connections is another important part of the Revolution Lifestyle for reducing the risk of AD.

By studying the brains of people who have been imprisoned, especially those who have been placed in solitary confinement, we have learned that social isolation can be profoundly detrimental and lead to neurological damage. Writing about such studies in the *New Yorker*, bestselling author and physician Atul Gawande, M.D. states, "Without sustained social interaction, the human brain may become as impaired as one that has incurred a traumatic injury." [1004]

Humans are hard-wired for a sense of community and meaningful connection with others. We thrive when we feel a connection with others. When we connect with others, we are more likely to remain mentally sharp and free of depression and anxiety, and also more likely to ward off physical illness and to reduce or eliminate conditions that give rise to illness, such as inflammation.

In Okinawa, one of the Blue Zone regions where the most long-lived and healthy people reside, residents practice a tradition called "moai," which refers to a healthy social support network. Individuals who are part of these social circles, which meet regularly, talk together about their lives, have shared experiences, offer one another advice, and assist each other in other ways, even including financial support in times of need. Traditionally, one's moai is consciously developed in childhood, and they often last for a lifetime. Some residents belong to more than one moai.

Many large studies affirm the health benefits of such social safety nets. They show us that people with extensive social networks who remain socially engaged see a reduction in risk of cognitive decline. In one study of 6,000 participants followed over a five-year period, individuals who had strong social networks enjoyed a 39 percent reduction in their risk of cognitive decline, while those who were most socially engaged saw a 91 percent reduction during the study period.[1005] It is one thing to know that you have a network of friends, but much more beneficial to engage with them frequently.

Despite the advent of Facebook, Twitter, Instagram, Nextdoor, and other forms of social media, we who live in Western countries are lonelier than ever. In a 2012 national survey some 20 to 40 percent of older adults in the US said they felt lonely, and five to seven percent reported feeling intense and persistent feelings of loneliness. [1006] The problem seems to be worsening. By 2018, a survey of 20,000 Americans conducted by Cigna Health found almost half reported they did not have meaningful interactions with family or friends on a daily basis, and 43 percent characterized their friendships as weak and experienced feelings of isolation. Fifty-four percent said that they sometimes or always feel that no one knows them well.[1007] This is not just sad, but harmful to one's well-being. People who feel isolated, left out, and lack companionship experience a more rapid rate of functional decline and they have a greater risk of mortality. In a meta-analysis that examined the results of 148 previous studies, the authors found that compared to those who are least socially connected, people who have the strongest social relationships, regardless of gender, age, or initial health status, have a 50 percent greater chance of survival. Individuals who lack significant social relationships also tend to have more major medical risk factors.[1008] Social isolation is linked to heart disease, high blood pressure, and depression, all of which are independent risk factors for AD.[1009]

When we form and sustain strong social bonds, our body produces more of the two neuropeptides, oxytocin and vasopressin. Oxytocin increases immune function, reduces recovery time from illness, reduces feelings of stress, and cuts the risk of depression. Vasopressin enhances memory and information processing and reduces anxiety.

GROUPS OF LIKE-MINDED PEOPLE

These days it's easier than ever to form friendships with like-minded individuals online, but we should also try to bring those connections to the real world. An easy way to make social connections and build community is to tap into the Meetup.com service online. Meetup groups provide a wonderfully effective way to find others in your community who enjoy the things that you do and who are also looking to make connections and build community around a hobby or activity. Another way to connect with others and find people with shared interests is to join your neighborhood Nextdoor social networking service at Nextdoor.com

VOLUNTEERING

Another option for enhancing social connections is to look for volunteer opportunities, whether at a local school, library, or nonprofit.

There are countless opportunities to offer support to those in need. Some volunteer opportunities send the adventuresome to a school in Nepal for a few months. A double-whammy experience awaits: learning through exposure to a new culture while you form community. Volunteermatch.com is a site that can assist with securing a rewarding volunteer position in your community.

By making human connection a top priority, you will not only be rewarded with a richer and more enjoyable life, but you will also help keep your brain in the best possible shape. Here's to a happy, healthful lifestyle that protects you and your family.

AFTERWORD

Alzheimer's is a uniquely devastating disease. The social, emotional, and economic costs associated with a diagnosis, for both patients and their families, are substantial. Added to these costs is the tendency for caregivers supporting Alzheimer's patients to experience anxiety, depression, and burnout.

The greatest tragedy related to the disease, however, is that we have allowed it to run rampant while ignoring prevention and giving too much attention to drug treatments that have repeatedly shown little or no benefit. As a society we have failed to do all that we can to dramatically reduce the chance that many of us will become victims of Alzheimer's.

Many citations in this book reference research that underscores the promise of lifestyle changes that can preserve cognitive health and prevent the onset of Alzheimer's. Yet most Americans—and too many in the medical community—aren't aware that there are modifiable risk factors that can lower their risk.[1010] That shouldn't be the case.

If this lack of awareness persists, the prognosis is bleak. We can expect a future with state and federal budgets significantly overburdened and nursing homes inundated with AD patients. There will be escalating costs to businesses dealing with lost productivity, the healthcare system will be overwhelmed, and Medicare may well go bankrupt. AD is also giving rise to a secondary population of victims—those millions of unpaid caregivers who themselves are traumatized by the experience of providing care under such discouraging circumstances and who develop illnesses as a result of the overwhelming stress they endure.

Currently, only three percent of Americans meet the four basic public health recommendations to ward off chronic disease, including neurological disease. These are consuming five or more servings of fruits and vegetables a day, not smoking, participating in 30 minutes of physical activity five times a week, and maintaining a healthy bodyweight.[1011]

Yet surveys show that people *do* want to know what they can do to protect their cognitive health.[1012] To reduce the development of new AD cases substantially, we must do a much better job of conveying the importance and effectiveness of lifestyle risk reduction strategies to the public—and the sooner in life these strategies are implemented, the better. Because pathological changes in the brain may begin in midlife before symptoms become apparent, for the best chance at prevention we should be getting the word out to people in their fifties and forties, and perhaps even younger.

Our best investment would be a public education campaign at the local, state, and federal levels aimed at changing the way Americans think about cognitive health. This would involve giving Americans the knowledge they need to make truly effective and protective lifestyle choices both for themselves and for the next generation.

In 2000, childhood lead poisoning was widespread, and constituted a significant public health burden costing society billions of dollars. A public health education campaign fostered a major jump in awareness of the problem, and the number of states with lead poisoning prevention laws on the books rose from just five prior to the campaign to 23 in 2010. The percentage of kids aged one to five whose blood lead level exceeded 10 μg/dL (micrograms per deciliter) was slashed from 88.2 percent in 2000 to 0.9 percent by 2008, and billions of dollars in healthcare costs related to lead exposure are now saved annually as a result.[1013] Whenever we have committed ourselves to affecting positive change through a public education campaign and encouraged action by lawmakers, impressive results have followed.

A blueprint for such a campaign to address Alzheimer's disease could include the following:

- Use of social media, TV, radio, and movie theater previews to publicize the latest findings about risk factors and how we can take steps to protect our cognitive health. Public health and safety campaigns of this type have been quite successful in the past. Examples include Mothers Against Drunk Driving, the Tobacco-Free America initiative, and others encouraging the use of seat belts or breastfeeding, and promoting HIV awareness. Each has contributed to changing behavior and the way we think about these health and safety issues.

- Continuing education and targeted campaigns directed at healthcare professionals to ensure that the medical community is aware of the latest scientific findings about lifestyle and the risk for AD.

- Incentivizing the healthcare community to disseminate information about important lifestyle choices that lower risk.

- Persuading state and federal lawmakers to appropriate significant funds for AD prevention research and education efforts focused on lifestyle, diet, and environmental factors.

- Encouraging health insurance providers to incentivize the adoption of science-based risk-reduction strategies on the part of their customers by offering discounts in return for changes in behavior that promote cognitive health.

- Ban neurotoxic chemicals currently used in agriculture and in schools, parks, and homes, and encourage chemical manufacturers through tax and other incentives to develop safer products.

- Require industry-funded and federally managed comprehensive neurotoxicology tests to be performed before any additional pesticides receive approval. Remove from the marketplace all pesticides that were granted regulatory approval in the absence of adequate neurotoxicology testing.

- Levy additional taxes on alcohol and cigarettes, as well as on large industrial polluters, to fund community-based public health programs and education centers that promote physical activity, social interaction, and awareness of other key lifestyle strategies for cognitive health and the prevention of AD.

It makes sense to do all of these things.

Because dietary and other lifestyle strategies that promote cognitive health also promote vascular health and reduce the risk for heart disease, stroke, diabetes, hypertension, obesity, osteoporosis, and depression, we can expect a substantial additional dividend in the form of a lower overall healthcare cost burden to society.

In 2011 Congress approved the National Alzheimer's Project Act (NAPA), which among other things called for an acceleration of the development of treatments that would "prevent, halt, or reverse the course of Alzheimer's." One sponsor of the bill was Representative Christopher H. Smith of New Jersey, who likened the bill to a declaration of "war on a dreaded disease." The language reminded me of the National Cancer Act, which was signed into law back in 1971 by President Richard Nixon. The president said the act amounted to a "war on cancer." Yet 45 years and $500 billion later, the death rate from cancer has changed only marginally and the incidence of breast and prostate cancer is now higher than ever before, striking one in eight and one in seven Americans respectively. Unfortunately, cancer remains the number two killer in the USA, the same as in 1971. One of the reasons why the National Cancer Act has had so little impact is that, like much of the Alzheimer's research that has been conducted so far, it largely focused on a cure while paying little attention to addressing the controllable causes of the disease.

The campaign to educate America about how to protect cognitive health must do better, and must begin to do so immediately. We can't afford to lose 45 years when it comes to Alzheimer's.

Ironically, NAPA calls for preventive treatments to be developed within the next 25 years. Why take so long? We already know what actions to take to reduce the incidence of Alzheimer's. As I've shown in this book, we have the information we need to take meaningful and effective steps that will reduce the incidence of Alzheimer's disease. Let's get serious about our commitment to take those steps.

ACKNOWLEDGMENTS

Thank you to the team at Hatherleigh Press for their terrific support. Thank you to my outstanding editor, Alison Owings, for her support and friendship. Special thanks to Jon Harrison for his editorial assistance and proofreading of the manuscript. Thanks also to Allison Hall for reviewing the manuscript. Special thanks to Beth Gonzales for reviewing the manuscript and offering valuable insights. I'm grateful to Laurent Valosek for sharing his insights about transcendental meditation and some of the TM research that is discussed in this book, and for being an inspiration to those seeking wellness through the practice of meditation. I'm grateful to Dr. Susanna Rosi for sharing her insights and remarkable research on traumatic brain injury. Thank you to Hootan Roozrokh, MD for his advisory role and friendship. I'm deeply grateful to Farrokh Farrokhi, MD for making the time to review the neuroscience. Finally, thank you to my agent, Katherine Boyle, who believed in this project and found it a good home.

RESOURCES

A list of resources, helpful products and informative reference material beneficial to better understanding, preventing and/or treating Alzheimer's disease can be found on the author's website at: www.josephkeon.com

ENDNOTES

1. Aune, D., et al., "Dairy products, calcium, and prostate cancer risk: a systematic review and meta-analysis of cohort studies," *American Journal of Clinical Nutrition* 101 (2015):87-117.

2. *The Fort Wayne Sentinel* "Edison Hails Era of Speed," 31 December 1902 (p. 49).

3. Rocca, Walter A., et al., "Risk of Cognitive Impairment or Dementia in Relatives of Patients with Parkinson Disease," *Archives of Neurology* 64 (2007):1458-64.

4. Pritchard, Colin, et al., "Neurological deaths of American adults (55–74) and the over 75's by sex compared with 20 Western countries 1989–2010: Cause for concern," *Surgical Neurology International* 6 (2015), published online July 2015: http://www.ncbi. nlm.nih.gov/pmc/articles/PMC4521226/; Pritchard, C., et al., "Changing patterns of neurological mortality in the 10 major developed countries—1979–2010," *Public Health*, accessed online, Apr. 2013: http://www.ncbi.nlm.nih.gov/pubmed/23601790.

5. Rizzi, Liara, et al., "Global Epidemiology of Dementia: Alzheimer's and Vascular Types," *BioMed Research International* 2014 (2014):908-915.

6. Pritchard, C., et al., "Changing patterns of neurological mortality in the 10 major developed countries--1979-2010," *Public Health* 127 (2013):357-68; Pritchard, Colin, et al., "Neurological deaths of American adults (55–74) and the over 75's by sex compared with 20 Western countries 1989–2010: Cause for concern," *Surgical Neurology International* 6 (2015):123. 10.4103/2152-7806.161420

7. The Young Dementia Network has merged with DementiaUK. www.dementiauk. org/the-young-dementia-network/

8. "Early-onset dementia and Alzheimer's diagnoses spiked 373 percent for generation X and millennials," Blue Cross Blue Shield Association, February 27, 2020; "Early-onset Alzheimer's rates grow for younger American adults," February 27, 2020.

9. Hebert, L. E, et al., "Alzheimer disease in the United States (2010–2050) estimated using the 2010 census," *Neurology* 80 (2013):1778–83; James, B.D., et al., "Contribution of Alzheimer disease to mortality in the United States," *Neurology* 82 (2014):1045-50.

10. "Alzheimer's incidence accelerates among the oldest old," in Proceedings of the Alzheimer's Association International Conference on Alzheimer's Disease (ICAD '09), Vienna, Austria, 2009, http://www.medpagetoday.com/MeetingCoverage/ICAD/ 15075.

11. Belluck, Pam, "Dementia care cost is projected to double by 2040," *New York Times* April 3, 2013.

12. Hurd, Michael D., et al., "Monetary costs of dementia in the United States," *New England Journal of Medicine 368* (2013):1326–34.

13. Carlton, Lindsey, "Could Alzheimer's really bankrupt Medicare and Medicaid?" *FOX News*, March 1, 2017.

14. Alzheimer's Association, "New Alzheimer's Association report examines racial and ethnic attitudes on Alzheimer's and dementia care," March 2, 2021.

15. Youssef H. El-Hayek et al. Tip of the Iceberg: Assessing the Global Socioeconomic Costs of Alzheimer's Disease and Related Dementias and Strategic Implications for Stakeholders, *Journal of Alzheimer's Disease* (2019). DOI: 10.3233/JAD-190426; "Costs of Alzheimer's to Medicare and Medicaid, Alzheimer's Association, March 2017; http://www.who.int/mental_health/neurology/chapter_3_a_neuro_disorders_public_h_challenges.pdf.

16. Belluck, Pam, "Dementia care costs is projected to double by 2040," *New York Times*, Apr. 3, 2013; Herbert, L. E., et al., "Alzheimer's disease in the United States (2010–2050) estimated using the 2010 census," *Neurology*, Feb. 6, 2013.

17. Caminiti, Susan, "A disease on track to bankrupt Medicare," CNBC.com, Nov. 10, 2015. http://www.cnbc.com/2015/11/09/a-disease-on-track-to-bankrupt-medicare.html, accessed online, Mar. 27, 2016.

18. Primary Care Physicians on the Front Lines of Diagnosing and Providing Alzheimer's and Dementia Care: Half Say Medical Profession Not Prepared to Meet Expected Increase in Demands," *Alzheimer's & Dementia: The Journal of the Alzheimer's Association* 16 (2020). Alz.org/facts

19. McCurry, Justin, "Dementia towns: how Japan is evolving for its ageing population." *The Guardian* January 14, 2018; "Japan's dementia crisis hits record levels as thousands go missing," *The Guardian* June 16, 2016; Ross, Eleanor, "Aging Japan Faces Rising Dementia and Caregivers Shortage," *Newsweek* June 6, 2017.

20. Burke, Maria, "Why Alzheimer's drugs keep failing," *Scientific American* July 14, 2014.

21. Bailey, Melissa, "Billions spent, but cure for Alzheimer's remains elusive," Kaiser Health News February 6, 2017. http://www.denverpost.com/2017/02/06/alzheimers-cure-elusive/

22. Dockrill, Peter, "One of World's Biggest Drug Companies Just Abandoned Alzheimer's And Parkinson's Research," *Science Alert* January 9, 2018

23. Bach, Peter B. and Redberg, Rita F., "Medicare needs to test the new Alzheimer's drug before paying," *Bloomberg* January 3, 2022. https://www.bloomberg.com/opinion/articles/2022-01-03/medicare-needs-to-test-the-new-alzheimer-s-drug-aduhelm-before-paying

24. Belluck, Pam, "Biogen slashes price of Alzheimer's drug Aduhelm, as it faces obstacles," *New York Times* December 20, 2021. https://www.nytimes.com/2021/12/20/health/alzheimers-aduhelm-price.html

25. Munro, Dan, "U.S. healthcare ranked dead last compared to 10 other countries," *Forbes* June 16, 2014; Khazan, Olga, "U.S. healthcare: Most expensive and worst performing," *The Atlantic* June 16, 2014.

26. Caminiti, Susan, "A disease on track to bankrupt Medicare," CNBC.com, Nov. 10, 2015. http://www.cnbc.com/2015/11/09/a-disease-on-track-to-bankrupt-medicare.html, accessed online, Mar. 27, 2016.

27. Barnes, Deborah E., "The projected impact of risk factor reduction on Alzheimer's disease prevalence," *Lancet Neurology* 10 (2011):819-28.

28. Ibid.

29. "Lifestyle interventions provide maximum memory benefit when combined, may offset elevated Alzheimer's risk due to genetics, pollution," Presented at the Alzheimer's Association International Conference, July 14, 2019.

30. Isaacson, Richard S., et al., "Individualized clinical management of patients at risk for Alzheimer's dementia," *Alzheimer's and Dementia* (2019): DOI: https://doi.org/10.1016/j.jalz.2019.08.198

31. Kivipelto, Miia, et al., "A 2 year multidomain intervention of diet, exercise, cognitive training, and vascular risk monitoring versus control to prevent cognitive decline in at-risk elderly people (FINGER): A randomized controlled trial," *The Lancet* 385 (2015). DOI: 10.1016/S0140-6736(15)60461-5

32. Grossman, David, "We can prevent dementia," Karolinska University Hospital. May 4, 2017.

33. Xureui, Jin, et al., "Association of *APOE* ε4 genotype and lifestyle with cognitive function among Chinese adults aged 80 years and older: A cross-sectional study," *PLoS Medicine* (2021). Doi.org/10.1371/journal.pmed.1003597

34. Hippius, Hans, "The discovery of Alzheimer's disease," *Dialogues in Clinical Neuroscience* 5 (2003):101-8.

35. Ibid.

36. Shaffer, Joyce, "Neuroplasticity and clinical practice: building brain power for health," *Frontiers in Psychology* 7 (2016):1118: doi: 10.3389/fpsyg.2016.01118

37. Sorells, Shawn F., et al., "Human hippocampal neurogenesis drops sharply in children to undetectable levels in adults," *Nature* 555 (2018):377; Frisen, Jonas, et al., "Dynamics of hippocampal neurogenesis in adult humans," *Cell* 153 (2013):1219-1227; Alvarez-Buylla, A., et al., "Identification of neural stem cells in the adult vertebrate brain," *Brain Research Bulletin* 57 (2002):751–758; Gould, E., "How widespread is adult neurogenesis in mammals?," *Nature Reviews Neuroscience* 8 (2008):481–88; Eriksson, Peter S., et al., "Neurogenesis in the adult human hippocampus," *Nature Medicine* 4 (1998):3113–17; Gould, Elizabeth, et al., "Neurogenesis in the Neocortex of Adult Primates," *Science* 286 (1999):548–52.

38. Christian, K.M., et al., "Functions and dysfunctions of adult hippocampal neurogenesis," *Annual Reviews in Neuroscience* 37 (2014):243–262.

39. Spalding, K.L., et al., "Dynamics of hippocampal neurogenesis in adult humans," *Cell* 153 (2017):1219–1227.

40. Moreno-Jiménez, E.P., et al., "Evidences for Adult Hippocampal Neurogenesis in Humans," *Journal of Neuroscience* 41 (2021):2541-2553. doi:10.1523/JNEUROSCI.0675-20.2020

41. Moreno-Jiménez, E.P., "Evidences for Adult Hippocampal Neurogenesis in Humans," *Journal of Neuroscience* 41 (2021):2541-2553. doi: 10.1523/JNEUROSCI.0675-20.2020. PMID: 33762406; PMCID: PMC8018741.

42. Salk Institute. "Memory capacity of brain is 10 times more than previously thought." *ScienceDaily* 20 January 2016; www.sciencedaily.com/releases/2016/01/160120201224.htm

43. Zimmer, Carl, "100 trillion connections: new efforts probe and map the brain's detailed architecture," *Scientific American* January 2011: https://www.scientificamerican.com/article/100-trillion-connections/

44. R. M. Koffie, et al., "Alzheimer's disease: synapses gone cold," *Molecular Neurodegeneration* 6 (2011):63.

45. Peters, R., Ageing and the brain," *Postgraduate Medicine* Journal 82 (2006):84-88.

46. Strauss, Neil, "Kris Kristofferson: An Outlaw at 80," *Rolling Stone* June 6, 2016.

47. Wolkowitz, O.M, et al., "Glucocorticoid medication, memory and Steroid Psychosis in medical illness," *Annals of the New York Academy of Science* 823 (1997):81-96.

48. Clare, Ryan, et al., "Synapse loss in dementias," *Journal of Neuroscience Research* 88 (2010):2083-2090.

49. Mitchell, A.J, et al., "Rate of progression of mild cognitive impairment to dementia: Meta-analysis of 41 robust inception cohort studies," *Acta Psychiatrica Scandinavica* 119 (2019):252-65.

50. Sweeney, Patrick et al., "Protein misfolding in neurodegenerative diseases: implications and strategies," *Translational Neurodegeneration* 66 (2017): doi:10.1186/s40035-017-0077-5

51. "Clearing amyloid beta from brain," Biomed Radio, Washington University School of Medicine in St. Louis, December 9, 2010. https://medicine.wustl.edu/news/podcast/clearing-amyloid-beta-from-brain/

52. O'brien, J.T., et al., "18F-FDG PET and perfusion SPECT in the diagnosis of Alzheimer and Lewy body dementias," *Journal of Nuclear Medicine* 55 (2014):1959-65.

53. Baker-Nigh, Alaina, et al., "Neuronal amyloid-β accumulation within cholinergic basal forebrain in ageing and Alzheimer's disease," *Brain* 138 (2015):1722-3; Bailey, Melissa, "Billions spent, but cure for Alzheimer's remains elusive," *Kaiser Health News* February 6, 2017.

54. Goedert, M., et al., "A century of Alzheimer's disease," *Science* 314 (2006):777–81.

55. Ising, Christina, et al., "NLRP3 inflammasome activation drives tau pathology," Nature (2019): doi:10.1038/s41586-019-1769-z.

56. Smith, Ruben, et al., "The accumulation rate of tau aggregates is higher in females and younger individuals," *Alzheimer's & Dementia* 16 (2020) https://doi.org/10.1002/alz.043876

57. Stern, Yaakov, "Cognitive reserve in ageing and Alzheimer's disease," *Lancet Neurology* 11 (2012):1006-1012; Schofield, P.W., et al., "An association between head circumference and Alzheimer's disease in a population-based study of aging," *Neurology* 49 (1997):30–37.

58. Katzman, R., et al., "Clinical, pathological, and neurochemical changes in dementia: a subgroup with preserved mental status and numerous neocortical plaques," *Annals of Neurology* 23 (1988):138-44.

59. Devasagayam, T. P. A. et al., "Free radicals and antioxidants in human health: Current status and future prospects," *Journal of Association of Physicians of India* 52 (2004):796.

60. Weiss RF, Fintelmann V., *Herbal Medicine* (Stuttgart: Thieme; 2000). pp. 3–20.

61. Stefanis, L., et al., "Apoptosis in neurodegenerative disorders," *Current Opinions Neurology* 10 (1997):299–305.

62. Feng, Ye, et al., "Antioxidant therapies for Alzheimer's disease," *Oxidative Medicine and Cellular Longevity 2012* (2012) Article ID 472932; https://www.hindawi.com/journals/omcl/2012/472932/#B27

63. Nunomura, A., et al., "RNA oxidation is a prominent feature of vulnerable neurons in Alzheimer's disease," *Journal of Neuroscience* 19 (1999):1959–64; Mecocci, P., et al., "Oxidative damage to mitochondrial DNA is increased in Alzheimer's disease," *Annals of Neurology* 36 (1994):747–51; Praticò, D., et al., "Lipid peroxidation and oxidative imbalance: Early functional events in Alzheimer's disease," *Journal of Alzheimer's Disease* 6 (2004):171–75; Feng, Ye, et al., "Antioxidant therapies for Alzheimer's disease," *Oxidative Medicine and Cellular Longevity 2012* (2012) Article ID 472932; https://www.hindawi.com/journals/omcl/2012/472932/#B27

64. Zhao, Yan, et al., "Oxidative stress and the pathogenesis of Alzheimer's disease," *Oxidative Medicine and Cellular Longevity* 2013 (2013):1–10.

65. Guglielmotto, Michela, et al., "Oxidative stress mediates the pathogenic effect of different Alzheimer's disease risk factors," *Frontiers in Aging and Neuroscience* 2 (2010):3.

66. Adibhatia, R. M., et al., "Lipid oxidation and peroxidation in CNS health and disease: From molecular mechanisms to therapeutic opportunities," *Antioxidant Redox Signal* 12 (2010):125–69.

67. Aschbacher, Kristin, et al., "Good Stress, Bad Stress and Oxidative Stress: Insights from Anticipatory Cortisol Reactivity," *Psychoneuroimmunology* 38 (2013):1698-1708.

68. Collins, T., "Acute and chronic inflammation," in Robbins Pathologic Basis of Disease, R. S. Cotran, V. Kumar, and T. Collins, Eds., pp. 50–88, (W.B. Saunders, Philadelphia, Pa, USA, 1999); Mrak, R.E., et al., "Glia and their cytokines in progression of neurodegeneration," *Neurobiology of Aging* 26 (2005):349–354.

69. Schmidt, R., et al., "Early inflammation and dementia: A 25-year follow-up of the Honolulu-Asia Aging Study," *Annals of Neurology* 59 (2002):168–74; Yaffe, K., et al., "Inflammatory markers and cognition in well-functioning African-American and white elders," *Neurology* 61 (2003):76–80; Dik, M. G., et al., "Serum inflammatory proteins and cognitive decline in older persons," *Neurology* 64 (2005):1371–77; Tan, Z. S., et al., Inflammatory markers and the risk of Alzheimer's disease: The Framingham Study," *Neurology* 68 (2007):1902–8; Rafnsson, S. B., et al., "Cognitive decline and markers of inflammation and homeostasis: the Edinburgh artery study," *Journal of the American Geriatric Society* 55 (2007):708–16; Because we can't see inflammation inside the body, we look for markers of inflammation in blood tests. Two such markers are c-reactive protein (CRP) and white blood cells.

70. Simen, Arthur, et al., "Cognitive dysfunction with aging and the role of inflammation," *Therapeutic Advances in Chronic Disease* 2 (2011):175-95.

71. McGeer, P. L. et al., "The inflammatory response system of brain: implications for therapy of Alzheimer and other neurodegenerative diseases," *Brain Research Reviews* 21 (1995):195–218.

72. Hoozemans J.J., et al., "Maximal COX-2 and ppRb expression in neurons occurs during early Braak stages prior to the maximal activation of astrocytes and microglia in Alzheimer's disease," *Journal of Neuroinflammation* 2 (2005):27.

73.   Craft, J. M., et al., "Human amyloid beta-induced neuroinflammation is an early event in neurodegeneration," *Glia* 53 (2006):484–90; Venegas, Carmen, et al., "Microglia-derived ASC specks cross-seed amyloid-β in Alzheimer's disease," *Nature* 552 (2017): 355 DOI: 10.1038/nature25158

74.   Walker, Keenan A., et al., "Midlife systemic inflammatory markers are associated with late-life brain volume: The ARIC study," *Neurology* 89 (2017): DOI.org/10.1212/WNL.0000000000004688

75.   Yaffe, K., et al., "The metabolic syndrome, inflammation, and risk of cognitive decline," *JAMA* 292 (2004):2237–2242.

76.   Leung, Rufina, et al., "Inflammatory Proteins in Plasma Are Associated with Severity of Alzheimer's Disease," *PLoS ONE* 8 (2013): e64971.

77.   Dietrich, M., et al., "The effect of weight loss on a stable biomarker of inflammation, C-reactive protein," *Nutrition Reviews* 2005; *63*: 22–28.

78.   Brown, G.C., et al., "Inflammatory neurodegeneration and mechanisms of microglial killing of neurons," *Molecular Neurobiology* 41 (2010):242-7: Brown, Guy, et al., "How microglia kill neurons," *Bain Research* 1628 (2015):288-97

        Emerit, J., et al., "Neurodegenerative diseases and oxidative stress," *Biomedicine & Pharmacotherapy* 58 (2004):9–46.

79.   Zimmer, Eduardo Rigon, et al., "Tracking neuroinflammation in Alzheimer's disease: the role of positron emission tomography imaging," *Journal of Neuroinflammation* 11 (2014); published online at: https://www.ncbi.nlm.nih.gov/pmc/articles/PMC4099095/

80.   Wirtz, P.H., et al., "Psychological stress, inflammation, and coronary heart disease," *Current Cardiology Reports* 19 (2017):111.

81.   Bourassa, M.W., et al., "Butyrate, neuroepigenetics and the gut microbiome: Can a high fiber diet improve brain health?" *Neuroscience Letters* 625 (2016):56-63; Matt, Stephanie, M., et al., "Butyrate and Dietary Soluble Fiber Improve Neuroinflammation Associated with Aging in Mice," *Frontiers in Immunology* (2018): doi: 10.3389/fimmu.2018.01832

82.   Lopez-Garcia, E., et al., "Major dietary patterns are related to plasma concentrations of markers of inflammation and endothelial dysfunction," *American Journal of Clinical Nutrition* 80 (2006):1029; Nettleton, J.A., et al., "Dietary patterns are associated with biochemical markers of inflammation and endothelial activation in the Multi-Ethnic Study of Atherosclerosis (MESA)," *American Journal of Clinical Nutrition* 83 (2006):1369; Esmaillzadeh, A., et al., "Fruit and vegetable intakes, C-reactive protein, and the metabolic syndrome," *American Journal of Clinical Nutrition* 84 (2006):1489; Salas-Salvad, J., et al., "Components of the mediterranean-type food pattern and serum inflammatory markers among patients at high risk for cardiovascular disease," *European Journal of Clinical Nutrition* 62 (2008):651; Nanri, A., et al., "Dietary patterns and C-reactive protein in Japanese men and women," *American Journal of Clinical Nutrition* 87 (2008):1488.

83.   Azadbakht, Leila, et al., "Red Meat Intake Is Associated with Metabolic Syndrome and Plasma C-Reactive Protein Concentrations in Women," *Journal of Nutrition* 139 (2008):335-9; Erridge, C., "The capacity of foodstuffs to induce innate immune activation of human monocytes in vitro is dependent on food content of stimulants of Toll-like receptors 2 and 4," *British Journal of Nutrition* 105 (2011):15–23; Yu, B.,

et al., "Lipopolysaccharide binding protein and soluble CD14 catalyze exchange of phospholipids," *Journal of Clinical Investigation* 99 (1997):315–24.

84. Spencer, Sarah, J., et al., "Food for thought: how nutrition impacts cognition and emotion," *Science of Food* 7 (2017): doi:10.1038/s41538-017-0008-y

85. Jenkins, D.J., et al., "Effects of a dietary portfolio of cholesterol-lowering foods vs lovastatin on serum lipids and C-reactive protein," *JAMA* 290 (2003):502-10.

86. Zheng, G, et al., "Effect of Aerobic Exercise on Inflammatory Markers in Healthy Middle-Aged and Older Adults: A Systematic Review and Meta-Analysis of Randomized Controlled Trials," *Frontiers in Aging and Neuroscience* 11 (2019):98. doi:10.3389/fnagi.2019.00098

87. Dimitrov, Stoyan, et al., "Inflammation and exercise: Inhibition of monocytic intracellular TNF production by acute exercise via B_2 adrenergic activation," *Brain, Behavior, and Immunity* 61 (2017):60-68.

88. Munoz, D. G., et al., "Causes of Alzheimer's disease," *Canadian Medical Association Journal* 162 (2000):65–72.

89. Chia-Chen, Liu, et al., "Apolipoprotein E and Alzheimer disease: risk, mechanisms, and therapy," *Nature Reviews Neurology* 9 (2013):106-118.

90. Corder, E.H., et al., "Protective effect of apolipoprotein E type 2 allele for late onset Alzheimer disease," *Nature Genetics* 7 (1994): 180–4.

91. Farrer, L. A., et al., "Effects of age, sex, and ethnicity on the association between apolipoprotein E genotype and Alzheimer disease. A meta-analysis. APOE and Alzheimer Disease Meta-Analysis Consortium," *JAMA* 278 (1997):1349–56; Raber, J., et al., "ApoE genotype accounts for the vast majority of AD risk and pathology," *Neurobiology Aging* 25 (2004):641–50; Haan, M. N., et al., "The role of APOE epsilon4 in modulating effects of other risk factors for cognitive decline in elderly persons," *JAMA* 282(1999):40–46.

92. Farrer, L. A., et al., "Effects of age, sex, and ethnicity on the association between apolipoprotein E genotype and Alzheimer disease. A meta-analysis. APOE and Disease Meta-Analysis Consortium," *JAMA* 278 (1997):1349–56.

93. Michaelson, D.M., "APOE epsilon4: the most prevalent yet understudied risk factor for Alzheimer's disease," *Alzheimer's and Dementia* 10 (2014):861-8; Yassine, N.H., et al., "Association of Docosahexaenoic Acid Supplementation with Alzheimer Disease Stage in Apolipoprotein E ε4 Carriers: A Review," *JAMA Neurology* 74 (2017):339-47.

94. Sepehrnia, B., et al., "Genetic studies of human apolipoproteins: The effect of the apolipoprotein E polymorphism on quantitative levels of lipoproteins in Nigerian blacks," *American Journal of Human Genetics* 45 (1989):586–91.

95. Hendrie, H. C., et al., "Incidence of dementia and Alzheimer disease in 2 communities: Yoruba residing in Ibadan, Nigeria, and African Americans residing in Indianapolis, Indiana," *JAMA* 285 (2001):739–47; Gureje, O., et al., "APOE epsilon 4 is not associated with Alzheimer's disease in elderly Nigerians," *Annals of Neurology* 59 (2006):182–85.

96. Bouchaerd-Mercier Annie, et al., "Associations between dietary patterns and gene expression profiles of healthy men and women: a cross-sectional study," *Nutrition*

Journal 12 (2013): doi: 10.1186/1475-2891-12-24; Morad, Renee, "How diet can change your DNA," *Scientific American* April 24, 2017.

97.   Tanner, C. M., et al., "Parkinson disease in twins: An etiologic study," *JAMA* (1999):281, 341–46.

98.   Brickell, K.L., et al., "Clinicopathological concordance and discordance in three monozygotic twin pairs with familial Alzheimer's disease," *Journal of Neurology Neurosurgery and Psychiatry* 78 (2007):1050-5; Gatz, M., et al., "Role of genes and environments for explaining Alzheimer disease," *Archives of General Psychiatry* 63 (2008):168-74.

99.   Mastroeni, Diego, et al., "Epigenetic Differences in Cortical Neurons from a Pair of Monozygotic Twins Discordant for Alzheimer's Disease," *PLOS One* 4 (2009); https://doi.org/10.1371/journal.pone.0006617

100. ALZForum, "Twin Study Suggests Epigenetic Differences in AD," August 21, 2009; http://www.alzforum.org/news/research-news/twin-study-suggests-epigenetic-differences-ad

101. White, L., et al., "Prevalence of dementia in older Japanese-American men in Hawaii: The Honolulu-Asia Aging Study," *JAMA* 276 (1996):955–60.

102. Hendrie, H.C., et al., "Incidence of dementia and Alzheimer disease in 2 communities: Yoruba residing in Ibadan, Nigeria, and African Americans residing in Indianapolis, Indiana," *JAMA* 285 (2001):739-47; Grant, William B., "Dietary links to Alzheimer's disease," *Alzheimer's Disease Review* 2 (1997):42–45.

103. Fainaru, Steve, and Fainaru-Wada, Mark. *ESPN.go.com*, "Brain impairment begins younger," Sept. 13, 2014. http://espn.go.com/nfl/story/_/id/11513442/data-estimates-3-10-nfl-retirees-face-cognitive-woes, accessed online, Mar. 29, 2016; Fleminger, S., et al., "Head injury as a risk factor for Alzheimer's disease: The evidence 10 years on; a partial replication," *Journal of Neurology, Neurosurgery and Psychiatry* 74 (2003):857–62; Lehman, Everett J., et al., "Neurodegenerative causes of death among retired National Football League players," *Neurology* 79 (2012):1970-74.

104. Farrer, Lindsay A., "Intercontinental epidemiology of Alzheimer disease: A global approach to bad gene hunting," *JAMA* 285 (2001):796–98.

105. Mangialasche, Francesca, et al., "Dementia prevention: Current epidemiological evidence and future perspective," *Alzheimer's Research & Therapies* 4 (2012):6; Kivipelto, M., et al., "Apolipoprotein E epsilon4 magnifies lifestyle risks for dementia: a population-based study," *Journal of Cellular and Molecular Medicine* 12 (2008):2762-2771. doi:10.1111/j.1582-4934.2008.00296.x

106. Virani, S.S., et al., "Heart disease and stroke statistics—2021 update: a report from the American Heart Association," *Circulation* 143 (2021): e254–e743.

107. Stelzmann, Rainulf A., et al., "An English translation of Alzheimer's 1907 paper, 'Uber eine eigenartige Erkankung der Hirnrinde,'" *Clinical Anatomy* 8 (1995):429–31.

108. Leenders, K. L., et al., "Cerebral blood flow, blood volume and oxygen utilization: Normal values and effect of age," *Brain* 113 (1990):27–47.

109. Ainslie, P.N., et al., "Elevation in cerebral blood flow velocity with aerobic fitness throughout healthy human ageing," *Journal of Physiology* 586 (2008):4005–4010;

Buijs P.C., "Effect of age on cerebral blood flow: measurement with ungated two-dimensional phase-contrast MR angiography in 250 adults," *Radiology* 209 (1998): 667–674.

110. de la Torre, J. C., "Critically attained threshold of cerebral hypoperfusion: The CATCH hypothesis of Alzheimer's pathogenesis," *Neurobiology of Aging* 21 (2000):331–42.

111. Albrecht, Daniel A. et al., "Associations between vascular function and tau PET are associated with global cognition and amyloid," *Journal of Neuroscience* (2020):1230-20; DOI: 10.1523/JNEUROSCI.1230-20.2020

112. Jefferson, A.L., et al., "Lower cardiac index levels relate to lower cerebral blood flow in older adults," Neurology (2017): https://www.ncbi.nlm.nih.gov/pubmed/29117962

113. Roher, A. E., et al., "Atherosclerosis of cerebral arteries in Alzheimer disease," *Stroke* 35 (2004):2623–27; Honig, L. S., et al., "Atherosclerosis and AD: Analysis of data from the U.S. National Alzheimer's Coordinating Center," *Neurology* 64 (2005):494–500.

114. Newsroom, University of Rochester Medical Center, "Study details brain damage triggered by mini-strokes," Dec. 12, 2012.

115. Erkinjuntti, T., et al., "Accuracy of the clinical diagnosis of vascular dementia: A prospective clinical and post-mortem neuropathological study," *Journal of Neurology Neurosurgery and Psychiatry* 51 (1998):1037–44.

116. Frazier, D. T, et al., "The role of carotid intima-media thickness in predicting longitudinal cognitive function in an older adult cohort," *Cerebrovascular Disease* 38 (2014):441–47.

117. Zhu, J., et al., "Intracranial artery stenosis and progression from mild cognitive impairment to Alzheimer's disease," *Neurology* 82 (2014):82–89.

118. Sun, X., et al., "Hypoxia facilitates Alzheimer's disease pathogenesis by up-regulating BACE1 gene expression," *Proceedings of the National Academy of Sciences* 103 (2006):18727-32.

119. Hughes, Timothy M., et al., "Pulse Wave Velocity Is Associated With Beta Amyloid Deposition in the Brains of Very Elderly Adults," *Neurology* 81 (2013): 1-8.

120. Strong, J.P., et al., "The pediatric aspects of atherosclerosis," *Atherosclerosis* 9 (1969):251-65.

121. Makoto, Ishi, "Apolipoprotein B as a New Link Between Cholesterol and Alzheimer Disease," *JAMA Neurology* (2019): doi:10.1001/jamaneurol.2019.0212

122. Puglielli, L., et al., "Alzheimer's disease: The cholesterol connection," *Nature Neuroscience* 6 (2003):345–51; Reed, B., et al., "Associations between serum cholesterol levels and cerebral amyloidosis," *JAMA Neurology* 71 (2014):195-200.

123. Matsuzaki, T., et al., "Association of Alzheimer's disease pathology with abnormal lipid metabolism: The Hisayama Study," *Neurology* 77 (2011):1068–75.

124. Notkola, I. L., et al., "Serum total cholesterol, apolipoprotein E epsilon 4 allele, and Alzheimer's disease," *Neuroepidemiology* 17 (1998):14–20.

125. Notkola, I. L., et al., "Serum total cholesterol, apolipoprotein E epsilon 4 allele, and Alzheimer's disease," *Neuroepidemiology* 17 (1998):14–20.

126. Solomon, A., et al., "Midlife serum cholesterol and increased risk of Alzheimer's and vascular dementia three decades later," *Dementia and Geriatric and Cognitive Disorders* 28 (2009):75-80. doi:10.1159/000231980

127. Kivipelto, M., "Apolipoprotein E epsilon4 allele, elevated midlife total cholesterol level, and high midlife systolic blood pressure are independent risk factors for late-life Alzheimer disease," *Annals of Internal Medicine* 137 (2002):149–155.

128. Bergeron, Nathalie, et al., "Effects of red meat, white meat, and nonmeat protein sources on atherogenic lipoprotein measures in the context of low compared with high saturated fat intake: a randomized controlled trial," *The American Journal of Clinical Nutrition* 110 (2019):783. doi.org/10.1093/ajcn/nqz143

129. Ferdowsian H.R., et al., "Effects of plant-based diets on plasma lipids," *American Journal of Cardiology* 104 (2009):947–956, 2009

130. Notkola, I.L., et al., "Serum total cholesterol, apolipoprotein E epsilon 4 allele, and Alzheimer's disease," *Neuroepidemiology* 17 (1998): 14–20; Corsinovi, Laura, "Dietary lipids and their oxidized products in Alzheimer's disease," *Molecular Nutrition & Food Research* 55 (2011):S161–72

131. Willcox, B.J., et al., "Siblings of Okinawan centenarians share lifelong mortality advantages," *The Journals of Gerontology Series A Biological Sciences and Medical Sciences* 61 (2006):345-54; Salaris, L., et al., "Height and survival at older ages among men born in an inland village in Sardinia (Italy), 1866-2006," 58 *Biodemography and Social Biology* (2012):1-13.

132. Kaplan, Hillard, et al., "Coronary atherosclerosis in indigenous South American Tsimane: a cross-sectional cohort study," *The Lancet* 389 (2017):1730-39.

133. Kaplan, H., et al., "Coronary atherosclerosis in indigenous South American Tsimane: a cross-sectional cohort study," *Lancet* 389 (2017):1730-39.

134. Kahleova, H., et al., "Vegetarian dietary patterns and cardiovascular disease," *Progress in Cardiovascular Disease* 61(2019):54-61. doi: 10.1016/j.pcad.2018.05.002.

135. Walker, K.A., et al., "Defining the relationship between hypertension, cognitive decline, and dementia: a review," *Current Hypertension Reports* 24 (2017). doi: 10.1007/s11906-017-0724-3; Iadecola, C., et al., "Impact of hypertension on cognitive function: a scientific statement from the American heart association," *Hypertension* 68 (2016): e67–94. doi: 10.1161/HYP.0000000000000005

136. Kolata Gina, "Under new guidelines, millions more Americans will need to lower blood pressure," *New York Times* November 13, 2017.

137. Riley, Margaret, et al., "High blood pressure in children and adults," *American Family Physician* 85 (2012):693-700; Kearney, P.M., et al., "Global burden of hypertension: analysis of worldwide data," *Lancet* 365 (2005):217–23.

138. Cassels, Alan, "Move over war on transfats; make way for the war on salt," *Canadian Medical Association Journal* 178 (2008):256.

139. "Low-dose quadruple antihypertensive combination: More efficacious than individual agents—a preliminary report," *Hypertension* 49 (2007):272-75.

140. Skoog, Gustafson, D., "Update on hypertension and Alzheimer's disease," *Neurological Research* 28 (2006):605–11.

141. Obisesan, Thomas Olabode, "Hypertension and Cognitive Function," *Clinics in Geriatric Medicine* 25 (2009):259-88.

142. Polidori, M. C., et al., "Heart disease and vascular risk factors in the cognitively impaired elderly: Implications for Alzheimer's dementia," *Aging* 13 (2001):231–39;

Savoia, C., et al., "Inflammation in hypertension," *Current Opinion in Nephrology and Hypertension* 15 (2006):152–158; Poulet, Roberta, et al., "Acute Hypertension Induces Oxidative Stress in Brain Tissues," *Journal of Cerebral Blood Flow & Metabolism* (2006): doi.org/10.1038/sj.jcbfm.9600188

143.   Sang Wong, Seo, et al., "Clinical Significance of Microbleeds in Subcortical Vascular Dementia," *Stroke* 38 (2007):1949-51; Henskens, Leon H.H., et al., "Brain Microbleeds Are Associated with Ambulatory Blood Pressure Levels in a Hypertensive Population," *Hypertension* 51 (2008):62-68.

144.   Arvanitakis, Zoe, et al., "Late-life blood pressure association with cerebrovascular and Alzheimer disease pathology," *Neurology* (2018): DOI: https://doi.org/10.1212/WNL.0000000000005951

145.   Fazekas, F., et al., "Histopathologic analysis of foci of signal loss on gradient-echo T2*-weighted MR images in patients with spontaneous intracerebral hemorrhage: evidence of microangiopathy-related microbleeds," *AJNR American Journal of Neuroradiology* 2- (1999):637– 642

146.   Kovacic, J.C., et al., "Atherosclerotic risk factors, vascular cognitive impairment, and Alzheimer disease," *Mt. Sanai Journal of Medicine* 79 (2012):554-73.

147.   Gilsanz, Paola, et al., "Female sex, early-onset hypertension, and risk of dementia," *Neurology* 10 (2017): doi: http://dx.doi.org/10.1212/WNL.0000000000004602

148.   Rodrigue, Karen, et al., "Risk Factors for β-Amyloid Deposition in Healthy Aging: Vascular and Genetic Effects," *JAMA Neurology* 70 (2013):600–606

149.   Yasar, Sevil, et al., "Antihypertensive drugs decrease risk of Alzheimer disease," *Neurology* 81 (2013):896-903; Forette, F., et al., "Prevention of dementia in randomized double-blind placebo-controlled Systolic Hypertension in Europe (Syst-Eur) trial," *Lancet* 352 (1998):1347–1351.

150.   Lipsitz, Lewis, et al., "Antihypertensive Therapy Increases Cerebral Blood Flow and Carotid Distensibility in Hypertensive Elderly Subjects," *Hypertension* 45 (2005):216-21.

151.   De Jomng, Daan L.K., et al., "Effects of Nilvadipine on cerebral blood flow in patients with Alzheimer's disease," *Hypertension* (2019): doi.org/10.1161/HYPERTENSIONAHA.119.12892

152.   Harvard Men's Health Watch, "Blood pressure and your brain," *Harvard Health Publishing*, October 2009.

153.   University of Alabama at Birmingham, "Blood pressure medications can lead to increased risk of stroke," *ScienceDaily* May 29, 2015. <www.sciencedaily.com/releases/2015/05/150529193554.ht; Masafumi, Oka, et al., "Chronic Stimulation of Renin Cells Leads to Vascular Pathology Novelty and Significance," *Hypertension* 70 (2017): doi: 10.1161/HYPERTENSIONAHA.117.09283

154.   Faras, Auda, "use of beta-blockers and risk of dementia in elderly patients," *Journal of Psychiatry and Neurosciences* (2012): doi.org/10.1176/appi.neuropsych.11100240

155.   Kempner, Walter "Treatment of heart and kidney disease and of hypertensive and arteriosclerotic vascular disease with rice diet," *Annals of Internal Medicine* 31 (1949):821-56.

156.   Symonds, B., "Blood pressure of healthy men and women," *JAMA* 8 (1923):232–236.

157.   Manson, J.E., et al., "Body weight and mortality among women," *New England Journal of Medicine* 333 (1995):677-85.

158.   Fabijana, Jakulj, et al., "A High-Fat Meal Increases Cardiovascular Reactivity to Psychological Stress in Healthy Young Adults," *Journal of Nutrition* 137 (2007):935-939.

159.   Hozumi, T., et al., "Change in Coronary Flow Reserve on Transthoracic Doppler Echocardiography after a Single High-Fat Meal in Young Healthy Men," *Annals of Internal Medicine* 136 (2002):523-28; Bui, C., et al., "Acute effect of a single high-fat meal on forearm blood flow, blood pressure and heart rate in healthy male Asians and Caucasians: a pilot study," *Southeast Asian Journal of Tropical Medicine and Public Health* 41 (201):490-500.

160.   McDougall John, et al., "effects of 7 days on an ad libitum low-fat vegan diet: the McDougall Program cohort," *Nutrition Journal* 16 (2017): doi: 10.1186/1475-2891-13-99.

161.   Appleby, P.N., et al., "Hypertension and blood pressure among meat eaters, fish eaters, vegetarians and vegans in EPIC-Oxford," *Public Health Nutrition* 5 (2002):645-54.

162.   Appleby, P.N., et al., "Hypertension and blood pressure among meat eaters, fish eaters, vegetarians and vegans in EPIC-Oxford," *Public Health and Nutrition* 5 (2002):645-54.

163.   Slag, M.D., et al., "Meal stimulation of cortisol secretion: a protein induced effect," *Metabolism* 30 (1981):1104-8.

164.   Appleby, P.N., et al., "Hypertension and blood pressure among meat eaters, fish eaters, vegetarians and vegans in EPIC-Oxford," *Public Health Nutrition* 5 (2002):645–54.

165.   Borgi L, et al., "Long-term intake of animal flesh and risk of developing hypertension in three prospective cohort studies," *Journal of Hypertension* 33 (2015):2231–2238.

166.   Lindahl, O., et al., "A vegan regimen with reduced medication in the treatment of hypertension," *British Journal of Nutrition* 52 (1984):11–20.

167.   Curran, James, "The Yellow Emperor's Classic of Internal Medicine" *BMJ* 336 2008):777.

168.   Farquhar, William, et al., "Dietary Sodium and Health: More Than Just Blood Pressure," *Journal of the American College of Cardiology* 65 (2015):1042-50.

169.   Bernstein, A.M, et al., "Trends in 24-h urinary sodium excretion in the United States, 1957-2003: a systematic review," *American Journal of Clinical* Nutrition 92 (2010):1172–80; DeNoon, Danie J., "90% in U.S. Get Too Much Sodium; 5 Foods Blamed," WebMD June 24, 2010

170.   Parker, Laura, "Microplastics found in 90 percent of table salt," *National Geographic* October 17, 2018.

171.   Cox, Kieran D., "Human consumption of microplastics," *Environmental Science & Technology* (2019): DOI: 10.1021/acs.est.9b01517

172.   Friedman, R., et al., "Hypertension—salt poisoning?" *Lancet* 2 (1978):584; Kaplan, H., et al., "Coronary atherosclerosis in indigenous South American Tsimane: a cross-sectional cohort study," *Lancet* 389 (2017):1730-39; Oliver, W.J., et al., "Blood pressure, sodium intake, and sodium related hormones in the Yanomamo Indians, a 'No-salt' culture," *Circulation* 52 (1975):146–151; Carvalho, J.J., et al., "Blood pressure in four remote populations in the INTERSALT study," *Hypertension* 14 (1989):238–246; Kaplan, Hillard, et al., "Coronary atherosclerosis in indigenous South American Tsimane: a cross-sectional cohort study," *The Lancet* 389 (2017): 1730-39; Kawasaki, T., et al., "Investigation of high salt intake in a Nepalese population with low blood pressure," *Journal of Human Hypertension* 7 (1993): 131–140;

173. Champagne, C.M., "Dietary interventions on blood pressure: the Dietary Approaches to Stop Hypertension (DASH) trials," *Nutrition Reviews* 64 (2006): S53-6.

174. Glushakova, O., "Fructose induces the inflammatory molecule ICAM-1 in endothelial cells," *Journal of the American Society of Nephrology* 19 (2008): 1712–1720; Jalal, Diana, et al., "Increased Fructose Associates with Elevated Blood Pressure" *Journal of the American Society of Nephrology* 21 (2010):1543-49.

175. Soleimani, M., "Dietary fructose, salt absorption and hypertension in metabolic syndrome: towards a new paradigm," *Acta Physiologica* 201 (2011):55–62.

176. Grasser, E.K, et al., "Cardio- and cerebrovascular responses to the energy drink Red Bull in young adults: a randomized cross-over study," *European Journal of Nutrition* 53 (2014):1561-71. doi: 10.1007/s00394-014-0661-8. Epub 2014 Jan 29. PMID: 24474552; PMCID: PMC4175045; Franks, A.M., et al., "Comparison of the effects of energy drink versus caffeine supplementation on indices of 24-hour ambulatory blood pressure," *Annals of Pharmacotherapy* 46 (2012):192-9. doi: 10.1345/aph.1Q555. Epub 2012 Jan 31. PMID: 22298600.

177. Chobanian, A.V., et al., "The seventh report of the joint national committee of prevention, detection, evaluation, and treatment of high blood pressure: The JNC 7 report," *JAMA* 289 (2003): 2560-2572.

178. Pescatello, L.S., et al., "Exercise and hypertension," *Medicine and Science in Sports and Exercise* 36 (2004): 533-553.

179. Kelly, J. J., et al., "Cortisol and hypertension," *Clinical and Experimental Pharmacology Physiology* 25 (1998): S51–56.

180. Schneider, Robert, et al., "Stress Reduction in the Secondary Prevention of Cardiovascular Disease: Randomized, Controlled Trial of Transcendental Meditation and Health Education in Blacks," *Circulation: Cardiovascular Quality and Outcomes* (2012): 10.1161/CIRCOUTCOMES.112.967406

181. Bruce-Keller, A.J et al., "Obesity and vulnerability of the cns," *Biochimica et Biophysica, Acta* 1792 (2009): 395–400; Beilharz, J. E., et al., "Diet-Induced Cognitive Deficits: The Role of Fat and Sugar, Potential Mechanisms and Nutritional Interventions," *Nutrients* 7 (2015):6719–6738.

182. Center for Disease Control and Prevention, Division of Nutrition, Physical Activity, and Obesity, National Center for Chronic Disease Prevention and Health Promotion, June 29, 2020.

183. Obesity and Overweight. World Health Organization. http://www.who.int/news-room/fact-sheets/detail/obesity-and-overweight.

   Finucane, M.M., et al., "National, regional, and global trends in body-mass index since 1980: Systematic analysis of health examination surveys and epidemiological studies with 960 country-years and 9.1 million participants," *Lancet* 377 (2011):557–567.

184. Steele, C.B., et al., "Vital Signs: trends in incidence of cancers associated with overweight and obesity—United States, 2005–2014," *MMWR Morbidity and Mortality Weekly* 66 (2017):1052-58.

185. Whitmer, R.A., et al., "Body mass index in midlife and risk of Alzheimer disease and vascular dementia," *Current Alzheimer Research* 4 (2007):103–109.

186. Whitmer, R.A., et al., "Central obesity and increased risk of dementia more than three decades later," *Neurology* 71 (2008):1057–1064.

187. Te Morenga L., et al., "Dietary sugars and body weight: systematic review and meta-analyses of randomized controlled trials and cohort studies," *British Medical Journal* 346 (2013):e7492.

188. Scarmeas, N., et al., "Physical Activity, Diet, and Risk of Alzheimer Disease," *JAMA* 302 (2009):627-637

189. Koenig, Debbie, "Quarantine weight gain not a joking matter," *WebMD* May 21, 2020.

190. United States Census Bureau. The 2012 Statistical Abstract. Health & Nutrition: Food Consumption and Nutrition. Table #217. Per Capita Consumption of Major Food Commodities: 1980 to 2009; PublicHealth.org, "Why are Americans obese?"

191. Ellulu, M.S., et al., "Obesity and inflammation: the linking mechanism and the complications," *Archives of Medical Science* 13 (2017):851-863. doi:10.5114/aoms.2016.58928

192. Kim, B., et al., "Insulin resistance as a key link for the increased risk of cognitive impairment in the metabolic syndrome," *Experimental and Molecular Medicine* 47 (2015):e149. doi:10.1038/emm.2015.3

193. Cournot, M., et al., "Relation between body mass index and cognitive function in healthy middle-aged men and women," *Neurology* 67 (2006):1208-14.

194. Amen, Daniel, G., et al., "Patterns of regional cerebral blood flow as a function of obesity in adults," *Journal of Alzheimer's Disease* (2020):1-7. DOI:10.3233/JAD-200655

195. Letra, Liliand, et al., "Obesity as a risk factor for Alzheimer's disease: The role of adipocytokines," *Metabolic Brain Disease* 29 (2014):563–68.

196. Letra, Liliand, et al., "Obesity as a risk factor for Alzheimer's disease: The role of adipocytokines," *Metabolic Brain Disease* 29 (2014):563–68.

197. Jagust, W., et al., "Central obesity and the aging brain," *Archives of Neurology* 62 (2005):1545-8; Ward, M.A., et al., "The effect of body mass index on global brain volume in middle-aged adults: a cross sectional study," *BMC Neurology* 5 (2005):23.

198. Cherbuin, N., et al., "Being overweight is associated with hippocampal atrophy: the PATH Through Life Study," *International Journal of Obesity* 39 (2015):1509–1514. https://doi.org/10.1038/ijo.2015.106

199. Cherbuin, N., et al., "Being overweight is associated with hippocampal atrophy: the PATH Through Life Study," *International Journal of Obesity* 39 (2015):1509-14.

200. Ronan, Lisa, et al., "Obesity associated with increased brain age from midlife," *Neurobiology of Aging* 47 (2016):63-70.

201. Macey, Paul M., et al., "Global Brain Blood-Oxygen Level Responses to Autonomic Challenges in Obstructive Sleep Apnea," *PLOS One* (2014): doi.org/10.1371/journal.pone.0105261

202. Body Mass Index (BMI) is a measure of body fat that is based upon a person's height and weight. The formula is BMI=kg/m^2. There are BMI calculators found on public health websites. The threshold for being overweight is a BMI of 25. A healthy range is considered to be between 18 and 24.

203. Chuang, Y. F., et al., "Midlife adiposity predicts earlier onset of Alzheimer's dementia, neuropathology and presymptomatic cerebral amyloid accumulation," *Molecular Psychiatry*, accessed online, Sept. 1, 2015: http://www.nature.com/mp/journal/v21/n7/full/mp2015129a.html.

204. Kivipelto, M., et al., "Obesity and vascular risk factors at midlife and the risk of dementia and Alzheimer disease," *Archives of Neurology* 62 (2005):1556–60.

205. Barnard N.D., et al., "The effects of a low-fat, plant-based dietary intervention on body weight, metabolism, and insulin sensitivity," *American Journal of Medicine* 118:991–997, 200; Kahleova, Hana, et al., "The Effect of a Vegetarian vs Conventional Hypocaloric Diabetic Diet on Thigh Adipose Tissue Distribution in Subjects with Type 2 Diabetes: A Randomized Study," *Journal of the American College of Nutrition* 36 (2017):364-69.

206. Tonstad, S., et al., "Type of vegetarian diet, body weight, and prevalence of type 2 diabetes," *Diabetes Care* 32 (2009):791-6.

207. Kahleova, Hana, et al., "A Plant-Based Diet Improves Beta-Cell Function and Insulin Resistance in Overweight Adult—A 16-Week Randomized Clinical Trial," *Diabetes* 67 (2018): doi.org/10.2337/db18-294-OR

208. https://www.diabetes.org/resources/statistics/cost-diabetes Retrieved Nov. 9, 2021.

209. Singh-Manoux, Archana, et al., "Association between age at diabetes onset and subsequent risk of dementia," *JAMA* 325 (2021):1640-1649.

Ohara, T., et al., "Glucose tolerance status and risk of dementia in the community: The Hisayama Study," *Neurology* 77 (2011): 1126 DOI: 10.1212/WNL.0b013e31822f0435

210. Zhao, W., et al., "Permissive role of insulin in the expression of long-term potentiation in the hippocampus of immature rats," *NeuroSignals* 18 (2011): 236–245; Chiu, S. L., et al., "Insulin receptor signaling regulates synapse number, dendritic plasticity, and circuit function in vivo," *Neuron* 58 (2008):708–719.

211. Marks, J. L., et al., "Localization of insulin and type 1 IGF receptors in rat brain by in vitro autoradiography and in situ hybridization," *Advances in Experimental Medicine and Biology* 293 (1991):459–70.

212. Fujisawa, Y., et al., "Increased insulin levels after OGTT load in peripheral blood and cerebrospinal fluid of patients with dementia of Alzheimer type," *Biological Psychiatry* 30 (1991):1219-1228

213. Janson, J., et al., "Increased risk of type 2 diabetes in Alzheimer disease," *Diabetes* 53 (2004):474.

214. McCaulley, M. E., et al., "Seeking a New Paradigm for Alzheimer's Disease: Considering the Roles of Inflammation, Blood-Brain Barrier Dysfunction, and Prion Disease," *International Journal of Alzheimer's Disease* (2017). doi: 10.1155/2017/2438901

215. Yang, Y., et al., "High glucose promotes Aβ production by inhibiting APP degradation," *PLoS One* 8 (2013). doi: 10.1371/journal.pone.0069824; Macauley SL, et al., "Hyperglycemia modulates extracellular amyloid beta concentrations and neuronal activity *in vivo*," *The Journal of Clinical Investigation* 125 (2015):2463-2467. doi:10.1172/JCI79742. Leistner, Juli, et al., "A changing landscape: Alzheimer's disease, research and the future of care," Washington University School of Medicine November 18, 2016; Kim, B., et. Al., "Insulin resistance as a key link for the increased risk of cognitive impairment in the metabolic syndrome," *Experimental Molecular Medicine* 47 (2015): e149: doi:10.1038/emm.2015.3

216. Vanhanen M., et al., "Cognitive function in an elderly population with persistent impaired glucose tolerance," *Diabetes Care* 21 (1998):398–402; Kalmijn, S., et al., "Glucose intolerance, hyperinsulinaemia and cognitive function in a general population of elderly men," *Diabetologia* 38 (1995):1096–102

217. Wardlaw, J.M., et al., "Mechanisms of sporadic cerebral small vessel disease: insights from neuroimaging," *Lancet Neurology 12* (2013):483–97.

218. Diabetes in Control, "Will type 2 diabetes shrink the brain?" May 1, 2014: http://www.diabetesincontrol.com/will-type-2-diabetes-shrink-the-brain/.

219. Moheet, A., et al., "Impact of diabetes on cognitive function and brain structure," *Annals of New York Academy of Science* 1353 (2015):60-71.

220. Krane, Paul K., et al., "Glucose levels and risk of dementia," *New England Journal of Medicine* 369 (2013):540-48.

221. Zheng, F., Yan, L., Yang, Z. et al. "HbA$_{1c}$, diabetes and cognitive decline: the English Longitudinal Study of Ageing," *Diabetologia* (2018). https://doi.org/10.1007/s00125-017-4541-7

222. Tilvis, R.S., et al., "Predictors of cognitive decline and mortality of aged people over a 10-year period," *Journal of Gerontology: Series A, Biological Sciences and Medical Sciences* 59 (2004):268–274

223. Hu, F.B., et al., "Walking compared with vigorous physical activity and risk of type 2 diabetes in women: a prospective study," *JAMA* 282 (1999):1433–1439.

224. Obesity Society, "Your weight and diabetes," http://tosconnect.obesity.org/obesity/content/weight-diabetes

225. Sears, Barry, et al., "The role of fatty acids in insulin resistance," *Lipids in Health and Disease* 14 (2015):10.1186/s12944-015-0123-1

226. Kazuaki, Ohtsubo., et al., "Pathway to diabetes through attenuation of pancreatic beta cell glycosylation and glucose transport," *Nature Medicine* (2011): doi: 10.1038/nm.2414

227. Samuel, V.T., et al., "Mechanisms for insulin resistance: common threads and missing links," *Cell* 148 (2012):852–871.

228. Newsholme, P., et al., "Life and death decisions of the pancreatic β-cell: the role of fatty acids," *Clinical Science* 112 (2007):27–42. doi: 10.1042/CS20060115

229. Guasch-Ferre, Marta, et al., "Total and subtypes of dietary fat intake and risk of type 2 diabetes mellitus in the Prevención con Dieta Mediterránea (PREDIMED) study," American *Journal of Clinical Nutrition* 105 (2017):723-35.

230. Menke, A., et al., "Prevalence of and Trends in Diabetes Among Adults in the United States, 1988-2012," *JAMA* 314 (2015):1021–1029. doi:10.1001/jama.2015.10029

231. McInnes, Natalia, et al., "*The Journal of Clinical Endocrinology & Metabolism* 102 (2017):1596-1605; Steven, Sarah, et al., "Very Low-Calorie Diet and 6 Months of Weight Stability in Type 2 Diabetes: Pathophysiological Changes in Responders and Nonresponders," *Diabetes Care* 39 (2016):808-15.

232. Anderson, J.W., et al., "High-carbohydrate, high-fiber diets for insulin-treated men with diabetes mellitus," *American Journal of Clinical Nutrition* 32 (1979):2312-21.

233. Tuomilehto, J., et al., "Finnish Diabetes Prevention Study Group: Prevention of type 2 diabetes mellitus by changes in lifestyle among subjects with impaired glucose tolerance," *New England Journal of Medicine* 344 (2001):1343–1350; Pan, X.R., et al., "Effects of diet and exercise in preventing NIDDM in people with impaired glucose tolerance: the Da Qing IGT and Diabetes Study," *Diabetes Care* 20 (1997):537–544; Marshall, Julie A., et al., "Dietary Fat and the Development of Type 2 Diabetes," *Diabetes Care* 25 (2002):620-22

234. Chan, J.M., et al., "Obesity, fat distribution, and weight gain as risk factors for clinical diabetes in men," *Diabetes Care* 17 (1994):961–969.

235. Snowdon, D.A., et al. "Does a vegetarian diet reduce the occurrence of diabetes?" *American Journal of Public Health* 75 (1985):507-12.

236. Tonstad, S., "Type of vegetarian diet, body weight, and prevalence of type 2 diabetes," *Diabetes Care* 32 (2009):791–796, 2009

237. Brinegar, C.H, et al., "Meats, processed meats, obesity, weight gain and occurrence of diabetes among adults: findings from Adventist Health Studies," *Annals of Nutrition and Metabolism* 52:96–104, 2008; Hu, F.B, et al., "Dietary patterns, meat intake, and the risk of type 2 diabetes in women," *Archives of Internal Medicine* 164 (2004):2235–2240; Pan, A., et al., "Red meat consumption and risk of type 2 diabetes: 3 cohorts of US adults and an updated meta-analysis," *American Journal of Clinical Nutrition* 94 (2011):1088–1096.

238. Bendinelli, B., et al., "Association between dietary meat consumption and incident type 2 diabetes: the EPIC-InterAct study," *Diabetologia* 56 (2013):46-59.

239. Tonstad, S., et al., "Vegetarian diets and incidence of diabetes in the Adventist Health Study," *Nutrition, Metabolism, and Cardiovascular Disease* 23 (2003):292-9.

240. Tonstad, S., et al., "Vegetarian diets and incidence of diabetes in the Adventist Health Study-2," *Nutrition, Metabolism and Cardiovascular Disease* 23 (2013):292-9.

241. Toumpanakis, A., et al., "Effectiveness of plant-based diets in promoting well-being in the management of type 2 diabetes: a systematic review.," *BMJ Open Diabetes Research & Care* (2018) doi:10.1136/bmjdrc-2018-000534

242. Goff, L.M., et al., Veganism and its relationship with insulin resistance and intramyocellular lipid," *European Journal of Clinical Nutrition* 59 (2005):291-8; McMacken, M., et al., "A plant-based diet for the prevention and treatment of type 2 diabetes," *Journal of Geriatric Cardiology* 14 (2017):342–354. doi: 10.11909/j.issn.1671-5411.2017.05.009

243. Rabinowitch, I.M., "Experiences with a high carbohydrate-low calorie diet for the treatment of diabetes mellitus," *Canadian Medical Association Journal* 23 (1930):489.

244. Rabinowitch, I.M., "Effects of the High Carbohydrate-Low Calorie Diet Upon Carbohydrate Tolerance in Diabetes Mellitus," *Canadian Medical Association Journal* 33 (1935)136-44.

245. Perseghin, G., et al., "Increased glucose transport-phosphorylation and muscle glycogen synthesis after exercise training in insulin-resistance subjects," *New England Journal of Medicine* 335 (1996):1357–1362.

246. Bird, S.R., et al., "Update on the effects of physical activity on insulin sensitivity in humans," *BMJ Open Sport & Exercise Medicine* 2 (2017):e000143. doi:10.1136/bmjsem-2016-000143

247. Gaitán, Julian M. et al. 'Brain Glucose Metabolism, Cognition, and Cardiorespiratory Fitness Following Exercise Training in Adults at Risk for Alzheimer's Disease' *Brain Plasticity* 5 2019: 83–95.

248. Barnard, R. James, et al., "Diet and Exercise in the Treatment of NIDDM: The need for early emphasis," *Diabetes Care* 17 (1994):1469-72.

249. Rockette-Wagner, B., et al., "The impact of lifestyle intervention on sedentary time in individuals at high risk of diabetes," *Diabetologia* 58 (2015):1198-202.

250. Heude, B., et al., "Cognitive decline and fatty acid composition of erythrocyte membranes—the EVA Study," *American Journal of Clinical Nutrition* 77 (2003):803–8; Beydoun, M. A, et al., "Plasma n-3 fatty acids and the risk of cognitive decline in older adults: The Atherosclerosis Risk in Communities Study," *American Journal of Clinical Nutrition* 85 (2007):1103–11; Eskelinen, M. H., et al., "Fat intake at midlife and cognitive impairment later in life: A population–based CAIDE study," *International Journal of Geriatrics Psychi*atry 23 (2008):741–47; Devore, E. E, et al., "Dietary antioxidants and long–term risk of dementia," *Archives of Neurology* 67 (2010):819–25.

251. Walker, Jennifer M., et al., "Shared neuropathological characteristics of obesity, Type 2 diabetes and Alzheimer's disease: Impacts on cognitive decline," *Nutrients* 7 (2015):7332–57; Berrino, F., et al., "Western diet and Alzheimer's disease." *Epidemiological Previews* 26 (2002):107–15; Grant, W.B., et al., "The significance of environmental factors in the etiology of Alzheimer's disease," *Journal of Alzheimer's Disease* 4 (2002):179–89; Pasinetti, G., "Metabolic syndrome and the role of dietary lifestyles in Alzheimer's disease," *Journal of Neurochemistry* 106 (2008):1503–14; Eskelinen, M., et al., "Fat intake at midlife and cognitive impairment later in life: a population-based CAIDE study," *International Journal of Geriatrics Psychiatry* 23 (2008):741–7; Scarmeas, N., et al., "Physical Activity, Diet, and Risk of Alzheimer Disease," *JAMA* 302 (2009):627-637.

252. Micha, R., et al., "Global, regional, and national consumption levels of dietary fats and oils in 1990 and 2010: a systematic analysis including 266 country-specific nutrition surveys," *BMJ* 348 (2014): doi: 10.1136/bmjopen-2015-008705

253. den Hartigh, L.J., et al., "Postprandial apoE isoform and conformational changes associated with VLDL lipolysis products modulate monocyte inflammation," *PLoS One* 7 (2012):e50513; Park, H. R., et al., "A high-fat diet impairs neurogenesis: Involvement of lipid peroxidation and brain-derived neurotrophic factor," *Neuroscience Letters* 482 (2010):235–39; Fabijana, Jakulj, et al., "A High-Fat Meal Increases Cardiovascular Reactivity to Psychological Stress in Healthy Young Adults," *The Journal of Nutrition* 137 (2007):935–939. doi.org/10.1093/jn/137.4.935

254. Morris, Martha Clare, et al., "Dietary fats and the risk of incident Alzheimer disease," *Archives of Neurology* 60 (2003):194–200; Laitinen, M. H., et al., "Fat intake at midlife and risk of dementia and Alzheimer's disease: A population-based study," *Dementia Geriatric Cognitive Disorders* 22 (2006): 99–107.

255. Kalmijn, S., et al., "Dietary fat intake and the risk of incident dementia in the Rotterdam Study," *Annals of Neurology* 42 (1997):776-82; Engelhart, M.J., et al., "Diet and risk of dementia: Does fat matter?: The Rotterdam Study," *Neurology* 59 (2002):1915-21; Laitinen, M.H., et al., "Fat intake at midlife and risk of dementia and disease: a population-based study," *Dementia and Geriatric Cognitive Disorders* 22

(2006):99-107; Morris, M.C., et al., "Dietary fat intake and 6-year cognitive change in an older biracial community population," *Neurology* 62 (2004):1573-9; Morris, M.C., et al., "Dietary fats and the risk of incident Alzheimer's disease," *Archives of Neurology* 60 (2003):194-200.

256. Okereke, Olivia I., et al., "Dietary fat types and 4-year cognitive change in community-dwelling older women," *Annals of Neurology* 72 (2012):124–34.

257. Molteni, R., et al., "Exercise reverses the harmful effects of consumption of a high-fat diet on synaptic and behavioral plasticity associated to the action of brain-derived neurotrophic factor," *Neuroscience* 123 (2004):429-440.

258. Barde, Y.A., et al., "Purification of a new neurotrophic factor from mammalian brain," *Embo Journal* 1 (1982):549–53.

259. Hanson, Angela J., et al., "Effect of Apolipoprotein E Genotype and Diet on Apolipoprotein E Lipidation and Amyloid Peptides," *JAMA Neurology* (2013): doi: 10.1001/jamaneurol.2013.396

260. https://libin.ucalgary.ca/node/1327.

261. Kiecolt-Glaser, Janice K., et al., "Afternoon distraction: a high-saturated-fat meal and endotoxemia impact postmeal attention in a randomized crossover trial," *The American Journal of Clinical Nutrition* (2020); DOI: 10.1093/ajcn/nqaa085

262. Molteni, R., et al., "A high-fat, refined sugar diet reduces hippocampal brain-derived neurotrophic factor, neuronal plasticity, and learning," *Neuroscience* 112 (2002):803-14.

263. Milanski, M., et al., "Saturated fatty acids produce an inflammatory response predominantly through the activation of TLR4 signaling in hypothalamus: implications for the pathogenesis of obesity," *Journal of Neuroscience* 29 (2009):359–370.

264. National Cancer Institute. Risk Factor Monitoring and Methods: Table 1. Top Food Sources of Saturated Fata among U.S. Population, 2005–2006. *NHANES*.

265. Morris, Martha Clare, "The role of nutrition in Alzheimer's disease: epidemiological evidence," *European Journal of Neurology* 16 (2009) (suppl 1):1-7; Morris, Martha Clare, et al., "Dietary fats and the risk of incident Alzheimer disease," *Archives of Neurology* 60 (2003):194–200.

266. Clapp, J., et al., "Prevalence of Partially Hydrogenated Oils in U.S. Packaged Foods, 2012," *Preventing Chronic Disease* 11 (2014): DOI: http://dx.doi.org/10.5888/pcd11.140161

267. Small Entity Compliance Guide: Trans Fatty Acids in Nutrition Labeling, Nutrient Content Claims, and Health Claims, Small Entity Compliance Guide, Food & Drug Administration, August 2003.

268. Mensink, R.P., et al., "Effect of dietary trans fatty acids on high-density and low-density lipoprotein cholesterol levels in healthy subjects," *New England Journal of Medicine* 323(1990):439–45.

269. Mozaffarian, D., et al., "Dietary intake of trans fatty acids and systemic inflammation in women," American *Journal of Clinical Nutrition* 79 (2004):606–12; Mozaffarian, D., "Trans fatty acids and systemic inflammation in heart failure," *American Journal of Clinical Nutrition* 80 (2004):1521–5; Tomey, K.M., et al., "Dietary fat subgroups, zinc, and vegetable components are related to urine F2a-isoprostane concentration, a measure of oxidative stress, in midlife women," *Journal of Nutrition* 137 (2007):2412–9.

270. De Schrijver, R., et al., "Interrelationship between dietary trans Fatty acids and the 6- and 9-desaturases in the rat," *Lipids* 17 (1982):27–34.

271. McCaddon, A., et al., "Total serum homocysteine in senile dementia of Alzheimer type," *International Journal of Geriatric Psychiatry* 13 (1998):235–39; Clarke, R., et al., "Vitamin B12, and serum total homocysteine levels in confirmed Alzheimer's disease," *Archives of Neurology* 55 (1998):1449–55.

272. Seshadri, S., et al., "Plasma homocysteine as a risk factor for dementia and Alzheimer's disease," *New England Journal of Medicine* 346 (2002):476-83. doi: 10.1056/NEJMoa011613. PMID: 11844848.

      NIH/National Institute on Aging. "High Homocysteine Levels May Double Risk of Dementia, Alzheimer's Disease, New Report Suggests," *ScienceDaily.* www.sciencedaily. com/releases/2002/02/020214075349.htm (accessed June 17, 2021).

273. Seshadri, Sudha, et al., "Plasma homocysteine as a risk factor for dementia and Alzheimer's disease," *New England Journal of Medicine* 346 (2002):476–83.

274. Jara-Prado, A., et al., "Homocysteine-induced brain lipid peroxidation: effects of NMDA receptor blockade, antioxidant treatment, and nitric oxide synthase inhibition," *Neurotoxin Research* 5 (2003):237–43.

275. Shin, J.Y., et al., "Elevated homocysteine by levodopa is detrimental to neurogenesis in parkinsonian model," *PLoS One* 7 (2012): e50496. doi: 10.1371/journal.pone.0050496

276. Hooshmand, B., et al., "Plasma homocysteine, Alzheimer and cerebrovascular pathology: a population-based autopsy study," *Brain* 136 (2013):2702-16.

277. Nurk, E., et al., "Plasma total homocysteine and memory in the elderly: the Hordaland Homocysteine Study," *Annals of Neurology* 58 (2005):847-57.

278. Smith, A.D., et al., "Homocysteine-lowering by B vitamins slows the rate of accelerated brain atrophy in mild cognitive impairment: a randomized controlled trial," *PLoS One* 5 (2010) e12244; Douaud, Gwenaelle, et al., "Preventing Alzheimer's disease-related gray matter atrophy by b-vitamin treatment," *PNAS* 110 (2013):9523-28.

279. Institute for Health Metrics and Evaluation. The State of U.S. Health: Innovations, Insights, and Recommendations from the Global Burden of Disease Study. Seattle, WA: IHME, 2013.

280. "The US Burden of Disease Collaborators. The state of US health, 1990-2016 burden of diseases, injuries, and risk factors among US states," *JAMA* 319 (2018):1444-1472.

281. Kalmijn, Set, al., "Metabolic cardiovascular syndrome and risk of dementia in Japanese-American elderly men: the honolulu-asia aging study," *Arteriosclerosis, Thrombosis and Vascular Biology* 20 (2000):2255-2260; Kalmijn, Set al., "Dietary fat intake and the risk of incident dementia in the Rotterdam Study," *Annals of Neurology* 42 (1997):776-782; Knopman, D., et al., "Cardiovascular risk factors and cognitive decline in middle-aged adults," *Neurology* 56 (2001):42-48.

282. Grant, W.B., "Trends in diet and Alzheimer's disease during the nutrition transition in Japan and developing countries," *Journal of Alzheimer's Disease* 38 (2014): 611–20.

283. Milne, Dave, "Alcohol consumption in Japan: different culture, different rules," *Canadian Medical Association Journal* 167 (2002):388.

284. Grant, W.B., "Trends in diet and Alzheimer's disease during the nutrition transition in Japan and developing countries," *Journal of Alzheimer's Disease* 38 (2014): 611–20.

285. Lubin, Gus and Mamta Badkar. "15 Facts about McDonald's that Will Blow Your Mind." *Business Insider*. December 17, 2010. Accessed: February 20,2020.

286. Krebs-Smith, S.M., et al., "Americans do not meet federal dietary recommendations," *Journal of Nutrition* 140 (2010):183-8.

287. Sobesky, J. L. et al., "High-fat diet consumption disrupts memory and primes elevations in hippocampal IL-1beta, an effect that can be prevented with dietary reversal or IL-1 receptor antagonism," Brain, Behavior, and Immunity 42 (2014): 22–32.

288. Godfrey S. et al., "Urban living in healthy Tanzanians is associated with an inflammatory status driven by dietary and metabolic changes," *Nature Immunology* 22 (2021): 287 DOI: 10.1038/s41590-021-00867-8

289. Kim, M.S., et al., "Strict vegetarian diet improves the risk factors associated with metabolic diseases by modulating gut microbiota and reducing intestinal inflammation," *Environmental Microbiology Reports* 5 (2013):765–775; Craddock, Joel C, et al., "Vegetarian-Based Dietary Patterns and their Relation with Inflammatory and Immune Biomarkers: A Systematic Review and Meta-Analysis," *Advances in Nutrition* 10 (2019):433–45; Franco-de-Moraes, A.C., et al., "Worse inflammatory profile in omnivores than in vegetarians associates with the gut microbiota composition," *Diabetology & Metabolic Syndrome* (2017):doi:10.1186/s13098-017-0261-x

290. Croll, Pauline H., et al., "Better diet quality relates to larger brain tissue volumes. The Rotterdam Study," *Neurology* 90 (2012): e2166-e173.

291. Jacka, Felice N., et al., "Western diet is associated with a smaller hippocampus: a longitudinal investigation," *BMC Medicine* (2015): https://doi.org/10.1186/s12916-015-0461-x

292. "The land of immortals: How and what Japan's oldest population eats," Chasing Life with Sanjay Gupta, CNN, May 21, 2019.

293. Sánchez-Villegas, Almudena, et al., "Mediterranean dietary pattern and depression: the PREDIMED randomized trial," *BMC Medicine* 11 (2013):208; Okereke, Olivia, et al., "Dietary fat types and 4-year cognitive change in community-dwelling older women," *Annals of Neurology 72* (2012): doi.org/10.1002/ana.23593; Gibson, E. Leigh, et al., "Habitual fat intake predicts memory function in younger women," *Frontiers in Human Neuroscience* 7 (2013): doi:10.3389/fnhum.2013.00838; Freeman, Linnea R., et al., "Damaging effects of a high-fat diet to the brain and cognition: A review of proposed mechanisms," *Nutrition Neuroscience* 17 (2014):241-51.

294. Perrone, L., et al., "Observational and ecological studies of dietary advanced glycation end products in national diets and Alzheimer's disease incidence and prevalence." *Journal of Alzheimer's Disease* 45 (2015): 965–79.

295. Grant, William B., "Using Multicountry Ecological and Observational Studies to Determine Dietary Risk Factors for Alzheimer's Disease," *Journal of the American College of Nutrition* 35 (2016): 476.

296. Giem, P., et al., "The Incidence of Dementia and Intake of Animal Products: Preliminary Findings from the Adventist Health Study," *Neuroepidemiology* 12 (1993): 28-36.

297. Mosconi, L., et al., "Nutrient intake and brain biomarkers of Alzheimer's disease in at-risk cognitively normal individuals: a cross-sectional neuroimaging pilot study," *BMJ* Open. 2014;4: e004850.

298. Azadbakht, L., et al., "Red meat intake is associated with metabolic syndrome and the plasma C-reactive protein concentration in women," *Journal of Nutrition* 139 (2009):335-9; Montonen J., et al., "Consumption of red meat and whole-grain bread in relation to biomarkers of obesity, inflammation, glucose metabolism and oxidative stress," *European Journal of Nutrition* 52 (2013):337-45.

299. Swann, P.F., "Carcinogenic risk from nitrite, nitrate and N-nitrosamines in food," *Proceedings of the Royal Society of Medicine* 70 (1977):113-115.

300. De la Monte, Suzanne M., et al., "Epidemilogical Trends Strongly Suggest Exposures as Etiologic Agents in the Pathogenesis of Sporadic Alzheimer's Disease, Diabetes Mellitus, and Non-Alcoholic Steatohepatitis," *Journal of Alzheimer's Disease*, 17 (2009):519-529

301. de la Monte, Suzanne, et al., "Mechanisms of nirosamine-mediated neurodegeneration: potential relevance to sporadic Alzheimer's disease," *Journal of Alzheimer's Disease* 17 (2009):817-25.

302. De la Monte, Suzanne M., et al., "Mechanisms of nitrosamine–mediated neurodegeneration: potential relevance to sporadic Alzheimer's disease," *Journal of Alzheimer's Disease* 17 (2009):817-25; Hongtao, Yu, "Environmental carcinogenic polycyclic aromatic hydrocarbons: photochemistry and phototoxicity," *Journal of Environmental Science and Health Part C* 20 (2002): doi: 10.1081/GNC-120016203; Mahsa, Ranjbar, et al., "Urinary Biomarkers of Polycyclic Aromatic Hydrocarbons Are Associated with Cardiometabolic Health Risk," *PLOS One* (2015): doi.org/10.1371/journal.pone.0137536

303. Ferguson, Kelly K., et al., "Urinary Polycyclic Aromatic Hydrocarbon Metabolite Associations with Biomarkers of Inflammation, Angiogenesis, and Oxidative Stress in Pregnant Women," *Environmental Science & Technology* 51 (2017):4652-4660.

304. Ko, S.Y., et al., "The Possible Mechanism of Advanced Glycation End Products (AGEs) for Alzheimer's Disease," *PLoS One* 10 (2015): doi: 10.1371/journal.pone.0143345. eCollection 2015.

       Sasaki, N., et al., "Advanced glycation end products in Alzheimer's disease and other neurodegenerative diseases," *American Journal of Pathology* 153 (1998):1149-55; Bailey, A.J., "Molecular mechanisms of ageing in connective tissues," *Mechanisms of Ageing and Development* 122 (2001):735–55

305. Alzheimer's Disease International, *World Alzheimer's Report, 2014*. http://www.alzint.org/u/WorldAlzheimerReport2014.pdf

306. Uribarri, J., et al., "Restriction of dietary glycotoxins reduces excessive advanced glycation end products in renal failure patients," *Journal of the American Society of Nephrology* 14 (203):728–31.

307. O'Brien, J. et al., "Nutritional and toxicological aspects of the Maillard browning reaction in foods," *Critical Reviews in Food Science and Nutrition* 28 (1989):211-48.

308. Solfrizzi, V., *et al.*, 'Metabolic syndrome, mild cognitive impairment, and progression to dementia. The Italian longitudinal study on aging," *Neurobiology and Aging 32*

(2011):1932–1941; Eskelinen, M. Het al., "Fat intake at midlife and cognitive impairment later in life: A population-based caide study," *International Journal of Geriatric Psychiatry 23* (2008): 741–747.

309. "Dietary fat types and 4-year cognitive change in community-dwelling older women," *Annals of Neurology* 72 (2012):124–34.

310. Goodman, L., "Alzheimer's disease; a clinico-pathologic analysis of twenty-three cases with a theory on pathogenesis," *Journal of Nervous and Mental Disorders* 118 (1953):97–130.

311. Crapper McLachlan, D.R., et al., "Intramuscular desferrioxamine in patients with Alzheimer's disease," *Lancet* 337 (1991):1304-8.

312. Crapper McLachlan, D.R., et al., "Intramuscular desferrioxamine in patients with Alzheimer's disease," *Lancet* 337 (1991):1304-8.

313. Genoud, S., et al., "Subcellular compartmentalisation of copper, iron, manganese, and zinc in the Parkinson's disease brain," *Metallomics* 9 (2017):1447–1455.

314. Sinha, R., et al., "Meat intake and mortality: a prospective study of over half a million people," *Archives of Internal Medicine* 169 (2009):562-71; Song, M., et al., "Association of Animal and Plant Protein Intake with All-Cause and Cause-Specific Mortality" *JAMA Internal Medicine* 176 (2016):1453-63; Yangbo, Sun, et al., "Association of Major Dietary Protein Sources With All-Cause and Cause-Specific Mortality: Prospective Cohort Study," *JAHA* 10 (2021). doi.org/10.1161/JAHA.119.015553

315. Willett, Walter, *Eat, Drink and Be Healthy* (New York: Free Press, 2001), p 159.

316. Feskanich, D., et al., "Milk, dietary calcium, and bone fractures in women: a 12-year prospective study," *American Journal of Public Health* 87 (1997):992-997. doi:10.2105/ajph.87.6.992

317. Michaëlsson Karl., et al., "Milk intake and risk of mortality and fractures in women and men: cohort studies," *BMJ* 349 (2014): doi: https://doi.org/10.1136/bmj.g6015; Freskanich, D., et al., "Milk, dietary calcium, and bone fractures in women: a 12-year prospective study," *American Journal of Public Health* 87 (1997):992-7.

318. Michaelsson, Karl, et al., "Milk intake and risk of mortality and fractures in women and men: cohort studies," *BMJ* 349 (2014): doi: https://doi.org/10.1136/bmj.g6015; Cui, X., et al., "Chronic systemic D-galactose exposure induces memory loss, neurodegeneration, and oxidative damage in mice: protective effects of R-alpha-lipoic acid," *Journal of Neuroscience Research* 83 (2006):1584-90; Cui, X., et al., "D-galactose-caused life shortening in Drosophila melanogaster and Musca domestica is associated with oxidative stress," *Biogerontology* 5 (2004):317-25.

319. Hellenbrand, W., et al. "Diet and Parkinson's disease. I: a possible role for the past intake of specific foods and food groups. Results from a self-administered food-frequency questionnaire in a case-control study," *Neurology* 47 (1996): 636–643; Chen, H., et al., "Diet and Parkinson's disease: a potential role of dairy products in men," *Annals of Neurology* 52 (2002):793–801; Park, M., et al., "Consumption of milk and calcium in midlife and the future risk of Parkinson disease," *Neurology* 64 (2005):1047–1051; Kyrozis, A., et al., "Dietary and lifestyle variables in relation to incidence of Parkinson's disease in Greece," *European Journal of Epidemiology* 28 (2013):67–77; Chen H., et al., "Consumption of dairy products and risk of Parkinson's disease," *American Journal of Epidemiology* 165 (2007):998–1006; Olsson, E., et al.,

Melao, Alice, "Milk linked to greater risk of Parkinson's, Swedish study shows," *Parkinson's News Today* March 27, 2019.

320. U.S. EPA. Evaluation Of Dioxin in U.S. Cow's Milk. https://cfpub.epa.gov/ncea/risk/era/recordisplay.cfm?deid=87623

321. "Per capita consumption of eggs in the United States from 2000 to 2020" Statista, https://www.statista.com/statistics/183678/per-capita-consumption-of-eggs-in-the-us-since-2000/, accessed February 15, 2020.

322. Komaroff, Anthony, "Are eggs risky for heart health?" *Harvard Health Publishing,* June 24, 2019.

323. Virani, Salim S.et al., "Heart Disease and Stroke Statistics—2019 Update: A Report From the American Heart Association," *Circulation* (2019): DOI: 10.1161/CIR.0000000000000659

324. Victor W. Zhong et al., "Associations of Dietary Cholesterol or Egg Consumption with Incident Cardiovascular Disease and Mortality," *JAMA* (2019). doi: 10.1001/jama.2019.1572

325. Siweon, Choi, et al., "Development and verification for analysis of pesticides in eggs and egg products using QuEChERS and LC–MS/MS," *Food Chemistry* 173 (2015):1236-42; Kahunyo, James, et al., "Organochlorine pesticide residues in chicken eggs: A survey," *Journal of Toxicology and Environmental Health* 24 (2009):543-50; Hamid, Almis, et al., "Assessment of human health risk associated with the presence of pesticides in chicken eggs," *Food Science and Technology,* Campinas, 2017. http://www.scielo.br/scielo.php?script=sci_arttext&pid=S0101-20612017005006102&lng=en&nrm=iso>. access on May 13, 2017.

326. "New Dietary Guidelines remove restriction on total fat and set limit for added sugars but censor conclusions of the scientific advisory committee," *The Nutrition Source,* Harvard T.H. Chan School of Public Health

327. The state of the world's fisheries and aquaculture," FAO 2018, http://www.fao.org/3/i9540en/I9540EN.pdf

328. Painter, Kim, "Americans are eating more fish, but still not enough," *USA Today* November 20, 2016.

329. Blondeau, Nicholas, et al., "Alpha-Linolenic Acid: An Omega-3 Fatty Acid with Neuroprotective Properties—Ready for Use in the Stroke Clinic?" *BioMed Research International* 2015 (2015): http://dx.doi.org/10.1155/2015/519830

330. Kwak, S. M., et al., "Efficacy of omega-3 fatty acid supplements (eicosapentaenoic acid and docosahexaenoic acid) in the secondary prevention of cardiovascular disease: A meta-analysis of randomized, double-blind, placebo-controlled trials," *Archives of Internal Medicine* 172 (2012):986–94; "Smith, D. A., "Review: Omega-3 polyunsaturated fatty acid supplements do not reduce major cardiovascular events in adults," *Annals of Internal Medicine* 157 (2012):837–45.

331. Rizos, E. C., et al., "Association between omega-3 fatty acid supplementation and risk of major cardiovascular disease events: a systematic review and meta-analysis," *JAMA* 308 (2012):1024–33.

332. Sunderland, E. M., et al., "Decadal changes in the edible supply of seafood and methylmercury exposure in the United States," *Environmental Health Perspectives* 126 (2018). doi: 10.1289/EHP2644.

333. Masley, S.C., et al., "Effect of mercury levels and seafood intake on cognitive function in middle-aged adults," *Integrative Medicine* 11 (2012):32-40; Danthiir, V., et al., "Cognitive performance in older adults is inversely associated with fish consumption but not erythrocyte membrane n-3 fatty acids," *Journal of Nutrition* 144 (2014):311–20.

334. Chen YW, et al., "Heavy metals, islet function and diabetes development," *Islets* 1 (2009):169–176; Chang, J.W., et al., "Simultaneous exposure of non-diabetics to high levels of dioxins and mercury increases their risk of insulin resistance," *Journal of Hazardous Materials* 185 (2011):749–755.

335. Schartup, Amina, et al., "Climate change and overfishing increase neurotoxicant in marine predators," *Nature* (2019): DOI: 10.1038/s41586-019-1468-9

336. Friedman, Lisa, et al., "The E.P.A. Is Weakening Controls on Mercury," *New York Times* April 16, 2020.

337. Pulster, E.L., *et al.,* "A First Comprehensive Baseline of Hydrocarbon Pollution in Gulf of Mexico Fishes," *Nature Science Reports* 10 (2020). https://doi.org/10.1038/s41598-020-62944-6

338. Urbina, Ian. *The Outlaw Ocean: Journeys Across the Last Untamed Frontier* New York, Alfred A. Knopf, 2019. P 276.

339. Smith, M., et al., "Microplastics in Seafood and the Implications for Human Health," *Current Environmental Health Reports* 5 (2018):375-386; Institute of Medicine (US) Committee on Evaluation of the Safety of Fishery Products; Ahmed FE, editor. Seafood Safety. Washington (DC): National Academies Press (US); 1991. 5, Occurrence of Chemical Contaminants in Seafood and Variability of Contaminant Levels. Available from: https://www.ncbi.nlm.nih.gov/books/NBK235723/

340. Thompson, Andrea, "From Fish to Humans, A Microplastic Invasion May Be Taking a Toll," *Scientific American* September 4, 2018; Gallo, F., et al., "Marine litter plastics and microplastics and their toxic chemicals components: the need for urgent preventive measures," *Environmental Science Europe* 30 (2018):13. doi:10.1186/s12302-018-0139-z

341. The Ocean Conference, United Nations, New York, June 5-9, 2017; www.oceanconference.un.org

342. Karami, Ali, et al., "Microplastics in eviscerated flesh and excised organs of dried fish," *Science Reports* (2017): doi: 10.1038/s41598-017-05828-6; Cox, Kieran D., et al., "Human Consumption of Microplastics," *Environmental Science & Technology* (2019): DOI: 10.1021/acs.est.9b01517

343. Thompson, Andrea, "From fish to humans, a microplastic invasion may be taking a toll," *Scientific American* September 4, 2018

344. Law, Karen Lavendar, et al., "Microplastics in the Seas," *Science* 345 (2014):144-45.

345. Hites, Ronald A. et al. "Global Assessment of Organic Contaminants in Farmed Salmon." *Science* 303 (2004):226-29.

346. Foran, J.A., et al., "Risk-based consumption advice for farmed Atlantic and wild Pacific salmon contaminated with dioxins and dioxin-like compounds," *Environmental Health Perspectives* 113 (2005):552-556. doi:10.1289/ehp.7626

347. Hites, et al., "Global assessment of organic contaminants in farmed salmon," *Science* 303 (2004):226-9.

348. Learn, Joshua Rapp, "Some rivers are so polluted their eels get high on cocaine," *National Geographic* June 20, 2018.

349. Miller, Thomas, H., et al., "Biomonitoring of pesticides, pharmaceuticals and illicit drugs in a freshwater invertebrate to estimate toxic or effect pressure," *Environment International* 129 (2019):595-606.

350. Meador, James P., et al., "Contaminants of emerging concern in a large temperate estuary," *Environmental Pollution* 213 (2016):254-67.

351. Capaldo, A., et al., "Effects of environmental cocaine concentrations on the skeletal muscle of the European eel (Anguilla anguilla)," *Science of the Total Environment* 640 (2018):862-73.

352. Kutcha, R., et al., "Tapeworm larvae in salmon from North America," *Emerging Infectious Diseases,* February 2017, Center for Disease Control and Prevention, https://wwwnc.cdc.gov/eid/content/23/2/pdfs/v23-n2.pdf; Scutti, Susan, "Unusual symptoms pointing to brain cancer turned into something completely different" CNN June 7, 2019.

353. Nylund, Are, et al., "Wild and farmed salmon (*Salmo salar*) as reservoirs for infectious salmon anaemia virus, and the importance of horizontal- and vertical transmission," *PLOS* (2019). doi.org/10.1371/journal.pone.0215478; Jansen, M.D., et. Al., "The epidemiology of pancreas disease in salmonid aquaculture: a summary of the current state of knowledge," *Journal of Fish Diseases* (2016): doi.org/10.1111/jfd.12478

354. Vidal, John, "Salmon farming in crisis: 'We are seeing a chemical arms race in the seas,'" *The Guardian* April 2017

355. Macaskill, Mark, "Salmon industry toxins soar by 1,000 per cent," *The Times* January 2017.

356. https://coronavirus.sepa.org.uk/media/1050/sea-lice-medicine-finfish-aqua-reg-position. pdf

357. U.S. Government Accountability Office. *Seafood Safety: FDA Needs to Improve Oversight of Imported Seafood and Better Leverage Limited Resources.* http://www.gao.gov/new. items/d11286.pdf (2011).

358. Hansa, Y., et al., "Reconnaissance of 47 Antibiotics and Associated Microbial Risks in Seafood Sold in the United States," *Journal of Hazardous Materials* (2014). DOI: 10.1016/j.jhazmat.2014.08.075

359. "5 Seafood staples to add to your grocery list this week," https://palm.southbeachdiet. com/seafood-staples/

360. Carrool, Linda, "Eating fish 2-3 times a week is recommended: What about every day?" Today.com; https://www.today.com/health/it-ok-eat-fish-every-day-t34261

361. "Study shows draft EPA/FDA mercury fish advice not protective nor beneficial enough," Mercury Policy Project, March 20, 2016; http://mercurypolicy.org/2016/03/20/study-shows-epafda-mercury-advice-not-protective/

362. Yaginuma-Sakurai, K., "Hair-to-blood ratio and biological half-life of mercury: experimental study of methylmercury exposure through fish consumption in humans,"

Journal of Toxicology and Science 37 (2012):123-30. doi: 10.2131/jts.37.123. PMID: 22293416.

363. Bilic, Case I., et al., "Relationship between the prenatal exposure to low-level of mercury and the size of a newborn's cerebellum," *Medical Hypothesis* 76 (2011):514–16.

364. LabDoor laboratory analysis of top-selling fish oil supplements. https://labdoor.com/rankings/fish-oil.

365. Varela-Lopez, Alfonso, et al., "Gene pathways associated with mitochondrial function, oxidative stress and telomere length are differentially expressed in the liver of rats fed lifelong on virgin olive, sunflower or fish oils" *Journal of Nutritional Biochemistry* 52 (2018):36-44.

366. Messori, A., et al., "w-3 fatty acid supplements for secondary prevention of cardiovascular disease: from "no proof of effectiveness" to "proof of no effectiveness," *JAMA Internal Medicine* 173 (2013):1466-68.

367. Abdelhamid, A.S., et al., "Omega 3 fatty acids for the primary and secondary prevention of cardiovascular disease," *Cochrane Database of Systematic Reviews* (2018). DOI: 10.1002/14651858.CD003177.pub3.

368. Witte, A.V., et al., "Long-chain omega-3 fatty acids improve brain function and structure in older adults," *Cerebral Cortex* 24 (2014):3059-68.

369. Harwood, J.L., "Algae: Critical Sources of Very Long-Chain Polyunsaturated Fatty Acids," *Biomolecules* 9 (2019):708. doi: 10.3390/biom9110708. PMID: 31698772; PMCID: PMC6920940.

370. Horrobin, D. F., "Fatty acid metabolism in health and disease: The role of Δ-6-Desaturase," *American Journal of Clinical Nutrition* 57 (1993):732S–37S.

371. Doughman, S. D., et al., "Omega-3 fatty acids for nutrition and medicine: Considering microalgae oil as a vegetarian source of EPA and DHA," *Current Diabetes Reviews* 3 (2007):198–203.

372. Arterburn, L.M., et al., "Algal-oil capsules and cooked salmon: nutritionally equivalent sources of docosahexaenoic acid," *Journal of the American Dietetic Association* 108 (2008):1204-9. doi: 10.1016/j.jada.2008.04.020. PMID: 18589030.

373. Lustig, Robert H., et al., "The toxic truth about sugar," *Nature* 482 (2012):27–29.

374. Te Morenga L., et al., "Dietary sugars and body weight: systematic review and meta-analyses of randomized controlled trials and cohort studies," *British Medical Journal* 346 (2013): e7492.

375. Gomez-Pinilla, Fernando, et al., 'Metabolic syndrome' in the brain: deficiency in omega-3 fatty acid exacerbates dysfunctions in insulin receptor signaling and cognition," *The Journal of Physiology* 590 (2012):2485-2599.

376. Pase, M., et al., "Sugar and artificially sweetened beverages and the risks of incident stroke and dementia a prospective cohort study" *Stroke* 48 (2017):1129-31.

377. Popkin, B.M., et al., "The sweetening of the world's diet," *Obesity Research* 11 (2003):1325-1332.

378. Popkin, Barry, M., et al., "The sweetening of the global diet, particularly beverages: patterns, trends and policy responses for diabetes prevention," *Lancet Diabetes & Endocrinology* 4 (2016):174-86.

379. Hsu, T.M., et al., "Effects of sucrose and high fructose corn syrup consumption on spatial memory function and hippocampal neuroinflammation in adolescent rats," *Hippocampus* 25 (2015):227–239.

380. Suez, J., et al., "Artificial sweeteners induce glucose intolerance by altering the gut microbiota," *Nature* 514 (2014):181-6.

381. Tey, S.L., et al., "Effects of aspartame-, monk fruit-, stevia- and sucrose-sweetened beverages on postprandial glucose, insulin and energy intake," *International Journal of Obesity* 41 (2017):450-57.

382. "A look at calorie sources in the American diet," Food Availability (per capita) Data System. U.S. Department of Agriculture. July 21. 2021.

383. Chang, Y. C., "Neurotoxic effects of n-hexane on the human central nervous system: evoked potential abnormalities in n-hexane polyneuropathy," *Journal of Neurology, Neurosurgery, and Psychiatry* 50 (1987): 269-74.

384. Azizian, H., et al., "A Rapid Method for the Quantification of Fatty Acids in Fats and Oil with Emphasis on trans Fatty Acids Using Fourier Transform Near Infrared Spectroscopy (FT-NIR)," *Lipids* 40 (2005):855-867; O'Keefe, Sean, et al., "Levels of *trans* geometrical isomers of essential fatty acids in some unhydrogenated US vegetable oils," *Journal of Food Lipids* (1994). doi.org/10.1111/j.1745-4522.1994.tb00244.

385. Bi, X., et al., "Plasticizer contamination in edible vegetable oil in a U.S. retail market," *Journal of Agriculture and Food Chemistry* 61 (2013):9502-9. doi: 10.1021/jf402576a.

386. Lin, C.Y., et al., "Association between levels of serum bisphenol A, a potentially harmful chemical in plastic containers, and carotid artery intima-media thickness in adolescents and young adults," *Atherosclerosis* 241 (2015):657-63; Weiss, Bernard, The intersection of neurotoxicology and endocrine disruption," *Neurotoxicology* 33 (2012):1410-19; Leranth, C., et al., "Bisphenol A prevents the synaptogenic response to estradiol in hippocampus and prefrontal cortex of ovariectomized nonhuman primates," Proceedings of the National Academy of Science USA Epub 2008 Sept. 3; Szychowski, K. A., et al., "Components of plastic disrupt the function of the nervous system," *Postepy Hig Med Dosw* (Online) 67 (2013):499–506; Kim, M. E., et al., "Exposure to bisphenol A appears to impair hippocampal neurogenesis and spatial learning and memory," *Food Chemistry and Toxicology* 49(2011):3383–89; Young, Jang, et al., "High dose bisphenol A impairs hippocampal neurogenesis in female mice across generations," *Toxicology* 296 (2012):73–82.

387. Moghe, A, et al., "Molecular mechanisms of acrolein toxicity: relevance to human disease," *Toxicological Sci*ences 143 (2015):242-255. doi:10.1093/toxsci/kfu233

388. Guillén, Maria, D., et al., "Aldehydes contained in edible oils of a very different nature after prolonged heating at frying temperature: Presence of toxic oxygenated α, β unsaturated aldehydes," *Food Chemistry* 131 (2012): DOI: 10.1016/j.foodchem.2011.09.079; Zhang Q, et al., "The changes in the volatile aldehydes formed during the deep-fat frying process," *Journal of Food Science and Technology* 52 (2015):7683-7696. doi:10.1007/s13197-015-1923-z

389. Uribarri, J., et al., "Advanced glycation end products in foods and a practical guide to their reduction in the diet," *Journal of the American Dietetic Association 110* (2010):911-16.

390. Frankel, E.N., et al., "Report: Evaluation of extra-virgin olive oil sold in California," U.C. Davis Olive Center, April 2011; Rodriguez, Cecelia, "The Olive Oil Scam: If 80% Is Fake, Why Do You Keep Buying It?" *Forbes* February 10, 2016.

391. "Pesticide residue assessment in different types of olive oil and preliminary exposure assessment of Greek consumers to the pesticide residues detected," *Food Chemistry* 113 (2009):253-261; DOI: 10.1016/j.foodchem.2008.06.073; Karanasios, E., et al., "Monitoring of glyphosate and AMPA in soil samples from two olive cultivation areas in Greece: aspects related to spray operators activities," *Environmental Monitoring and Assessment* 361 (2018): https://doi.org/10.1007/s10661-018-6728-x

392. "Worst fast-food meals for sodium" CNN January 23, 2014. http://www.cnn.com/2013/01/04/health/gallery/fast-food-worst-sodium-meals

393. National Institute on Aging, "Blood Vessels and Aging: The Rest of the Journey," *Aging Hearts & Arteries* https://www.nia.nih.gov/health/publication/aging-hearts-and-arteries/chapter-4-blood-vessels-and-aging-rest-journey

394. Grant, Bridget F., et al., "Prevalence of 12-Month Alcohol Use, High-Risk Drinking, and *DSM-IV* Alcohol Use Disorder in the United States, 2001-2002 to 2012-2013: Results from the National Epidemiologic Survey on Alcohol and Related Conditions," *JAMA Psychiatry* 74 (2017):911-23.

395. National Institute of Alcohol Abuse and Alcoholism, "Alcohol-related deaths increasing in the United States," News Release January 8, 2020.

396. "Alcohol Alert: National epidemiologic survey on alcohol and related conditions," National Institutes of Health, U.S. Department of Health and Human Services. https://pubs.niaaa.nih.gov/publications/AA70/AA70.htm; Ingraham, Christopher, "Think you drink a lot? This chart will tell you," *Washington Post* September 25, 2014.

397. Millwood, Iona, Y., et al., "Conventional and genetic evidence on alcohol and vascular disease aetiology: a prospective study of 500 000 men and women in China," *Lancet* (2019): doi.org/10.1016/S0140-6736(18)31772-0

398. Topiwala, Anya, et al., "No safe level of alcohol consumption for brain health: observational cohort study of 25,378 UK Biobank participants," 2021. https://doi.org/10.110½2021.05.10.21256931

399. Gorky, J., et al., "The role of the gut-brain axis in alcohol use disorders," *Progress in Neuro-Psychopharmacology & Biological Psychiatry* 65 (2016):234–241; Szabo, G., et al., "Converging actions of alcohol on liver and brain immune signaling," *International Review of Neurobiology* 118 (2014):359–380.

400. Cannon, Abigail, R., et al., "Alcohol, inflammation, and depression: the gut-brain axis," *Inflammation and Immunity in Depression* (2018). doi.org/10.1016/B978-0-12-811073-7.00029-5: Wang, H.J, et al., "Alcohol, inflammation, and gut-liver-brain interactions in tissue damage and disease development," *World Journal of Gastroenterology* 16 (2010):1304–1313. doi:10.3748/wjg.v16.i11.1304

401. Sergey, Kalinin, et al., "Transcriptome analysis of alcohol-treated microglia reveals down regulation of beta amyloid phagocytosis," *Journal of Neuroinflammation* 15 (2018): DOI:10.1186/s12974-018-1184-7; Athanasopoulos, Dimitrios, et al., "Recent Findings in Alzheimer Disease and Nutrition Focusing on Epigenetics," *Advances in Nutrition* 7 (2016):917-27.

402. Frontier C., et al., "Widespread effects of alcohol on white matter microstructure," *Alcoholism: Clinical & Experimental Research* 38 (2014):2925–33.

403. Edenberg, H.J., "The genetics of alcohol metabolism: Role of alcohol dehydrogenase and aldehyde dehydrogenase variants," *Alcohol Research & Health* 30 2007):5–13.

404. Eigenbrodt, Marsha L., et al., "Alcohol Intake and Cerebral Abnormalities on Magnetic Resonance Imaging in a Community-Based Population of Middle-Aged Adults. The Atherosclerosis Risk in Communities (ARIC) Study," *Stroke* 35 (2004):16-21; Paul, Carol Anne, et al., May 1, 2007, presentation, American Academy of Neurology annual meeting, Boston, MA.

405. Paul, C.A., et al., "Association of Alcohol Consumption with Brain Volume in the Framingham Study," *Archives of Neurology* 65 (2008):1363-67.

406. Topiwala, Anya, et al., "Moderate alcohol consumption as risk factor for adverse brain outcomes and cognitive decline: longitudinal cohort study," *BMJ* 357 (2017): doi.org/10.1136/bmj.j2553

407. Mukamal, Kenneth J., et al., "Alcohol Consumption and Subclinical Findings on Magnetic Resonance Imaging of the Brain in Older Adults," *Stroke* 32 (2001):1939-46.

408. Amber Bahorik, PhD, et al. Alcohol Use Disorders in Female Veterans and the Impact on Dementia Risk. Presented at the Alzheimer's Association International Conference, July 14, 2019.

409. Schwarzinger, Michael, et al., "Contribution of alcohol use disorders to the burden of dementia in France 2008–13: a nationwide retrospective cohort study," *Lancet* (2018): doi.org/10.1016/S2468-2667(18)30022-7.

410. Rock, C.L., et al., "American Cancer Society guideline for diet and physical activity for cancer prevention," *CA A Cancer Journal for Clinicians* 70 (2020):245-271. doi:10.3322/caac.21591

411. University of Pennsylvania School of Medicine. "One in four Americans develop insomnia each year: 75 percent of those with insomnia recover," *ScienceDaily* June 5, 2018: www.sciencedaily.com/releases/2018/06/180605154114.htm

412. Benedict, C., et al., "Acute sleep deprivation increases serum levels of neuron-specific enolase (NSE) and S100 calcium binding protein B (S-100B) in healthy young men," *Sleep* 37 (2014):195–198.

413. Hsie-Ling, Chen, et al., "Systemic inflammation and alterations to cerebral blood flow in obstructive sleep apnea," *Journal of Sleep Research* 26 (2017) doi.org/10.1111/jsr.12553

414. Huang, Y., et al., "Effects of age and amyloid deposition on Abeta dynamics in the human central nervous system," *Archives of Neurology* 69 (2012):51–58

415. Ibid.

416. Sprecher, Kate E., et al., "Poor sleep is associated with CSF biomarkers of amyloid pathology in cognitively normal adults," *Neurology* (2017). Published online: doi: http://dx.doi.org/10.1212/WNL.0000000000004171

417. Holth, Jerrah, K., et al., "The sleep-wake cycle regulates brain interstitial fluid tau in mice and CSF tau in humans," *Science* 363 (2019):880-84.

418. Holth, J.K, et al., "The sleep-wake cycle regulates brain interstitial fluid tau in mice and CSF tau in humans," *Science* (2019): DOI: 10.1126/science.aav2546

419. Spira, Adam, et al., "Self-reported Sleep and β-Amyloid Deposition in Community-Dwelling Older Adults," *JAMA Neurology*, 21 (2013):4258.

420. Kang, J.E., et al., "Amyloid-beta dynamics are regulated by orexin and the sleep-wake cycle," *Science* 326 (2009):1005–1007.

421. Shokri-Kojori, E., et al., "β-Amyloid accumulation in the human brain after one night of sleep deprivation," *Proceedings of the National Academy of Sciences* 115 (2018):4483-88.

422. Ogawa Y, et al,. "Total sleep deprivation elevates blood pressure through arterial baroreflex resetting: A study with microneurographic technique," *Sleep* 26 (2003):986–9.

423. Lac, G., et al., "Elevated salivary cortisol levels as a result of sleep deprivation in a shift worker," *Occupational Medicine* 53 (2003):143–5.

424. Spiegel K, et al., "Sleep loss: A novel risk factor for insulin resistance and type 2 diabetes," *Journal of Applied Physiology* 99 (2005):2008–19.

425. Xie, L., et al., "Sleep drives metabolite clearance from the adult brain," *Science* 342 (2013):373–7.

426. Mendelsohn, A.R., et al., "Sleep facilitates clearance of metabolites from the brain: glymphatic function in aging and neurodegenerative diseases," *Rejuvenation Research* 16 (2013):518-23; Xie, L., et al., "Sleep drives metabolite clearance from the adult brain," *Science* 342 (2013):373–377.

427. Xie, Lulu, et al., "Sleep drives metabolite clearance from the Adult Brain," *Science* 342 (2013):373-377.

428. Xie, Lulu, et al., "Sleep drives metabolite clearance from the adult brain," *Science* 2013, 342 (2013):373–77.

429. Stickgold R., "Sleep-dependent memory consolidation," *Nature* 437 (2005):1272–8.

430. Rasch, B., et al., "About sleep's role in memory," *Physiological Reviews* 93 (2013):681–766.

431. Bukalo, Olena, et al., "Synaptic plasticity by antidromic firing during hippocampal network oscillations," *Proceedings of the National Academy of Sciences* 110 (2013):5175-80.

432. Yuan T. F., et al., "Adult neurogenesis in the hypothalamus: evidence, functions, and implication," *CNS and Neurological Disorders - Drug Targets* 10 (2011): 433–439

433. Fernandes, Carina, et al., "Detrimental role of prolonged sleep deprivation on adult neurogenesis," *Frontiers in Cellular Neuroscience* (2015):140.

434. Cheng, Wei, "Sleep duration, brain structure, and psychiatric and cognitive problems in children," *Molecular Psychiatry* (2020): DOI: 10.1038/s41380-020-0663-2

435. Daghlas, Iyas, et al., "Genetically Proxied Diurnal Preference, Sleep Timing, and Risk of Major Depressive Disorder," *JAMA Psychiatry* 2021; DOI: 10.1001/jamapsychiatry.2021.0959

436. Deal, J.A., et al., "Hearing impairment and incident dementia and cognitive decline in older adults: The Health ABC Study," *The Journals of Gerontology* 2016; (published online April 12.) DOI:10.1093/gerona/glw069

437. Lin Fret al., "Hearing loss and incident dementia," *Archives of Neurology* 68 (2011):214-220. doi:10.1001/archneurol.2010.362

438. McCormack, A., et al., "Why do people fitted with hearing aids not wear them?" *International Journal of Audiology* 52 (2013):360-368. doi:10.3109/14992027.2013.769066

439. Su, BM, et al., "Prevalence of Hearing Loss in US Children and Adolescents: Findings from NHANES 1988-2010," *JAMA Otolaryngology Head Neck Surgery* 143 (2017):920–927. doi:10.1001/jamaoto.2017.0953

440. Mosnier, Isabelle, et al., "Improvement of Cognitive Function After Cochlear Implantation in Elderly Patients," *JAMA Otolaryngology Head Neck Surgery* 141 (2015):442-450.

441. Deal, J.A., et al., "Hearing impairment and incident dementia and cognitive decline in older adults: The Health ABC Study," *The Journals of Gerontology* 2016; (published online April 12.) DOI:10.1093/gerona/glw069

442. Wells, T.S., et al., "Hearing loss associated with US military combat deployment," *Noise Health* 17 (2015):34-42. doi:10.4103/1463-1741.149574

443. Warszawa, A., et al., "Noise exposure in movie theaters: a preliminary study of sound levels during the showing of 25 films," *Ear, Nose, & Throat Journal* 89 (2010):444-50.

444. Bridges, C.C., et al., "Transport of inorganic mercury and methylmercury in target tissues and organs," *Journal of Toxicology and Environmental Health—Part B* 13 (2010):385–410.

445. James, S.J., et al., "Thimerosal neurotoxicity is associated with glutathione depletion: protection with glutathione precursors," *Neurotoxicology* 26 (2005):1-8.

446. Atchison, W.D., et al., "Mechanisms of methylmercury-induced neurotoxicity," *FASEB J* 8 (1994):622-9.

447. Azevedo, Bruna Fernandes, et al., "Toxic Effects of Mercury on the Cardiovascular and Central Nervous Systems," *Journal of Biomedicine and Biotechnology* 2012, Published online.

448. Main, Douglas, "The surprising source of most mercury pollution," *Livescience* Sept. 26, 2013. www.livescience.com/39982-surprising-mercury-pollution-sources.html.

449. Szpir, Michael, "New thinking on neurodevelopment," *Environmental Health Perspectives* 114 (2006): A100-A107.

450. Eskes, C., et al., "Microglial reaction induced by noncytotoxic methylmercury treatment leads to neuroprotection via interactions with astrocytes and IL-6 release," *Glia* 37 (2002):43-52.

451. Mingwei, Ni, et al., "Methylmercury Induces Acute Oxidative Stress, Altering Nrf2 Protein Level in Primary Microglial Cells," *Toxicological Sciences* 116 (2010):590-603; Kempuraj, Duraisamy, et al., "Mercury induces inflammatory mediator release from human mast cells," *Journal of Neuroinflammation* 7 (2010):20.

452. Monnet-Tschudi, F., et al., "Involvement of environmental mercury and lead in the etiology of neurodegenerative diseases," *Reviews of Environmental Health* 21 (2006):105–17.

453. International POPs Elimination Network, "Mercury in Women of Child-bearing Age in 25 Countries," https://ipen.org/site/mercury-women-child-bearing-age-25-countries

454. U.S. Environmental Protection Agency, 1997, "Mercury study report to congress, Volume II: An inventory of anthropogenic mercury emissions in the United States," table ES-3, sum of Utility boilers and Commercial/industrial boilers. Report EPA-452/R-97-004.

455. Urbina, Ian. *The Outlaw Ocean: Journeys Across the Last Untamed Frontier* (New York, Alfred A. Knopf, 2019.)

456. Drevnick, Paul E., et al., "Increase in mercury in Pacific yellowfin tuna," Environmental Toxicology and Chemistry 34 (2015):931–34; Schartup, Amina, et al., "Climate change and overfishing increase neurotoxicant in marine predators," *Nature* (2019): DOI: 10.1038/s41586-019-1468-9

457. Sunderland, Elsie M., et al., "Decadal changes in the edible supply of seafood and methylmercury exposure in the United States," *Environmental Health Perspectives* 126 (2018) doi.org/10.1289/EHP2644

458. Weise, Elizabeth, Traci Watson, "Warnings on river, lake fish jump," *USA Today*, Aug. 25, 2004.

459. Kay, Jane, "Doctors urge mercury labels for fish: Resolution warns public of poisonous chemical found in tuna, swordfish, shark," *San Francisco Chronicle*, Apr. 2, 2003.

460. Kay, Jane, "Rich folks eating fish feed on mercury too: Healthy clearly isn't," *San Francisco Chronicle* Nov. 5, 2002.

461. *Now with Bill Moyers*, "Mercury in fish"; Allchin, Douglas, "The Poisoning of Minimata," www.pbs.org/now/science/mercuryinfish/html, July 18, 2003; also see *Ishimure*, 1972, 1975, 1990, a book by *Life* photographer Eugene Smith and his wife, Aileen, documenting the Minimata tragedy.

462. Kay, Jane, "Rich folks eating fish feed on mercury too: 'Healthy diet' clearly isn't," *San Francisco Chronicle* Nov. 5, 2002.

463. Hightower, Jane, et al., "Mercury levels in high-end consumers of fish," *Environmental Health Perspectives* 111 (2003):604–8.

464. Kay, Jane, "Rich folks eating fish feed on mercury too: 'Healthy diet' clearly isn't," *San Francisco Chronicle*, Nov. 5, 2002.

465. Whitty, Julia, "The fate of the ocean," *Mother Jones*, Mar./Apr. 2006, p. 40.

466. Levy, M., "Dental Amalgam: Toxicological evaluation and health risk assessment". *J Canadian Dental Association* 61 (1995):667–68.

467. Alfrey, A. C., et al., "The dialysis encephalopathy syndrome: Possible aluminum intoxication," *New England Journal of Medicine* 294 (1976):184–88.

468. Solfrizzi, V., et al., "The role of diet in cognitive decline," *Journal of Neural Transmission* 110 (2003):95–110.

469. Joshi, J. G., "Aluminum, a neurotoxin which affects diverse metabolic reactions," *Biofactors* 2 (1990):163–69.

470. Yokel, R.A., et al., "The distribution of aluminum into and out of the brain," *Journal of Inorganic Biochemistry* 76 (1999):127-32.

471. Edwardson, J. A., et al., "Aluminum accumulation, beta amyloid deposition and neurofibrillary changes in the central nervous system," *Ciba Foundation Symposium* 169 (1992):165–79; Yumoto, S., "Demonstration of aluminum in amyloid fibers in the cores of senile plaques in the brains of patients with Alzheimer's disease," *Journal of Inorganic Biochemistry* 103 (2009):1579–84.

472. Campbell, A., et al., "Chronic exposure to aluminum in drinking water increases inflammatory parameters selectivelyin the brain," *Journal of Neuroscience Research* 75 (2004):565-72.

473. Praticò, D., et al., "Aluminum modulates brain amyloidosis through oxidative stress in APP transgenic mice," *FASEB J* 16 (2002):1138–40.

474. Murakami, K., et al., "Aluminum decreases the glutathione regeneration by the inhibition of NADP-isocitrate dehydrogenase in mitochondria," *Journal of Cell Biochemistry* 93 (2004):1267-71; Jovanova-Nesic, K., et al., "Aluminum excytotoxicity and neuroautotoimmunity: the role of the brain expression of CD32+ (FcγRIIa), ICAM-1+ and CD3ξ in aging," *Current Aging Science* 5 (2012):209-17.

475. Mirza, A., et al., "Aluminum in brain tissue in familial Alzheimer's disease," *Journal of Trace Elements in Medicine and Biology* 40 (2017):30-36. doi:10.1016/j.jtemb.2016.12.001. Epub 2016 Dec 9. PMID: 28159219.

476. Martyn, C.N, et al., "Geographical relation between Alzheimer's disease and aluminum in drinking water," *The Lancet* 8629 (1989):59–62; Flaten, T.P., "Aluminum as a risk factor in Alzheimer's disease, with emphasis on drinking water," *Brain Research Bulletin* 55 (2001):187–196; Martyn, C.N., et al., "Geographical relation between Alzheimer's disease and aluminum in drinking water," *The Lancet* 8629 (1989):59–62; Rondeau, V., et al., "Aluminum and silica in drinking water and the risk of Alzheimer's disease or cognitive decline: findings from 15-year follow-up of the PAQUID cohort," *American Journal of Epidemiology* 169 (2009):489–496; Frecker, M.F., "Dementia in Newfoundland: identification of a geographical isolate?" *Journal of Epidemiology and Community Health* 45 (1991):307–311.

477. Zumkley, H., et al., "Aluminium konzentration in Knochen und Gehirn nach Antazidagabe," *Fortschritte der Medizin* 105 (1987):15–18.

478. Whiting, S. J., "Safety of some calcium supplements questioned," *Nutrition Reviews* 52 (1994):95–97.

479. Saiyed, Salim, et al., "Aluminium content of some foods and food products in the USA, with aluminium food additives," *Food Additives & Contaminants* 22 (2004):234-44.

480. Bassioni, Ghada, et al., "Risk Assessment of Using Aluminum Foil in Food Preparation," *International Journal of Electrochemical Science* 7 (2012):4498-4509.

481. Bárcena-Padilla, Diego Armando, et al., "Aluminum contents in dry leaves and infusions of commercial black and green tea leaves: Effects of sucrose and ascorbic acid added to infusions," *Natural Resources* 2 (2011):141–45.

482. Malik, J., et al., "Aluminum and other elements in selected herbal tea plant species and their infusions," *Food Chemistry* 139 (2013):728-34.

483. Rondeau, Virginie, et al., "Relation between aluminum concentrations in drinking water and Alzheimer's disease: An 8-year follow-up study," *American Journal of Epidemiology* 152 (2000):59–66.

484. McLachlan, D. R. C., et al., "Risk for neuropathologically confirmed Alzheimer's disease and residual aluminum in municipal drinking water employing weighted residential histories," *Neurology* 46 (1996):401–5; Campbell, A., et al., "Chronic exposure to aluminum in drinking water increases inflammatory parameters selectively in the brain," *Journal of Neuroscience Research* 75 (2004):565-72.

485. Fimreite, N., et al., "Aluminum concentrations in selected foods prepared in aluminum cookware, and its implications for human health," *Bulletin of Environmental Contamination and Toxicology* 58 (1997):1–7.

486. United States Food and Drug Administration, "Common ingredients in U.S. licensed vaccines," May 1, 2014: http://www.fda.gov/BiologicsBloodVaccines/SafetyAvailability/VaccineSafety/ucm187810.htm.

487. Bucossi, S., et al., "Copper in Alzheimer's disease: A meta-analysis of serum, plasma, and cerebrospinal fluid studies," *Journal of Alzheimer's Disease* 24 (2011):175–85.

488. Singh, I., et al., "Low levels of copper disrupt brain amyloid-β homeostasis by altering its production and clearance," *PNAS* 110 (2013):14771–76.

489. "Elevated serum copper levels and cognitive decline in Alzheimer's disease," *Alzheimer's & Dementia* 10 (2014):564; Squitti, R., et al., "Low-copper diet as a preventive strategy for Alzheimer's Disease," *Neurobiology & Aging* 35 (2014): S40–S50; Gouping, Zhou, et al., "Association between Serum Copper Status and Working Memory in Schoolchildren," *Nutrients* 7 (2015):7185-96.

490. Morris, M.C., et al., "Dietary copper and high saturated and trans fatsintakes associated with cognitive decline," *Archives of Neurology* 63 (2006):1085–1088.

491. Dwyer, Barney E., et al., "Getting the iron out: Phlebotomy for Alzheimer's disease?" *Medical Hypothesis* 72 (2009):504-509.

492. Ibid.

493. Zecca, L., et al., "Iron, brain ageing and neurodegenerative disorders," *Nature Reviews Neuroscience* 5 (2004):863-73; Ward, R.J., et al., "The role of iron in brain ageing and neurodegenerative disorders," *Lancet Neurology* 13 (2014):1045-60.

494. Sayre, L.M., et al., "In situ oxidative catalysis by neurofibrillary tangles and senile plaues in Alzheimer's disease: a central role for bound transition metals," *Journal of Neurochemistry* 74 (2000):270-9.

495. Rouault, T.A., "Iron on the brain," *Nature Genetics* 28 (2001):299–300; Richardson, D.R., "Novel chelators for central nervous system disorders that involve alterations in the metabolism of iron and other metal ions," *Annals of New York Academy of Science* 1012 (2004): 326–341.

496. Ayton, Scott, et al., "Ferritin levels in the cerebrospinal fluid predict Alzheimer's disease outcomes and are regulated by APOE," *Nature Communications* 6 (2015).

497. Perry, George, et al., "Alzheimer disease and oxidative stress," *Journal of Biomedical Biotechnology* 2 (2002):120–23.

498. Stankiewicz, J., et al., "Iron in chronic brain disorders: Imaging and neurotherapeutic implications," *Neurotherapeutics* 4 (2007):371–86.

499. Raven, Erika P., et al., "Increased iron levels and decreased tissue integrity in hippocampus of Alzheimer's disease detected in vivo with magnetic resonance imaging," *Journal of Alzheimer's Disease* 37 (2013):127-36.

500. Ayton, S., et al., "Ferritin levels in the cerebrospinal fluid predict Alzheimer's disease outcomes and are regulated by APOE," *Nature Communications* 19 (2015): 6760. doi:10.1038/ncomms7760. http://dx.doi.org/10.1038/ncomms7760.

501. Kontoghiorghes, G. J., et al., "Molecular factors and mechanisms affecting iron and other metal excretion or absorption in health and disease: the role of natural and synthetic chelators," *Current Medicinal Chemistry* 12 (2005):2695-709.

502. Shersten, Killip, et al., "Iron deficiency anemia," *American Family Physician* 75 (2007):671-678.

503. http://www.hemochromatosis.org/#overview

504. Needleman, H., "Low level lead exposure: History and discovery," *Annals of Epidemiology* 19 (2009):235–38.

505. Cradock, AL, et al., "State approaches to testing school drinking water for lead in the United States. Boston, MA: Prevention Research Center on Nutrition and Physical Activity at the Harvard T.H. Chan School of Public Health; 2019. Available at https://www.hsph.harvard.edu/prc/projects/ school-research/early-adopters.

506. Dart, R. C, et al., Lead, in R. C. Dart, ed., *Medical Toxicology* (Philadelphia: Lippincott Williams & Wilkins, 2004).

507. Walker Jr., B., "Neurotoxicity in human beings," *Journal of Laboratory and Clinical Medicine* 136 (2000):168–180.

508. Lopes, A.C., et al., "Lead Exposure and Oxidative Stress: A Systematic Review," *Reviews of Environmental Contamination and Toxicology* 236 (2016):193-238.

509. Mason, Lisa H., et al., "Pb Neurotoxicity: Neuropsychological Effects of Lead Toxicity," *BioMed Research International* 2014 (2014) Article ID 840547

510. Stewart, W., et al., "ApoE genotype, past adult lead exposure, and neurobehavioral function," *Environmental Health Perspectives* 110 (2002); Weisskopf, M. G., et al., "Cumulative lead exposure and cognitive performance among elderly men," *Epidemiology* 18 (2007):59–66; Basha, M. R., et al., "Lead exposure and its effect on APP proteolysis and AB aggregation," *FASEB J* 19 (2005):2083–84.

511. Shih, R. A., et al., "Environmental lead exposure and cognitive function in community-dwelling older adults," *Neurology* 67 (2006):1556–62.

512. Weisskopf, M. G., et al., "Cumulative lead exposure and cognitive performance among elderly men," *Epidemiology* 18 (2007):59–66.

513. Basha, M. R., et al., "The fetal basis of amyloidogenesis: Exposure to lead and latent overexpression of amyloid precursor protein and beta amyloid in the aging brain," *Journal of Neuroscience* 25 (2005):823–29; Kim, J., et al., "Environmental exposure to lead (Pb) and variations in its susceptibility," *Journal of Environmental Science and Health* Part C: *Environmental* Carcinogenesis and *Ecotoxicology* Reviews 32 (2014):159–85.

514. Rankin, Charley, W., et al., "Lead contamination in cocoa and cocoa products: Isotopic evidence of global contamination," *Environmental Health Perspectives* 113 (2005):1344–48; Bernstein, Lenny, "How much lead is in your chocolate?" *Washington Post*, Feb. 11, 2015. https://www.washingtonpost.com/news/to-your-health/wp/2015/02/11/lead-and-cadmium-in-chocolate-noooooooooooo, accessed online, Mar. 27, 2015.

515. Bourgoin, B. P., et al., "Lead content in 70 brands of dietary calcium supplements," *American Journal of Public Health* 83 (1993):1155–60.

516. Scelfo, G. M., et al., "Lead in calcium supplements," *Environmental Health Perspectives* 108 (2000):309–19.

517. Ferrari, F., et al., "Predicting and measuring environmental concentration of pesticides in air after soil application," *Journal of Environmental Quality* 32 (2003):1623-33.

518. Klarich, Kathryn, L., et al., "Occurrence of Neonicotinoid Insecticides in Finished Drinking Water and Fate during Drinking Water Treatment," *Environmental Science & Technology Letters* 5 (2017):168-73.

519. Hussain, Sarfraz, et al., "Impact of Pesticides on Soil Microbial Diversity, Enzymes, and Biochemical Reactions," *Advances in Agronomy* 102 (2009):159-200.

520. Rossman, Sean, "Strawberries and these other foods have the most pesticides," *USA Today* March 10, 2017; "Eat the peach, not the pesticide," *Consumer Reports* March 19, 2015.

521. Ross, Z., et al., "Poisoning the air: Airborne pesticides in California," *California Public Interest Research Group and Californians for Pesticide Reform* (San Francisco, 1999); Glotfelty, Pearce, Fred, et al., "Pesticides in fog," *Nature* 325 (1987):602–5.

522. United States Geological Survey, "Pesticides in the nation's streams and ground water, 1992–2001: A summary." http://pubs.usgs.gov/fs/2006/3028.

523. Goodman, Sara, "Tests find more than 200 chemicals in newborn umbilical cord blood," *Scientific American* December 2, 2009.

524. National Center for Healthy Housing. Pesticides. https://nchh.org/information-and-evidence/learn-about-healthy-housing/health-hazards-prevention-and-solutions/pesticides/

525. Goodman, Sara, "Tests find more than 200 chemicals in newborn umbilical cord blood," *Scientific American* December 2, 2009.

526. Yan, Dandan, et al., "Pesticide exposure and risk of Alzheimer's disease: a systematic review and meta-analysis," *Nature* Scientific Reports 6 (2016). Published online: http://www.nature.com/articles/srep32222

527. Bosma, H., et al., "Pesticide exposure and risk of mild cognitive dysfunction," *Lancet* 356 (2000):912–913; Bosma, H., et al., "Pesticide exposure and risk of mild cognitive dysfunction," *Lancet* 356 (2000): 912–913.

528. Lindsay, J., et al., "The Canadian Study of Health and Aging: risk factors for vascular dementia," *Stroke; A Journal of Cerebral Circulation* 28 (1997): 526–530.

529. Kamel, F., et al., "Pesticide exposure and amyotrophic lateral sclerosis," *Neurotoxicology* 33 (2012):457–62.

530. Betarbet, Ranjita, et al., "Chronic systemic pesticide exposure reproduces features of Parkinson's disease," *Nature Neuroscience* 3 (2000):1301-06; Fong, Chin-Shih, et al., "Pesticides exposure and genetic polymorphism of paraoxonase in the susceptibility of Parkinson's disease," *Acta Neurlogica Taiwanica* 14 (2005):55-60; Priyadarshi, A., et al., "A metaanalysis of Parkinson's disease and exposure to pesticides," *Neurotoxicology* 21 (2000):435-40; Lai, B.C., et al., "Occupational and environmental risk factors for Parkinson's disease," *Parkinsonism & Related Disorders* 8 (2002):297-309; Gorell, J.M., et al., "The risk of Parkinson's disease with exposure to pesticides, farming, well water, and rural living," *Neurology* 50 (1998):1346-50.

531. Hayden, K. M. et al., "Occupational exposure to pesticides increases the risk of incident AD: the Cache County study," *Neurology* 74 (2010): 1524–1530; Baldi, I. et al., "Neurodegenerative diseases and exposure to pesticides in the elderly," *American Journal of Epidemiology* 157 (2003): 409–414; Parron, T., Requena, M., Hernandez, A. F. & Alarcon, R. "Association between environmental exposure to pesticides and neurodegenerative diseases," *Toxicology and Applied Pharmacology* 256 (2011): 379–385.

532. Cicchetti, F., et al., "Systemic exposure to paraquat and maneb models early Parkinson's disease in young adult rats," *Neurobiology* of Disease 20 (2005):360–71; Costello., S., et al., "Parkinson's disease and residential exposure to maneb and paraquat from agricultural applications in the central valley of California," *American Journal of Epidemiology* 169 (2009):918–26.

533. Yadav, Sunishtha Singh, et al., "Organophosphates Induced Alzheimer's Disease: An Epigenetic Aspect," *Journal of Clinical Epigenetics* (2016): DOI: 10.21767/2472-1158.100010

534. Hamblin, James, "The toxins that threaten our brains," *The Atlantic*, Mar. 18, 2014. http://www.theatlantic.com/health/archive/2014/03/the-toxins-that-threaten-our-brains/284466/.

535. Ann M. Blacker and Bruce M. Young, *Hayes' Handbook of Pesticide Toxicology* (Third Edition), 2010

536. E. Todd, Carbamates, *Encyclopedia of Food Sciences and Nutrition* (Second Edition), 2003.

537. Parron, T., et al., "Association between environmental exposure to pesticides and neurodegenerative diseases," *Toxicology & Applied Pharmacology* 256 (2011):379–385. 10.1016/j.taap.2011.05.006

538. Baldi, I., et al., "Neurodegenerative diseases and exposure to pesticides in the elderly," *American Journal of Epidemiology* 157 (2003):409–14.

539. Tyas, S. L., et al., Risk factors for Alzheimer's disease: A population-based, longitudinal study in Manitoba, Canada," *International Journal of Epidemiology* 30 (2001):590–97.

540. Richardson, Jason R., et al., "Elevated serum pesticide levels and risk for Alzheimer's disease," *JAMA Neurology* 71 (2014)284-290.

541. Toxicology Profile for DDT, DDE, and DDD. United States Department of Health and Human Services, Agency for Toxic Substances and Disease Registry, September 2002.

542. Paley, Joy, "Researchers find PCBs, other chemicals in food," *Food Safety News*, Sept. 15, 2010. http://www.foodsafetynews.com/2010/09/researchers-find-pcbs-and-other-chemicals-in-food/#.V0XABJMrJBw.

543. Van den Berg, Henk, "Global Status of DDT and Its Alternatives for Use in Vector Control to Prevent Disease," *Environmental Health Perspectives* 117 (2009):1656–1663.

544. Lally, Robin, "Pesticide exposure linked to Alzheimer's disease," *Rutgers Today*, Jan. 27, 2014. http://news.rutgers.edu/research-news/pesticide-exposure-linked-alzheimer's-disease/20140127#.VVesoFy4lAY, accessed online, May 16, 2015.

545. Kamel, Freya, et al., "Association of pesticide exposure with neurologic dysfunction and disease," *Environmental Health Perspectives* (2004):950–58.

546. Thiruchelvam, M., et al., "Age-related irreversible progressive nigrostriatal dopaminergic neurotoxicity in the paraquat and maneb model of the Parkinson's disease phenotype," *European Journal of Neuroscience* 18 (2003):589–600.

547. McCormack, A. L., et al., "Environmental risk factors and Parkinson's disease: Selective degeneration of nigral dopaminergic neurons caused by the herbicide paraquat," *Neurobiology of Disease* 10 (2002):119–27; "Link between pesticides and Parkinson's strengthened with family study," *Science Daily* Mar. 29, 2008.

548. *Pesticide National Synthesis Project*, 2002 Pesticide Use Maps, USGS.

549. Costa, L. G., et al. "Neurotoxicity of pesticides: A brief review," *Frontiers in Bioscience* 13 (2008):1240–49.

550. Zaganas, Ioannis, et al., "Linking pesticide exposure and dementia: What is the evidence?" *Toxicology* 307 (2013):3–11.

551. Emory University Health Sciences Center. "Several commonly used pesticides are toxic to mitochondria in laboratory experiments," *Science Daily* Nov. 10, 2003. www.sciencedaily.com/releases/2003/11/031110054609.htm.

552. Copely, Caroline, "German beer purity in question after environment group finds weed killer traces," Reuters February 25, 2016; http://www.reuters.com/article/us-germany-beer-idUSKCN0VY222

553. Gillam Carey, "Tests show monsanto's weed killer in Cheerios, other popular foods," *Huffington Post* November 14, 2016.

554. Strom, Stephanie, "Traces of Controversial Herbicide Are Found in Ben & Jerry's Ice Cream," *New York Times*, July 25, 2017.

555. Almeida, Isis, et al., "Nestle steps up testing after weed killer found in coffee beans," *Bloomberg* September 26, 2019.

556. Mills, Paul J., et al., "Excretion of the Herbicide Glyphosate in Older Adults Between 1993 and 2016," *JAMA* 318 (2017):1610-1611.

557. EcoWatch, Organic Consumer's Association, "Glyphosate found in urine of 93% of Americans tested," May 29, 2016. https://www.ecowatch.com/glyphosate-found-in-urine-of-93-percent-of-americans-tested-1891146755.html

558. Cattani, D., et al., "Mechanisms underlying the neurotoxicity induced by glyphosate-based herbicide in immature rat hippocampus: Involvement of glutamate excitotoxicity," *Toxicology* 320 (2014):34–45; Hawkins M., Updated Review of Glyphosate (103601). Incident Reports. Memorandum, EPA Toxicology and Epidemiology Branch. February 26. 2009. Available from: http://www.epa.gov/pesticides/chemical/foia/cleared-reviews/reviews/103601/103601-2009-02-26a.pdf.

559. Donley, N., "The USA lags behind other agricultural nations in banning harmful pesticides." *Environmental Health* 44 (2019). doi.org/10.1186/s12940-019-0488-0

560. Circle of Poison, November 15, 2016. Aljazeera, https://www.aljazeera.com/program/featured-documentaries/2016/11/15/circle-of-poison/ (the film can be viewed on Amazon and Google Pla)

561. "What's on My Food," Pesticide Action Network North America, searchable database for pesticides on food products. http://www.whatsonmyfood.org/food.jsp?food=ST;

Pesticide Action Network, North America, 49 Powell Street, Suite 500, San Francisco, CA 94102; phone: 415-981-1771.

562. U.S. Food and Drug Administration, Pesticide Residue Monitoring Program Fiscal Year 2017 Pesticide Report, www.fda.gov/food/chemicals-metals-pesticides-food/pesticides; Schecter, Arnold, et al., "Perfluorinated compounds, polychlorinated biphenyls, and organochlorine pesticide contamination in composite food samples from Dallas, Texas, USA," *Environmental Health Perspectives* 118 (2010):796–802.

563. Editorial, "Congress moves, finally, on toxic chemicals," *New York Times*, May 24, 2016, p. A20.

564. Kurland, L. T., et al., "Epidemiologic investigations of amyotrophic lateral sclerosis. I. Preliminary report on geographic distribution, with special reference to the Mariana Islands, including clinical and pathological observations," *Neurology* 4 (1954):355–78.

565. Bell, E. A., et al., "Toxicity of Cycads: Implications for neurodegenerative diseases and cancer, Fifth Cycad Conference 1967" (M.G. Whiting, ed.). New York: Third World Medical Research Foundation, 1988; Holtcamp, Wendee, "The emerging science of BMAA: Do cyanobacteria contribute to neurodegenerative disease?," *Environmental Health Perspectives* 120 (2012):110–16. ; Seawright, A. A., et al., "Selective degeneration of cerebellar cortical neurons caused by cycad neurotoxin, L-B-methylaminoalanine (L-BMAA), in rats," *Neuropathology Applied Neurobiology* 16 (1990):153–69; Spencer, P. S., et al., "Guam amyotrophic lateral sclerosis-parkinsonism-dementia linked to plant excitant neurotoxin," *Science* 237 (1987):517–22.

566. Banack, S. A., et al., "Biomagnification of cycad neurotoxins in flying foxes: Implications for ALS-PDC in Guam," *Neurology* 61 (2003):387–89.

567. Murch, S. J., et al., "Occurrence of B-methylamino-L-alanine (BMAA) in ALS-PDC disease in Guam," *Acta Neurologica Scandinavica* 110 (2004):267–69.

568. Mash, D., et al., "Neurotoxic non-protein amino acid BMAA in brain from patients dying with ALS and Alzheimer's disease," presented at American Academy of Neurology Annual Meeting, Chicago, IL, Apr. 17, 2008, *Neurology* 70 (2008): A329; Pablo, J., et al., "Cyanobacterial neurotoxin BMAA in ALS and Alzheimer's disease," *Acta Neurologica Scandinavica* 120 (2009):216–25.

569. Cox, Paul Alan, et al., "Dietary exposure to an environmental toxin triggers neurofibrillary tangles and amyloid deposits in the brain," *Proceedings of The Royal Society B* 283 (2016), accessed online: http://rspb.royalsocietypublishing.org/content/283/1823/20152397.

570. Karlsson, O., et al., "Selective brain uptake and behavioral effects of the cyanobacterial toxin BMAA (beta-N-methylamino-L-alanine) following neonatal administration to rodents," *Toxicological Science* 109 (2009):286–95.

571. Nunes-Costa, Danilea, et al., "Microbial BMAA and the Pathway for Parkinson's Disease Neurodegeneration," *Frontiers of Aging and Neuroscience* 07 February 2020 | https://doi.org/10.3389/fnagi.2020.00026

572. Dunlop, R. A., et al., "The non-protein amino acid BMAA is misincorporated into human proteins in place of l-serine causing protein misfolding and aggregation," *PLoS ONE* 8 (2013):1371.

573. http://www.ucmp.berkeley.edu/bacteria/cyanointro.html, accessed online, May 20, 2016.

574. Brand, L. E., "The transport of terrestrial nutrients to South Florida coastal waters, in J. W. Porter and K. G. Porter, eds., *The Everglades, Florida Bay, and Coral Reefs of the Florida Keys* (Boca Raton, FL: CRC Press, 2002).

575. Brand, L. E., et al., "Cyanobacterial blooms and the occurrence of the neurotoxin, beta-N-methylamino-L-alanine (BMAA), in South Florida aquatic food webs," *Harmful Algae* 9 (2010):620–35; Jiang, Liying, et al., "Quantification of neurotoxin BMAA (β-*N*-methylamino-L-alanine) in seafood from Swedish markets," *Nature* (Scientific Reports) 4 (2014). http://www.nature.com/srep/2014/141106/srep06931/full/srep06931.html. "Neurotoxins in shark fins: A human health concern," Rosenthal School of Marine & Atmospheric Science, Feb. 23, 2012, http://www.rsmas.miami.edu/news-events/press-releases/2012/neurotoxins-in-shark-fins-a-human-health-concern; Jonasson, Sara, et al., "Transfer of a cyanobacterial neurotoxin within a temperate aquatic ecosystem suggests pathways for human exposure," *PNAS* 107 (201):9252–57.

576. Jiang, Let al., "Quantification of neurotoxin BMAA (β-N-methylamino-L-alanine) in seafood from Swedish markets," *Science Reports* 6931 (2014). doi:10.1038/srep06931

577. Seafood sold in Sweden contains BMAA: A study of free and total concentrations with UHPLC–MS/MS and dansyl chloride derivatization," *Toxicology Reports* 2 (2015):1473-81.

578. Al-sammak, Maitham Ahmed, et al., "Co-occurrence of the cyanotoxins BMAA, DABA and anatoxin-a in Nebraska resevoirs, fish and aquatic plants," *Toxins* 6 (2014):488-508; Al-Sammak, Maitham, "Occurrence and effect of algal neurotoxins in Nebraska freshwater ecosystem," dissertation, University of Nebraska, Lincoln, 2012, 163 pages; 3518908. http://search.proquest.com/docview/1034575257.

579. Press Association, "100 million sharks killed each year, say scientists," *The Gaurdian* March 1, 2013; Clarke, S. C., et al., "Global estimates of shark catches using trade records from commercial markets," *Ecology Letters* 9 (2006):1115–26.

580. FAO, Rome, Italy: Food and Agriculture Organization of the United Nations, 1999. "Shark utilization, marketing and trade," Fisheries Technical Paper. http://www.fao.org/docrep/005/x3690e/x3690e1g.htm, accessed online, May 19, 2012.

581. Mondo, K., et al., Cyanobacterial neurotoxin B-N-methylamino-L-alanine (BMAA) in shark fins," *Marine Drugs* 10 (2012):509–20.

582. Pablo, J., et al., Cyanobacterial neurotoxin BMAA in ALS and Alzheimer's disease," *Acta Neurologica Scandia* 120 (2009):216–25.

583. Mondo, Kiyo, et al., Environmental neurotoxins β-*N*-methylamino-l-alanine (BMAA) and mercury in shark cartilage dietary supplements," *Food and Chemical Toxicology* 70 (2014):26–32.

584. Dietrich, D. R., et al., "Toxin mixture in cyanobacterial blooms—a critical comparison of reality with current procedures employed in human health risk assessment," *Advances in Experimental Medicine and Biology* 619 (2008):885–912.

585. Lobner, Doug, et al., "Synergistic toxicity of the environmental neurotoxins methylmercury and B-N-methylamino-L-alanine," *NeuroReport* 23 (2012):216–19.

586. Davis, D.A., et al., "Cyanobacterial neurotoxin BMAA and brain pathology in stranded dolphins," *PLoS ONE* 14 (2019): e0213346. https://doi.org/10.1371/journal.pone.0213346

587. Davis, D.A., et a.l., "L-serine reduces spinal cord pathology in a vervet model of preclinical ALS/MND," *Journal of Neuropathology and Experimental Neurology* 79 (2020):396–406.

588. Gilbert, P.M., et al., "The Role of Eutrophication in the Global Proliferation of Harmful Algal Blooms New Perspectives and New Approaches," *Oceanography* 18 *(*2005):198-209; Herman, Rob, "Toxic algae blooms are on the rise," *Scientific American* September 7, 2016.

589. Pendrod, Emma, "Additional waters closed as 'unprecedented' Utah Lake algal bloom moves north," *Salt Lake Tribune* July 21, 2016, http://archive.sltrib.com/article.php?id=4134873&itype=CMSID

590. Barnard, Anne, "Algae bloom fouls N.J.'s largest lake, indicating broader crisis," *New York Times* August 5, 2019.

591. Cecco, Leyland, "Whistleblower warns baffling illness affects growing number of young adults in Canadian province," *The Guardian* January 2, 2022.

592. Lance, E., et al., "Occurrence of β-*N*-methylamino-L-alanine (BMAA) and Isomers in Aquatic Environments and Aquatic Food Sources for Humans," *Toxins* 10 (2018):83. doi.org/10.3390/toxins10020083

593. Parry, Wynne, "Blame Hitchcock's crazed birds on toxic algae," *LiveScience* January 3, 2012.

594. Bates, S. S., et al., "Pennate diatom Nitzschia pungens as the primary source of domoic acid, a toxin in shellfish from eastern Prince Edward Island, Canada," *Canadian Journal of Fisheries and Aquatic Sciences* 46 (1989):1203-1215.

595. Channel Islands National Marine Sanctuary Management Plan, Volume 2, November 2008, p. 448; Flatow, Ira, "Toxin triggers epilepsy in sea lions and humans," NPR, KQED Public Media, February 19, 2010.

596. Teitelbaum, J.S., et al., "Neurologic sequelae of domoic acid intoxication due to the ingestion of contaminated mussels," *New England Journal of Medicine* 322 (1990):1781-7.

597. Wekell, J. C., et al., "The origin of the regulatory limits for PSP and ASP toxins in shellfish," *Journal of Shellfish Research* 23 (2004):927-930.

598. Fields, R. Douglas, "How a neurotoxin in crabs causes brain damage," *Scientific American* November 11, 2015.

599. Barlow, Jeffrey B., et al., "Amnesic shellfish poison," *Food Chemistry & Toxicology* 42 (2004):545-57.

600. Yuhas, Alan, "Experts puzzled as 30 whales stranded in 'unusual mortality event' in Alaska," *The Guardian* August 22, 2015.

601. Trainer, V. L., et al., "Toxic Diatoms. In Oceans and Human Health: Risks and Remedies from the Sea" (P. J. Walsh, S. L. Smith, L. E. Fleming, H. Solo-Gabriele, and W. H. Gerwick, Eds.), 2008. pp. 219-238. Elsevier Science Publishers, New York.

602. Carr, Teresa, "Too many meds? America's love affair with prescription medication," *Consumer Reports* August 3, 2917.

603. Risacher, S.L., et al., "Association Between Anticholinergic Medication Use and Cognition, Brain Metabolism, and Brain Atrophy in Cognitively Normal Older

Adults," *JAMA Neurology* 73 (2016):721-32; Gray, Shelly, L., et al., "Cumulative Use of Strong Anticholinergics and Incident Dementia: A Prospective Cohort Study," *JAMA Internal Medicine* 175 (2015):401-7.

604. "Antimuscarinic Drugs and Memory Loss in Patients with Overactive Bladder: An Expert Interview with Dr. Gary Kay," *Medscape* March 27, 2021; https://www.medscape.org/viewarticle/533083

605. Gray, Shelly L., et al, "Cumulative use of strong anticholinergic medications and incident dementia: A prospective cohort study." *JAMA Internal Medicine* 175 (2015):401–7.

606. Weigand, Alexandra J., et al., "Association of anticholinergic medication and AD biomarkers with incidence of MCI among cognitively normal older adults," *Neurology* (2020) DOI: 10.1212/WNL.0000000000010643

607. Mayo Clinic. "Nearly 7 in 10 Americans are on prescription drugs," *ScienceDaily* 19 June 2013.

608. Billioti de Gage, Sophie, et al., "Benzodiazepine use and risk of Alzheimer's disease: case-control study," *BMJ* 349 (2014):349.

609. Ibid.

610. Billioti de Gage, Sophie, et al., "Benzodiazepine use and risk of Alzheimer's disease: case control study," *BMJ* 349 (2014):349.

611. Torjesen, Ingrid, "Statins are overprescribed for primary prevention, study suggests," *BMJ* 363 (2018). doi: https://doi.org/10.1136/bmj.k5110; Akyea, R.K., et al., "Suboptimal cholesterol response to initiation of statins and future risk of cardiovascular disease," *Heart* 105 (2019):975-981.

612. Beng-Choon, Ho, et al., Long-term antipsychotic treatment and brain volumes: A longitudinal study of first-episode schizophrenia," *Archives of General Psychiatry* 68 (2011):128–37; O'Meara, Kelly Patricia, "Honey, they shrunk my brain—study confirms antipsychotics decrease brain tissue," *CCHR International* Sept. 12, 2013.

613. The Week Staff, "America's 'startling use' of mental-illness drugs: By the numbers," *The Week*, Nov. 18, 2011.

614. Coupland, Carol A. C., et al., "Anticholinergic Drug Exposure and the Risk of Dementia: A Nested Case-Control Study," *JAMA Internal Medicine* (2019): doi:10.1001/jamainternmed.2019.0677

615. Terret, G., et al., "Prospective memory impairment in long-term opiate users," *Psychopharmacology* 231 (2014):2623-32.

616. Leng, Yue, et al., "Sleep Medication Use and Risk of Dementia in a Biracial Cohort of Older Adults. Presented at: Alzheimer's Association International Conference; July 14-18, 2019; Los Angeles.

617. Gray, Shelly L., et al., "Cumulative Use of Strong Anticholinergics and Incident Dementia: A Prospective Cohort Study," *JAMA Internal Medicine* 175 (2015):401-07.

618. Paul, Marla, "Marijuana users have abnormal brain structure and poor memory," Dec. 16, 2013. http://www.northwestern.edu/newscenter/stories/2013/12/marijuana-users-have-abnormal-brain-structure--poor-memory.html#!.

619. Louis Bengyella, et al., "Global impact of trace non-essential heavy metal contaminants in industrial cannabis bioeconomy," *Toxin Reviews* (2021). DOI: 10.1080/15569543.2021.1992444 <http://dx.doi.org/10.1080/155

620. Meier, Madeline, et al., "Persistent cannabis users show neuropsychological decline from childhood to midlife," *PNAS* (2012): https://doi.org/10.1073/pnas.1206820109

621. Lautieri, Amanda, American Addiction Centers, CIA, "Cocaine History and Statistics." Updated August 20, 2021

622. Ersche, K. D., et al., "Cocaine dependence: A fast-track for brain ageing?" *Molecular Psychiatry* 18 (2013):134–35.

623. Cataldo, Janine, et al., "Cigarette smoking is a risk factor for Alzheimer's disease: An analysis controlling for tobacco industry affiliation," *Journal of Alzheimer's disease* 19 (201):465–80.

624. Almeida, O. P, et al., "Smoking as a risk factor for Alzheimer's disease: Contrasting evidence from a systematic review of case-control and cohort studies," *Addiction* 97 (2002):15–28; Anstey, K. J, et al., "Smoking as a risk factor for dementia and cognitive decline: A meta-analysis of prospective studies," *American Journal of Epidemiology* 166 (2007):367–78; Hernan, M. A, et al., "Cigarette smoking and dementia: Potential bias in the elderly," *Epidemiology* 19 (2008):448–50; Purnell, C., et al., "Cardiovascular risk factors and incident Alzheimer disease," *Alzheimer's Disease and Associated Disorders* 23 (2009):1–10.

625. World Health Organization, *Tobacco and Dementia,* June 2014. http://apps.who.int/iris/bitstream/10665/128041/1/WHO_NMH_PND_CIC_TKS_14.1_eng.pdf.

626. Bahorik, A., et al., "Early adult to mid-life cigarette smoking and cognitive function: findings from the Cardia study," Presented at: The Alzheimer's Association International Conference; July 14-18, 2019; Los Angeles, CA. Abstract P3-572.

627. Durazzo, T.C., et al., "Smoking and increased Alzheimer's disease risk: a review of potential mechanisms," *Alzheimer's & Dementia: The Journal of the Alzheimer's Association* 10, S122-145.

628. Lapenna, D., et al., "Cigarette smoke, ferritin, and lipid peroxidation," *American Journal of Respiratory and Critical Care Medicine* 151 (1995): 431–35.

629. Ashraf, Muhammad Waqar, "Levels of heavy metals in popular cigarette brands and exposure to these metals via smoking," *The Scientific World Journal* 2012 (2012). http://www.hindawi.com/journals/tswj/2012/729430/abs/.

630. Rabin, Roni Caryn "A glut of antidepressants." http://well.blogs.nytimes.com/2013/08/12/a-glut-of-antidepressants/?_r=0, accessed online, Sept. 27, 2015.

631. National Institutes of Mental Health. http://www.nimh.nih.gov/health/statistics/prevalence/major-depression-among-adults.shtml.

632. Ownby, R. L., et al. "Depression and risk for Alzheimer's disease: Systematic review, meta-analysis, and metaregression analysis," *Archives of General Psychiatry* 63 (2006):530–38.

633. Wilson, R. S., et al., "Chronic psychological distress and risk of Alzheimer's disease in old age," *Neuroepidemiology* 27 (2006):143053.

634. Blue Cross Blue Shield. The Health of America: Early-onset dementia and Alzheimer's rates grow for younger American adults, February 27, 2020.

635. Hashmi, A. M., et al., "Is depression an inflammatory condition? A review of available evidence," *Journal of the Pakistani Medical Association* 63 (2013):899–905.

636. Yang, Tao, et al., "The Role of BDNF on Neural Plasticity in Depression," *Frontiers in Cellular Neuroscience* April 15, 2020, https://doi.org/10.3389/fncel.2020.00082

637. Videbech, P., "Hippocampal volume and depression: a meta-analysis of MRI studies. *American Journal of Psychiatry* 161 (2004):1957–66.

638. Lai, J.S., et al., "A systematic review and meta-analysis of dietary patterns and depression in community-dwelling adults," *American Journal of Clinical Nutrition* 99 (2013):181–97.

639. Jacka F., et al. "Association of Western and traditional diets with depression and anxiety in women," *American Journal of Psychiatry* 167 (2010):305–11; Jacka, F.N., et al. "The association between habitual diet quality and the common mental disorders in community-dwelling adults: the Hordaland Health study," *Psychosomatic Medicine* 73 (2011):483–90; Jacka, F.N., et al., "Dietary patterns and depressive symptoms over time: examining the relationships with socioeconomic position, health behaviors and cardiovascular risk," *PLoS One* 2014: 9: e87657.

640. Psaltopoulou, T., et al., "Mediterranean diet, stroke, cognitive impairment, and depression: a meta-analysis," *Annals of Neurology* 74 (2013):580–91.

641. Lucas, Michel, et al., "Inflammatory dietary pattern and risk of depression among women," *Brain, Behavior and Immunity* 36 (2014):46-53.

642. Agarwal, U., et al., "A multicenter randomized controlled trial of a nutrition intervention program in a multiethnic adult population in the corporate setting reduces depression and anxiety and improves quality of life: the GEICO study," *American Journal of Health Promotion* 29 (2015):245-54. doi: 10.4278/ajhp.130218-QUAN-72. Epub 2014 Feb 13. PMID: 24524383.

643. White, B.A., et al., "Many apples a day keep the blues away – daily experiences of negative and positive affect and food consumption in young adults," *British Journal of Health Psychology* 18 (2013):782-298.

644. Harvey, Samuel B., et al., "Exercise and the Prevention of Depression: Results of the HUNT Cohort Study," *American Journal of Psychiatry* (2017): doi.org/10.1176/appi.ajp.2017.16111223

645. Cooney, G.M., et al., "Exercise for depression," *Cochrane Database of Systematic Reviews* 12 (2013): doi: 10.1002/14651858.CD004366.pub6.

646. Moulton, P.V, et al., "Air pollution, oxidative stress, and Alzheimer's disease," *Journal of Environment and Public Health* (2012) doi:10.1155/2012/472751; Peters, R., "Air Pollution and Dementia: A Systematic Review," *Journal of Alzheimer's Disease* 70 (2019):S145-S163. doi:10.3233/JAD-180631

647. Cacciottolo, M., et al., "Particulate air pollutants, APOE alleles and their contributions to cognitive impairment in older women and to amyloidogenesis in experimental models," *Translational Psychiatry* 7 (2017). Doi.org/10.1038/tp.2016.280

648. Calderón-Garcidueñas L, et al., "Brain inflammation and Alzheimer's-like pathology in individuals exposed to severe air pollution," *Toxicologic Pathology* 32 (2004):650–658; Brook, Craig L., et al., "Air pollution and public health: a guidance document for risk managers," *Journal of Toxicology and Environmental Health* 71 (2008):588–698;

Kampa, M., "Human health effects of air pollution," *Environmental Pollution* 151 (2008):362–367.

649. Carey, Iain, M., et al., "Are noise and air pollution related to the incidence of dementia? A cohort study in London, England," *British Medical Journal* 8 (2018).doi:10.1136/bmjopen-2018-022404.

650. Hong, Chen, et al., "Living near major roads and the incidence of dementia, Parkinson's disease, and multiple sclerosis: a population-based cohort study," *The Lancet* (2017). DOI: 10.1016/S0140-6736(16)32399-6

651. Calderon-Garciduenas L., "Urban air pollution: Influences on olfactory function and pathology in exposed children and young adults," *Experimental Toxicology and Pathology* 62 (2010): 91–102.

652. Ranft, U, et al., "Long-term exposure to traffic-related particulate matter impairs cognitive function in the elderly," *Environmental Research* 109 (2009):1004–1011.

653. Alzheimer's Association, "Improving air quality reduces risk, multiple studies suggest," *Science Daily* July 26, 2021.

654. Wilson, Ryan, "Ex-Jets great Mark Gastineau: Diagnosed with dementia, Alzheimer's and Parkinson's," cbssports.com January 20, 2017.

http://www.cbssports.com/nfl/news/ex-jets-great-mark-gastineau-diagnosed-with-dementia-alzheimers-and-parkinsons/

655. Belson, Ken, "Brain trauma to affect one in three players, N.F.L. agrees," *New York Times*, Sept. 12, 2014, *http://www.nytimes.com/2014/09/13/sports/football/actuarial-reports-in-nfl-concussion-deal-are-released.html?_r=0.*

656. Breslow, James, "New: 87 deceased NFL players test positive for brain disease," *Frontline*, Sept. 18, 2016. http://www.pbs.org/wgbh/frontline/article/new-87-deceased-nfl-players-test-positive-for-brain-disease, accessed online, Mar. 29, 2016.

657. Beck, Julie, "The NFL's continuing concussion nightmare," *The Atlantic*, Sept. 21, 2015.

658. Nehls, Michael, "Unified theory of Alzheimer's disease (UTAD): implications for prevention and curative therapy," *Journal of Molecular Psychiatry* (2016) DOI 10.1186/s40303-016-0018-8

659. Centers for Disease Control and Prevention, "National Institute for Occupational Safety and Health (NIOSH) National Football League Players Mortality Study," Cincinnati, OH: NIOSH, Health Hazard Evaluation. (1994):88–085.

660. Mackay, Daniel F., et al., "Neurodegenerative Disease Mortality among Former Professional Soccer Players," *New England Journal of* Medicine (2019):1801-08

661. Fleminger, S., et al., "Head injury as a risk factor for Alzheimer's disease: The evidence 10 years on; a partial replication," *Journal of Neurology, Neurosurgery* and *Psychiatry* 74 (2003):857–62; Plassman, B.L., et al., "Documented head injury in early adulthood and risk of Alzheimer's disease and other dementias," *Neurology* 55 (2000):1158–66.

662. Fleminger, S., et al., "Head injury as a risk factor for Alzheimer's disease: The evidence 10 years on; a partial replication," *Journal of Neurology, Neurosurgery and Psychiatry* 74 (2003):857–62.

663. Yuhas, Daisy, "Veterans of Iraq, Afghanistan Show Brain Changes Related to Explosion Exposure," *Scientific American* January 15, 2016, https://www.scientificamerican.com/article/veterans-of-iraq-afghanistan-show-brain-changes-related-to-explosion-exposure/

664. Yaffe, K., et al., "Military-related risk factors in female veterans and risk of dementia," *Neurology* 92 (2019):e205-e211.

665. Plassman, B.L, et al., "Documented head injury in early adulthood and risk of Alzheimer's disease and other dementias," *Neurology* 55 (2000):1158–66.

666. McKee, A.C, et al., "The neuropathology of sport," *Acta Neuropathology* 127 (2014):29–51.

667. Mohamed, Abdalla Z., et al., "Traumatic brain injury fast-forwards Alzheimer's pathology: evidence from amyloid positron emission tomography imaging," *Journal of Neurology* (2021) DOI:10.1007/s00415-021-10669-5

668. Aspry, Karen, et al., "Medical Nutrition Education, Training, and Competencies to Advance Guideline-Based Diet Counseling by Physicians: A Science Advisory from the American Heart Association," *Circulation* (2018). doi.org/10.1161/CIR.0000000000000563 Circulation.2018;137: e821–e841

669. Barnard, N.D., "Ignorance of nutrition is no longer defensible," *JAMA Internal Medicine* Published online July 1, 2019.

670. "How much does your doctor actually know about nutrition?" *American Heart Association*, May 3, 2018.

671. Gustaw-Rothenberg, K., "Dietary patterns associated with Alzheimer's disease: Population based study," *International Journal of Environmental Research and Public Health* 6 (2009):1335–40.

672. Brand-Miller, J.C., et al., "Australian Aboriginal plant foods: a consideration of their nutritional composition and health implications," *Nutrition Research Reviews* 11 (1998):23

672. Morris, M.C., et al., "Association of vegetable and fruit consumption with age-related cognitive change," *Neurology* (2006):1370-76.

673. Engelhart, M. J., "Dietary antioxidants and risk of Alzheimer's disease," *JAMA* 287 (2002):3223–29.

674. Barnard N.D., et al., "Vegetarian and vegan diets in type 2 diabetes management," *Nutrition Reviews* 67 (2009):255–263. Ferdowsian HR, "Effects of plant-based diets on plasma lipids," *American Journal Cardiology* 104 (2009):947–956; Appleby PN, et al., "Hypertension and blood pressure among meat eaters, fish eaters, vegetarians and vegans in EPIC-Oxford," *Public Health Nutrition*5 (2002):645–654; Berkow SE., et al., "Vegetarian diets and weight status," *Nutrition Reviews* 64 (2006):175–188; Turner-McGrievy, G.M., et al., "A two-year randomized weight loss trial comparing a vegan diet to a more moderate low-fat diet," *Obesity* 15 (2007):2276–2281.

675. Ahmad, MI, et al., "The Role of Meat Protein in Generation of Oxidative Stress and Pathophysiology of Metabolic Syndromes," *Food Science of Animal Resources* 40 (2020):1-10. doi:10.5851/kosfa.2019.e96

676. Sun, L.J., et al., "Gut hormones in microbiota-gut-brain cross-talk," *Chinese Medical Journal (Engl)* 133 (2020):826-833. doi:10.1097/CM9.0000000000000706

677. Faintuch, Joel, Faintuch Salomao. *Microbiome and Metabolome in Diagnosis, Therapy, and other Strategic Applications* (Cambridge: Academic Press; 2019).

678. Clapp, M., et al., "Gut microbiota's effect on mental health: The gut-brain axis.," *Clinical Practice* 7 (2017):987. doi:10.4081/cp.2017.987; Daulatzai, M.A., et al., "Non-celiac

gluten sensitivity triggers gut dysbiosis, neuroinflammation, gut-brain axis dysfunction, and vulnerability for dementia," *CNS & Neurological Disorders* 14 (2015):110-31; Oriach, Clara Seira, et al., "Food for thought: The role of nutrition in the microbiota-gut-brain axis," *Clinical Nutrition Experimental* 6 (2016):25-38.

679. De Filippo, C., et al., "Impact of diet in shaping gut microbiota revealed by a comparative study in children from Europe and rural Africa," *Proceedings of the National Academy of Science* 107 (2010):14691-14696; Murphy, E.A., et al., "Influence of high-fat diet on gut microbiota: a driving force for chronic disease risk," *Current Opinion in Clinical Nutrition and Metabolic Care* 18 (2015):515-20. Novotný, M., et al., "Microbiome and Cognitive Impairment: Can Any Diets Influence Learning Processes in a Positive Way?" *Frontiers in Aging and Neuroscience* 170 (2019). doi:10.3389/fnagi.2019.00170

680. Asnicar, F., et al., "Microbiome connections with host metabolism and habitual diet from 1,098 deeply phenotyped individuals," *Nature Medicine* 27 (2021):321-332. doi: 10.1038/s41591-020-01183-8; Glick-Bauer, M., et al., "The health advantage of a vegan diet: exploring the gut microbiota connection," *Nutrients* 6 (2014):4822-38.

681. Melina, V., et al., "Position of the Academy of Nutrition and Dietetics: vegetarian diets," *Journal of the Academy of Nutrition and Dietetics* 116 (016):1970-1980.

682. http://www.fao.org/docrep/004/Y2809E/y2809e00.HTM

683. Craig W.J., et al., "Position of the American Dietetic Association: vegetarian diets," *Journal of the American Diet Association* 109 (2009):1266–1282; American Diabetes Association, "Standards of medical care in diabetes," *Diabetes Care* 35 (2012): (Suppl. 1):S11–S58, 2012

684. Tusso, Philp J., et al., "Nutrition update for physicians: Plant-based diets," *Permanente Journal* 17 (2013):6166.

685. Chan, Andrew T., et al., "Diet quality and risk and severity of COVID-19: a prospective cohort study," *Gut* 2021).

686. Kim, H., *et al.*, "Plant-based diets, pescatarian diets and COVID-19 severity: a population-based case–control study in six countries," *BMJ Nutrition, Prevention & Health* (2021). doi: 10.1136/bmjnph-2021-000272

687. Carddock J.C., et al., "Vegetarian-based dietary patterns and their relation with inflammatory and immune biomarkers: a systematic review and meta-analysis," *Advances in Nutrition* 10 (2019):433-451; Malter, M., et al., "Natural killer cells, vitamins, and other blood components of vegetarian and omnivorous men," *Nutrition and Cancer* 12 (1989):271-278.

688. Moosmann, B., et al., "Antioxidants as treatment for neurodegenerative disorders," *Expert Opinion on Investigational Drugs* 11 (2002):1407–35.

689. Heid, Markham, "Experts say lobbying skewed the U.S. dietary guidelines," *Time* January 8, 2016.

690. Watson, Elaine, "Food, politics, and the 2020 dietary guidelines for Americans," *Food Navigator* May 14, 2019.

691. Wu, Jing, et al., "Dietary pattern in midlife and cognitive impairment in late life: a prospective study in Chinese adults," *American Journal of Clinical Nutrition* 110 (2019):912-20; Kang, J. H., et al., "Fruit and vegetable consumption and cognitive decline in aging women," *Annals of Neurology* 57 (2005):713–20.

692. Lourida, Illianna, et al., "Mediterranean diet, cognitive function, and dementia: A systematic Review," *Epidemiology* 24 (2013):479–89.

693. Scarmeas, N., et al., "Mediterranean diet and risk for Alzheimer's disease," *Annals of Neurology* 59 (2006):912-21.

694. Pelletier, A., et al., "Mediterranean diet and preserved brain structural connectivity in older subjects," *Alzheimer's and Dementia* 11 (2015):1023–1031. doi:10.1016/j.jalz.2015.06.1888; Titova, O.E., et al., "Mediterranean diet habits in older individuals: associations with cognitive functioning and brain volumes," *Experimental Gerontology* 48 (2013):1443–1448. doi:10.1016/j.exger.2013.10.002

695. Morris, Martha Clare, et al., "MIND diet associated with a reduced incidence of Alzheimer's disease," *Alzheimer's & Dementia*, accessed online, Feb. 11, 2015.

696. Bergeron, Nathalie, et al., Effects of red meat, white meat, and nonmeat protein sources on atherogenic lipoprotein measures in the context of low compared with high saturated fat intake: a randomized controlled trial," *American Journal of Clinical Nutrition* (2019): doi.org/10.1093/ajcn/nqz035

697. Yang, S.Y., et al., "Chinese lacto-vegetarian diet exerts favorable effects on metabolic parameters, intima-media thickness, and cardiovascular risks in healthy men," *Nutrition in Clinical Practice* 27 (2012):392-398; Kim, M.K., "Long-term vegetarians have low oxidative stress, body fat, and cholesterol levels," *Nutrition Research and Practice* (2012):155-161; Trapp, D., et al., "Could a vegetarian diet reduce exercise-induced oxidative stress? A review of the literature," *Journal of Sports Sciences* 28 (2010):1261-1268.; Yokoyama, Y., et al., "Vegetarian diets and blood pressure: a meta-analysis," *JAMA* 174 (2014):577-587.

698. Harvey, A.L., "Medicines from nature: Are natural products still relevant to drug discovery?" *Trends in Pharmacological Sciences* 20 (1999):196–8.

699. Kumar, G. Phani, et al., "Neuroprotective potential of phytochemical," *Pharmacognosy Reviews* 6 (2002): 81–90.

700. Barberger-Gateau P., et al., "Dietary patterns and risk of dementia: The Three-City cohort study," *Neurology* 69 (2007):1921–30; von Amim, C.A., et al., "Dietary antioxidants and dementia in a population-based case-control study among older people in South Germany," *Journal of Alzheimer's Disease* 31 (2012):717-24; Devore, Elizabeth E., et al., "Dietary antioxidants and long-term risk of dementia," *Archives of Neurology* 67 (201):819-25; Engelhardt, Marianne J., et al., "Dietary Intake of Antioxidants and Risk of Alzheimer Disease," *JAMA* 287 (2002):3223-29; Luchsinger, Jose A., et al., "Dietary factors and Alzheimer's disease" *The Lancet* 3 (2004):579-87; Dai, Q., et al., "Fruit and vegetable juices and Alzheimer's disease: the Kame Project," *American Journal of Medicine* 119 (2006): 751-9; Liu, Rui Hai, "Health benefits of fruit and vegetables are from additive and synergistic combinations of phytochemicals," *American Journal of Clinical Nutrition* 78 (2003):517S-520S.

701. Mandel, S.A., et al., "Multifunctional activities of green tea catechins in neuroprotection. Modulation of cell survival genes, iron-dependent oxidative stress and PKC signaling pathway," *Neurosignals* 14 (2005):46–60; Xu, Y., et al., "Curcumin reverses impaired hippocampal neurogenesis and increases serotonin receptor 1A mRNA and brain-derived neurotrophic factor expression in chronically stressed rats," *Brain Research* 1162 (2007):9–18; Choi, D-Y, et al., "Antioxidant properties of natural polyphenols and

THE ALZHEIMER'S REVOLUTION

their therapeutic potentials for Alzheimer's disease," *Brain Research Bulletin* 87 (2012):144–53.

702. Carlsen, Monica H., et al., "The total antioxidant content of more than 3100 foods, beverages, spices, herbs and supplements used worldwide," *Nutrition Journal* 9 (2010):3–11.

703. Letenneur, L., et al., "Flavonoid intake and cognitive decline over a 10-year period," *American Journal of Epidemiology* 165 (2007):1364–71; Scarmeas, N., et al., "Mediterranean diet and Alzheimer disease mortality," *Neurology* 69 (2007):1084–1093; Dai, Q., et al., "Fruit and vegetable juices and Alzheimer's disease: the Kame Project," *American Journal of Medicine* 119 (2006):751–759.

704. Aquilano, K., et al., "Role of nitric oxide synthases in Parkinson's disease: a review on the antioxidant and anti-inflammatory activity of polyphenols," *Neurochemistry Research* 33 (2008):2416–2426.

705. Dubick, M.A., et al., "Evidence for grape, wine and tea polyphenols as modulators of atherosclerosis and ischemic heart disease in humans," *Journal of Nutraceuticals, Functional & Medicinal Foods* 3 (2001):67–93; Nardini, M., et al., "Role of dietary polyphenols in platelet aggregation. A review of the supplementation studies," *Platelets* 18 (2007):224–243; Vita, J.A., "Polyphenols and cardiovascular disease: effects on endothelial and platelet function," *American Journal of Clinical Nutrition* 81 (2005):292–297.

706. Pandey, Kanti Bhooshan, et al., "Plant polyphenols as dietary antioxidants in human health and disease," *Oxidative Medicine and Cellular Longevity* 2 (2009):270-78.

707. Yang, C.S., et al., "Inhibition of carcinogenesis by dietary polyphenolic compounds," *Annual Review of Nutrition* 21 (2001):381-406; Johnson, I.T., et al., "Anticarcinogenic factors in plant foods: A new class of nutrients?" *Nutrition Research Reviews* 7 (1994):175-204.

708. Xu Y, et al., "Curcumin reverses impaired hippocampal neurogenesis and increases serotonin receptor 1A mRNA and brain-derived neurotrophic factor expression in chronically stressed rats," *Brain Research* 1162 (2007):9–18.

709. Gerszon, J., et al., "Antioxidant properties of resveratrol and its protective effects in neurodegenerative diseases," *Advances in Cell Biology* 4 (2014): Chiu, S., et al., "The role of nutrient-based epigenetic changes in buffering against stress, aging, and Alzheimer's disease," *Psychiatric Clinics North America* 37 (2014):591–623.

710. Kumar, G. Phani, et al., "Neuroprotective potential of phytochemicals," *Pharmacognosy Reviews* 6 (2012):81-90.

711. Yoo, K. Y, et al., "Epigallocatechin-3-gallate increases cell proliferation and neuroblasts in the subgranular zone of the dentate gyrus in adult mice," *Phytotherapy Research* 24 (2010):1065–70; Commenges, D., et al., "Intake of flavonoids and risk of dementia," *European Journal of Epidemiology* 165 (2000):357–63; Letenneur, L., et al., "Flavonoid intake and cognitive decline over a 10-year period," *American Journal of Epidemiology* 16 (2007):1364–71; Bakoyiannis, Ioannis, et al., "Phytochemicals and cognitive health: Are flavonoids doing the trick?" *Biomedicine and Pharmacology* 109 (2019):1488-97.

712. Commenges, D., et al., "Intake of flavonoids and risk of dementia," *European Journal of Epidemiology* 165 (2000):357–63; Letenneur, L., et al., "Flavonoid intake and cognitive decline over a 10-year period," *American Journal of Epidemiology* 16 (2007):1364–71.

713. Holland, Thomas, J., et al., "Dietary flavonols and risk of Alzheimer dementia," *Neurology* 2020: doi: 10.1212/WNL.0000000000008981

714. Jacques, Paul F., "Long-term dietary flavonoid intake and risk of Alzheimer disease and related dementias in the Framingham Offspring Cohort," *The American Journal of Clinical Nutrition* (2020): DOI: 10.1093/ajcn/nqaa079

715. Renzi, L.M., et al., "Hammond B.R. Relationships between macular pigment optical density and cognitive function in unimpaired and mildly cognitively impaired older adults," *Neurobiology and Aging* 35 (2014):1695–1699.

716. Johnson, E.J., et al., "Relationship between serum and brain carotenoids, α-tocopherol, and retinol concentrations and cognitive performance in the oldest old from the Georgia centenarian study," *Journal of Aging Research* 2013 (2013): doi: 10.1155/2013/951786.

717. Obulesu, M., et al., "Carotenoids and Alzheimer's disease: an insight into therapeutic role of retinoids in animal models," *Neurochemistry International* 59 (2011):535-41.

718. Chakroborty, Shreaya, et al., "Early calcium dysregulation in Alzheimer's disease: setting the stage for synaptic dysfunction," *Science China Life Sciences* 54 (2011):752-62.

719. Soutif-Veillon, A., et al., "Increased dietary vitamin K intake is associated with less severe subjective memory complaint among older adults," *Maturitas* 93 (2016):131-136. doi: 10.1016/j.maturitas.2016.02.004.; Presse, N., et al., "Vitamin K status and cognitive function in healthy older adults," *Neurobiology of Aging* 34 (2013):2777-83. doi: 10.1016/j.neurobiolaging.2013.05.031.

720. Bruno, E.J., "The prevalence of vitamin K deficiency / insufficiency, and recommendations for increased intake," *Journal of Human Nutrition and Food Science* 4 (2016):1077; Presse, N., et al., "Low vitamin K intakes in community-dwelling elders at an early stage of Alzheimer's disease," *Journal of the American Dietetic Association* 108 (2008):2095-9.

721. Fulgoni, V.L., "Current protein intake in America: analysis of the National Health and Nutrition Examination Survey, 2003–2004," *The American Journal of Clinical Nutrition* 87 (2008):1554S–1557S.

722. Rizzo, N.S., et al., "Nutrient profiles of vegetarian and nonvegetarian dietary patterns," *Journal of the Academy of Nutrition and Dietetics* 113 (2013):1610-9.

723. Aune, D., et al., "Whole grain consumption and risk of cardiovascular disease, cancer, and all cause and cause specific mortality: systematic review and dose-response meta-analysis of prospective studies," *BMJ* 353 (2016): doi: 10.1136/bmj.i2716; World Cancer Research Fund, "Diet, nutrition, physical activity and colorectal cancer," Revised 2018.

724. Twaddell, Iona, "Stone-age people were making porridge 32,000 years ago," *NewScientist* September 7, 2015.

725. Capannolo, A., et al., "Non-Celiac Gluten Sensitivity among Patients Perceiving Gluten-Related Symptoms," *Digestion* 92 (2015):8-13.

726. Catassi, C., et al., "Diagnosis of Non-Celiac Gluten Sensitivity (NCGS): The Salerno Experts' Criteria," *Nutrients* 7 (2015):4966-4977. doi:10.3390/nu7064966

727. Ros, E., "Health benefits of nut consumption," *Nutrients* 2 (2010):652–82; Sabate, J., et al., "Nuts: nutrition and health outcomes," *British Journal of Nutrition* 96 (2006):S1–2; Ros, E., et al., "Nuts and berries for heart health," *Currents Atherosclerosis Reports* 12 (2010):397–406; Estruch, R., et al., "Primary prevention of cardiovascular disease with a Mediterranean diet," *New England Journal of Medicine* 368 (2013):1279–90; Pan, A., et al., "Walnut consumption is associated with lower risk of type 2 diabetes

in women," *Journal of Nutrition* 143 (2013):512–8; Davis, P.A., et al., "A high-fat diet containing whole walnuts (Juglans regia) reduces tumour size and growth along with plasma insulin-like growth factor 1 in the transgenic adenocarcinoma of the mouse prostate model," *British Journal of Nutrition* 108 (2012):1764–72; Hardman, W.E., et al., "Dietary walnut suppressed mammary gland tumorigenesis in the C(3)1 TAg mouse," *Nutrition and Cancer* 63 (2011):960–70; Parker, E.D., et al., "Nut consumption and risk of type 2 diabetes," *JAMA* 290 (2003):38–9.

728.   Pribis, Peter, et al., "Cognition: the new frontier for nuts and berries," *American Journal of Clinical Nutrition* 100 (2014):347S-352S.

729.   Nooyens, Astrid, et al., "Fruit and vegetable intake and cognitive decline in middle-aged men and women: the Doetinchem Cohort Study," *British Journal of Nutrition* 106 (2011):752-761; O'Brien, J., et al., "Long-term intake of nuts in relation to cognitive function in older women," *Journal of Nutrition, Health and Aging* 18 (2014):496-502.

730.   Berryman, Claire E., et al., "Inclusion of Almonds in a Cholesterol-Lowering Diet Improves Plasma HDL Subspecies and Cholesterol Efflux to Serum in Normal-Weight Individuals with Elevated LDL Cholesterol," *Journal of Nutrition* 147 (2017):1517-23.

731.   Berryman, C.E., et al., "Effects of almond consumption on the reduction of LDL-cholesterol: a discussion of potential mechanisms and future research directions," *Nutrition Reviews* 69 (2011):171-85.

732.   Cardoso, B. R, et al., "Nutritional status of selenium in Alzheimer's disease patients," *British Journal of Nutrition* 103 (2010):803–6.

733.   Salas-Salvado, J., et al., "The effect of nuts on inflammation," *Asia Pacific Journal of Clinical Nutrition* 17 Suppl (2008):333-6.

734.   Yingying, Ma., et al., "Effect of walnut consumption on endothelial function in type 2 diabetic subjects," *Diabetes Care* 33 (2010):227-32; Ros, Emilio, et al., "A walnut diet improves endothelial function in hypercholesterolemic subjects," *Circulation* 109 (2004):1609-14; Cortes, B., et al., "Acute effects of high-fat meals enriched with walnuts or olive oil on postprandial endothelial function," *Journal of the American College of Cardiology* 48 (2006):1666-71.

735.   Arab. Lenore, et al., "A Cross Sectional Study of the Association Between Walnut Consumption and Cognitive Function Among Adult U.S. Populations Represented in NHANES," *Journal of Nutrition Health & Aging* 19 (2015):284-90.

736.   Reynolds, E. H., "Folic acid, ageing, depression, and dementia," *BMJ* 324 (2002):1512–15.

737.   Arab, L., et al., "A cross sectional study of the association between walnut consumption and cognitive function among adult us populations represented in NHANES," *Journal of Nutrition, Health and Aging* 19 (2015):284-90.

738.   Gemmea, Flores-Mateo, et al., "Nut Intake and Adiposity: Meta-Analysis of Clinical Trials," *American Journal of Clinical Nutrition* 97 (2013):1346-55.

739.   King, J.C., "Supplement: 2007 Nuts and Health Symposium," *Journal of Nutrition* 138 (2008):1734S-1765S; Fraser, G.E., "A possible protective effect of nut consumption on risk of coronary heart disease. The Adventist Health Study," *Archives of Internal Medicine* 152 (1992):1416–1424; Sabaté, J., et al., "Effects of walnuts on serum lipid levels and blood pressure in normal men," *New England Journal of Medicine* 328

(1993):603–607; Ros, E., et al., "Fatty acid composition of nuts. Implications for cardiovascular health," *British Journal of Nutrition* 9(2006): S29S35.

740. Schlörmann, W., et al., "Influence of roasting conditions on health-related compounds in different nuts," *Food Chemistry* 180 (2015):77-85. doi: 10.1016/j.foodchem.2015.02.017. Epub 2015 Feb 11. PMID: 25766804.

741. Açar, O. C., et al., "Direct evaluation of the total antioxidant capacity of raw and roasted pulses, nuts and seeds," *European Food Research and Technoogy* 229 (2009): 961–969. https://doi.org/10.1007/s00217-009-1131-z

742. Yaacoub, R., "Formation of lipid oxidation and isomerization products during processing of nuts and sesame seeds," *Journal of Agriculture and Food Chemistry* 56 (2008):7082-90. doi: 10.1021/jf800808d. Epub 2008 Aug 5. PMID: 18680380.

743. Illian, T.G., et al., "Omega 3 Chia seed loading as a means of carbohydrate loading," *Journal of Strength & Conditioning Research* 25 (2011):61-5; Vuksan, V., et al., "Reduction in postprandial glucose excursion and prolongation of satiety: possible explanation of the long-term effects of whole grain Salba (Salvia Hispanica L.)," *European Journal of Clinical Nutrition* 64 (2010):436-8; Martinez-Cruz, O., et al., "Phytochemical profile and nutraceutical potential of chia seeds (Salvia hispanica L.) by ultra high performance liquid chromatography," *Journal of Chromatography* 13 (2014):43-8.

744. Djoussé L, et al., "Dietary linolenic acid is inversely associated with calcified atherosclerotic plaque in the coronary arteries. The NHLBI Family Heart Study," *Circulation* 111 (2005):2921–6; Kris-Etherton, Penny M., "Walnuts Decrease Risk of Cardiovascular Disease: A Summary of Efficacy and Biologic Mechanisms," *Journal of Nutrition* 113 (2014):547S-554S; Khabbazi, T., et al., "Effects of alpha-lipoic acid supplementation on inflammation, oxidative stress, and serum lipid profile levels in patients with end-stage renal disease on hemodialysis," *Journal of Renal Nutrition* 22 (2012):244-50; Franz, Mary, "Nutrition, inflammation, and disease," *Today's Dietician* 16 (2014):44; Webb, A.L., et al., "Dietary lignans: potential role in cancer prevention," *Nutrition and Cancer* 51 (2005):117-31; Pandey, Kanti Bhooshan, et al., "Plant polyphenols as dietary antioxidants in human health and disease," *Oxidative Medicine and Cell Longevity* 2 (2009):270-278; Fukumistu, S., et al., "Flaxseed lignan lowers blood cholesterol and decreases liver disease risk factors in moderately hypercholesterolemic men," *Nutrition Research* 30 (2010):441-6.

745. Rodriguez-leyva, D., et al., "Potent antihypertensive action of dietary flaxseed in hypertensive patients," *Hypertension* 62 (2013):1081-1089.

746. Hyson, Dianne A., "A Comprehensive Review of Apples and Apple Components and Their Relationship to Human Health," *Advances in Nutrition* 2 (2011):408-20.

747. Federation of American Societies for Experimental Biology. " 'Apple a day' advice rooted in science," *ScienceDaily* May 3, 2011.

748. Knekt, P., et al., "Quercetin intake and the incidence of cerebrovascular disease," *European Journal of Clinical Nutrition* 54 (2000):415-7.

749. López, Ledesma R, et al., "Monounsaturated fatty acid (avocado) rich diet for mild hypercholesterolemia," *Archives of Medical Research* 27 (1996):519-23.

750. Li, Z., et al., "Hass avocado modulates postprandial vascular reactivity and postprandial inflammatory responses to a hamburger meal in healthy volunteers," *Food and Function* 26 (2013):384-91. doi: 10.1039/c2fo30226h.

751. Scott, Tammy M., et al., "Avocado Consumption Increases Macular Pigment Density in Older Adults: A Randomized, Controlled Trial," *Nutrients* 9 (2017). doi:10.3390/nu9090919

752. Becerra, Tomás, et al., "Legume consumption is inversely associated with type 2 diabetes incidence in adults: A prospective assessment from the PREDIMED study," *Clinical Nutrition* 37 (2018):906-913.

      Mattei, Josiemer, et al., "A higher ratio of beans to white rice is associated with lower cardiometabolic risk factors in Costa Rican adults," *The American Journal of Clinical Nutrition* 94 (2011):869-76.

753. Krikorian, R. et al., "Blueberry supplementation improves memory in older adults," *Journal of Agriculture and Food Chemistry* 58 (2010):3996–4000; Miller, M. et al., "Dietary blueberry improves cognition among older adults in a randomized, double-blind, placebo-controlled trial," *European Journal of Nutrition* (2017): doi.org/10.1007/s00394-017-1400-8; Bowtell, J., et al., "Enhanced task related brain activation and resting perfusion in healthy older adults after chronic blueberry supplementation," *Applied Physiology Nutrition and Metabolism* 42 (2017):773–779; Whyte, A. R. et al., "Effects of a single dose of a flavonoid-rich blueberry drink on memory in 8 to 10 y old children," *Nutrition* 31 (2015):531–534; Krikorian, R., et al., "Blueberry supplementation improves memory in older adults," *Journal of Agriculture and Food Chemistry* 58 (2010):3996–4000. doi:10.1021/jf9029332

754. Bowtell, J.L., et al., "Enhanced task-related brain activation and resting perfusion in healthy older adults after chronic blueberry supplementation," *Applied Physiology, Nutrition, and Metabolism* 42 (2017):773-79.

755. Krikorian R, Shidler MD, Nash TA, Kalt W, Vinquist-Tymchuk MR, Shukitt-Hale B, Joseph J. Blueberry Supplementation Improves Memory in Older Adults," *Journal of Agriculture and Food Chemistry* 58 (2010):3996-4000; Krikorian, R., et al., "Concord grape juice supplementation improves memory function in older adults with mild cognitive impairment," *British Journal of Nutrition* 103 (2010):730–734

756. Curtis, Peter J., et al., "Blueberries improve biomarkers of cardiometabolic function in participants with metabolic syndrome—results from a 6-month, double-blind, randomized controlled trial," *American Journal of Clinical Nutrition* 109 (2019):1535–1545.

757. Williams, C. M., et al., "Blueberry-induced changes in spatial working memory correlate with changes in hippocampal CREB phosphorylation and brain-derived neurotrophic factor (BDNF) levels," *Free Radical Biology and Medicine* 45 (2008):295-305.

758. http://www.whatsonmyfood.org/food.jsp?food=BB

759. Kimira, M., et al., "Japanese intake of flavonoids and isoflavonoids from foods," *Journal of Epidemiology* 8 (1998):168–175.

760. Maher, P., et al., "Flavonoid fisetin promotes ERK-dependent long-term potentiation and enhances memory," *PNAS* 103 (2006):16568-15573.

7611. Chuang, J.Y., et al, "Regulatory effects of fisetin on microglial activation," *Molecules* 19 (2014):8820-8839.

762. Ahmad, A., et al., "Neuroprotective Effect of Fisetin Against Amyloid-Beta-Induced Cognitive/Synaptic Dysfunction, Neuroinflammation, and Neurodegeneration in Adult Mice," 54 *Molecular Neurobiology* (2017):2269-2285.

763. Kelley, Darshan S., et al., "Consumption of bing sweet cherries lowers circulating concentrations of inflammation markers in healthy men and women," *Journal of Nutrition* 136 (2006):981-86.

764. Vuksan, V., et al., "Supplementation of conventional therapy with the novel grain Salba (Salvia hispanica L.) improves major and emerging cardiovascular risk factors in type 2 diabetes: results of a randomized controlled trial," *Diabetes Care* 30 (2007):2804-10.

765. Klomparens, E. A., et al., "The neuroprotective mechanisms and effects of sulforaphane," *Brain Circulation* 5 (2019):74–83. doi:10.4103/bc.bc_7_19

766. Blekklenhorst, Lauren C., et al., "Total Vegetable Intakes Are Inversely Associated with Subclinical Atherosclerosis in Older Adult Women," *JAHA* (2018): doi.org/10.1161/JAHA.117.008391

767. Greenwood, P. M., et al., "Neuronal and cognitive plasticity: A neurocognitive framework for ameliorating cognitive aging," *Frontiers in Aging Neuroscience* 2 (2010):150; Chiu, S., et al., "The role of nutrient-based epigenetic changes in buffering against stress, aging, and Alzheimer's disease," *Psychiatric Clinics of North America* 37 (2014):591–623.

768. Tao Yuan, et al., "Pomegranate's Neuroprotective Effects against Alzheimer's Disease Are Mediated by Urolithins, Its Ellagitannin-Gut Microbial Derived Metabolites," *ACS Chemical Neuroscience* (2015). DOI: 10.1021/acschemneuro.5b00260

769. Sohrab, G., et al., "Effects of pomegranate juice consumption on inflammatory markers in patients with type 2 diabetes: A randomized, placebo-controlled trial," *Journal of Research in Medical Sciences* 19 (2014):215-20.

770. Bookheimer, Susan Y., et al., "Pomegranate Juice Augments Memory and fMRI Activity in Middle-Aged and Older Adults with Mild Memory Complaints," *Evidence-Based Complimentary and Alternative Medicine* (2013): doi.org/10.1155/2013/946298

771. Braidy, Nady, et al., "Consumption of pomegranates improves synaptic function in a transgenic mice model of Alzheimer's disease," *Oncotarget* 7 (2016):64589-64604.

772. Sedigheh, Asgary, et al., "Clinical Evaluation of Blood Pressure Lowering, Endothelial Function Improving, Hypolipidemic and Anti-Inflammatory Effects of Pomegranate Juice in Hypertensive Subjects," *Phytotherapy Research* 28 (2013): doi.org/10.1002/ptr.4977; Stowe, C.B., "The effects of pomegranate juice consumption on blood pressure and cardiovascular health," *Complimentary Therapies in Clinical Practice* 17 (2011):113-5.

773. Esmaillzadeh, A., et al., "Cholesterol-lowering effect of concentrated pomegranate juice consumption in type 2 diabetic patients with hyperlipidemia," *International Journal of Vitamin and Nutrition Research* 76 (2006):147-51.

774. Johnson, E.J., et al., "Relationship between serum and brain carotenoids, α-tocopherol, and retinol concentrations and cognitive performance in the oldest old from the georgia centenarian study," *Journal of Aging Research* 2013 (2013):951786. doi: 10.1155/2013/951786; Feeney, J., et al., "Low macular pigment optical density is associated with lower cognitive performance in a large, population-based sample of older adults," *Neurobiology of Aging* 34 (2013):2449–2456; doi: 10.1016/j.neurobiolaging.2013.05.007; Renzi,

L.M., et al., "Relationships between macular pigment optical density and cognitive function in unimpaired and mildly cognitively impaired older adults," *Neurobiology of Aging* 35 (2014):1695–1699.

775. Presley, T.D., et al., "Acute effect of a high nitrate diet on brain perfusion in older adults," *Nitric Oxide* 24 (2011):34–42. doi:10.1016/j.niox.2010.10.002

776. Morris, Martha Clare, et al., *"Nutrients and bioactives in green leafy vegetables and cognitive decline" Neurology* (2017): DOI: https://doi.org/10.1212/WNL.0000000000004815; Morris, Martha Clare, et al., "Relations to cognitive change with age of micronutrients found in green leafy vegetables," *FASEB* 29 suppl. (2015).

777. https://fox8.com/2015/09/22/cleveland-heights-woman-turns-111-reveals-sweet-secret-to-long-life/

778. Willcox, Donald Craig, et al., "Healthy aging diets other than the Mediterranean: A Focus on the Okinawan Diet," *Mechanisms of Aging and Development* 136-137 (2014):148-162

779. Qun, Shan, et al., "Purple Sweet Potato Color Ameliorates Cognition Deficits and Attenuates Oxidative Damage and Inflammation in Aging Mouse Brain Induced by D-Galactose," *Journal of Biomedicine and Biotechnology* 2009 (2009): doi:10.1155/2009/564737

780. Taylor, David A., "Lead in Cocoa Products: Where Does Contamination Come From?," *Environmental Health Perspectives* 113 (2005):A687-A688; Zhang, Liang, et al., "The Effects of Gene-Environment Interactions Between Cadmium Exposure and Apolipoprotein E4 on Memory in a Mouse Model of Alzheimer's Disease," *Toxicological Sciences* (2019): doi.org/10.1093/toxsci/kfz218.

781. https://www.asyousow.org/environmental-health/toxic-enforcement/toxic-chocolate

782. Brandt, K., et al., "Agroecosystem Management and Nutritional Quality of Plant Foods: The Case of Organic Fruits and Vegetables," *Critical Reviews in Plant Sciences* 30 (2011):177-97; Hunter, D., et al., "Evaluation of the micronutrient composition of plant foods produced by organic and conventional agricultural methods," *Critical Reviews of Food Science and Nutrition* 51 (2011):571-82; Asami, D.K., et al., "Comparison of the total phenolic and ascorbic acid content of freeze-dried and air-dried marionberry, strawberry, and corn grown using conventional, organic, and sustainable agricultural practices," *Journal of Agriculture and Food Chemistry* 51 (2003):1237-41; Baranski, M., et al., "Higher antioxidant and lower cadmium concentrations and lower incidence of pesticide residues in organically grown crops: a systematic literature review and meta-analyses," *British Journal of Nutrition* 112 (2014):794-811.

783. Oates, Liza, et al., "Reduction in urinary organophosphate pesticide metabolites in adults after a week-long organic diet," *Environmental Research* 132 (2014):105–11; "Effect of organic diet intervention on pesticide exposures in young children living in low-income urban and agricultural communities," *Environmental Health Perspectives* 123 (2015). http://ehp.niehs.nih.gov/1408660/.

784. Swedish Environmental Research Institute, "Human exposure to pesticides from food: A pilot study," Jan. 2015. https://www.coop.se/PageFiles/429812/ Coop%20 Ekoeffekten_Report%20ENG.pdf.

785. Hyland, Carly, et al., "Organic diet intervention significantly reduces urinary pesticide levels in U.S. children and adults," *Environmental Research* 171 (2019):568-75; Fagan,

John, et al., "Organic diet intervention significantly reduces urinary glyphosate levels in U.S. children and adults," *Environmental Research* 189 (2020). doi.org/10.1016/j.envres.2020.109898

786. Environmental Working Group. Shoppers Guide to Pesticides in Produce. 2015. www.ewg.org

787. Russell, Robert M., "Factors in aging that affect bioavailabilty of nutrients," *The Journal of Nutrition* 131 (2001):1359S–61S.

788. Solfrizzi, V., et al., "The role of diet in cognitive decline," *Journal of Neural Transmission* 110 (2003):95–110.

789. Smith, A. D., "Prevention of dementia: A role for B vitamins?" *Nutrition and Health* 18 (2006):225–26; Blazquez, Enrique, et al., "Insulin in the Brain: Its Pathophysiological Implications for States Related with Central Insulin Resistance, Type 2 Diabetes and Alzheimer's Disease," *Frontiers in Endocrinology* 5 (2014):161.

790. Douaud, Gwenaelle, et al., "Preventing Alzheimer's disease-related gray matter atrophy by B-vitamin treatment," *PNAS* 110 (2013):9523–28; de Jager, C.A., et al., "Cognitive and clinical outcomes of homocysteine-lowering B-vitamin treatment in mild cognitive impairment: a randomized controlled trial," *International Journal of Geriatrics and Psychiatry* 27 (2012):592–600.

791. Aroda V.R., et al., "Long-term Metformin Use and Vitamin B12 Deficiency in the Diabetes Prevention Program Outcomes Study," *Journal of Clinical Endocrinology and Metabolism* 101 (2016):1754-61.

792. deJager, C.A., et al., "cognitive and clinical outcomes of homocysteine-lowering B-vitamin treatment in mild cognitive impairment: a randomized controlled trial," *International Journal of Geriatric Psychiatry* 27 (2012):592-600.

793. Ikeda, T., et al., "Treatment of Alzheimer-type dementia with intravenous mecobalamin," *Clinical Therapeutics* 14 (1992):426–437.

794. Goodwin, J.S, et al., "Association between nutritional status and cognitive functioning in a healthy elderly population," *JAMA* 249 (1983):2917–2921.

795. Kato, Y., et al., "Trends in dietary intakes of vitamins A, C and E among Japanese men and women from 1974 to 2001," *Public Health and Nutrition* 12 (2009):1343-50.

796. Forrest, K. Y., et al., "Prevalence and correlates of vitamin D deficiency in U.S. adults," *Nutrition Research* 31 (2010):48–54.

797. Forrest, K.Y., et al., "Prevalence and correlates of vitamin D deficiency in US adults," *Nutrition Research* 31 (2011):48–54. doi:10.1016/j.nutres.2010.12.001; Zhou, Ang, et al., "Non-linear Mendelian randomization analyses support a role for vitamin D deficiency in cardiovascular disease risk," *European Heart Journal* (2021). DOI: 10.1093/eurheartj/ehab809

798. McCann, J. C., et al., "Is there convincing biological or behavioral evidence linking vitamin D deficiency to brain dysfunction?" *FASEB J* 22 (2008):982–1001; Grant, William B., "Does vitamin D reduce the risk of dementia?" *Journal of Alzheimer's Disease* 17 (2009):151–59.

799. Zhou, Ang, et al., "Non-linear Mendelian randomization analyses support a role for vitamin D deficiency in cardiovascular disease risk," *European Heart Journal*, 2021 DOI: 10.1093/eurheartj/ehab809

800. Littlejohns, T. J., et al., "Vitamin D and dementia," *The Journal of Prevention of Alzheimer's Disease* (Clinical Trials Service Unit and Epidemiological Studies Unit, Nuffield Department of Population Health, University of Oxford, Oxford, UK; 2. University of Exeter Medical School, University of Exeter, Exeter, UK). http://www.jpreventionalzheimer.com/1232-vitamin-d-and-dementia.html, accessed online, May 19, 2016.

801. Marie-France Nissou, et al., "Additional clues for a protective role of vitamin D in neurodegenerative diseases: 1,25- dihydroxyvitamin D3 triggers an anti-inflammatory response in brain pericytes," *Journal of Alzheimer's Disease* (2014):789–99.

802. Darwish H., et al., "Serum 25-hydroxyvitamin D predicts cognitive performance in adults," *Neuropsychiatric Disease and Treatment* 11 (2015):2217–23.

803. Littlejohns, Thomas J., et al., "Vitamin D and the risk of dementia and Alzheimer disease," *Neurology* 83 (2014):920–28; Soni, M., et al., "Vitamin D and cognitive function," *Scandanavia Journal of Clinical and Laboratory Investigation* (Suppl) 243 (2012):79–82; Grant, B., "Using multicountry ecological and observational studies to determine dietary risk factors for Alzheimer's disease," *Journal of the American College of Nutrition* 35 (2016):476-89.

804. Alipio, Mark, "Vitamin D Supplementation Could Possibly Improve Clinical Outcomes of Patients Infected with Coronavirus-2019 (COVID-19)," April 9, 2020. dx.doi.org/10.2139/ssrn.3571484

805. Nishida, Y., et al., "Depletion of vitamin E increases amyloid beta accumulation by decreasing its clearances from brain and blood in a mouse model of Alzheimer disease," *Journal of Biological Chemistry* 284 (2009):33400-8.

806. Dysken, Maurice W., et al., "Effect of vitamin E and memantine on functional decline in Alzheimer disease: The TEAM-AD VA Cooperative Randomized Trial," *JAMA* 311 (2014):33–44.

807. Sano, M., et al., "A controlled trial of selegiline, alpha-tocopherol, or both as treatment for Alzheimer's disease," *The New England Journal of Medicine* 336 (1997):1216–1222, 1997.

808. Wallace, Taylor C., et al., "Assessment of Total Choline Intakes in the United States. *Journal of the American College of Nutrition* 35 (2016): DOI: 10.1080/07315724.2015.1080127;

809. Niki, E., "Mechanisms and dynamics of antioxidant action of ubiquinol," *Molecular Aspects of Medicine* 18 (1997):S63–S70.

810. Deichmann, R., et al., "Coenzyme q10 and statin-induced mitochondrial dysfunction," *The Ochsner Journal* 10 (2010):16–21.

811. Arterburn, Linda M., et al., "Algal-oil capsules and cooked salmon: Nutritionally equivalent sources of docosahexaenoic acid," *Journal of the American Dietetic Association* 108 (2008):1204–9.

812. Hoption, Cann S. A., "Hypothesis: Dietary iodine intake in the etiology of cardiovascular disease," *Journal of the American College of Nutrition* 25 (2006):1–11.

813. Oldfiled, Eileen, "Task Force Recommends Against Vitamin D, Calcium Supplements," *Pharmacy Times* June 21, 2012.

814. Curhan, Gary C., et al., "Comparison of Dietary Calcium with Gary. C. Supplemental Calcium and Other Nutrients as Factors Affecting the Risk for Kidney Stones in Women," *Annals of Internal Medicine* 126 (1997):497-504. doi:10.7326/0003-4819-126-7-199704010-00001

815. Rehman, S., et al., "Calcium supplements: an additional source of lead contamination," *Biological Trace Element Research* 143 (2011):178-87. doi: 10.1007/s12011-010-8870-3. Epub 2010 Oct 15. PMID: 20953844; Bourgoin, B.P., et al., "Lead content in 70 brands of dietary calcium supplements," *America Journal of Public Health* 83 (1993):1155-1160. doi:10.2105/ajph.83.8.1155

816. Bolland, M. J., et al., "Effect of calcium supplements on risk of myocardial infarction and cardiovascular events: meta-analysis," *BMJ* 341 (2010):c3691 doi:10.1136/bmj.c3691; Bolland, M.J, et al., "Calcium supplements and cardiovascular risk: 5 years on," *Therapeutic Advances in Drug Safety* 4 (2013):199-210. doi:10.1177/2042098613499790

817. Lee, M. K., et al., "Asicatic acid derivatives protect cultured cortical neurons from glutamate-induced excitotoxicity," *Research Communications in Molecular Pathology and Pharmacology* 108 (2000):75–86.

818. Wattanathorn, J., et al., "Positive modulation of cognition and mood in the healthy elderly volunteer following the administration of centella asiatica," *Journal of Ethnopharmacology* 116 (2008):325–32.

819. Tiwari, S., et al., "Effect of centella asiatica on mild cognitive impairment (MCI) and other common age-related clinical problems," *Digest Journal of Nanomaterials and Biostructures* 3 (2008):215–20.

820. Akhondzadeh, Basti A., et al., "Comparison of petal of Crocus sativus L and fluoxetine in the treatment of depressed outpatients: A pilot double-blind randomized trial," *Progress in Neuropsychopharmacoloy Biological Psychiatry* 31 (2007):439–442.

821. Purushothuman, S., et al., "Saffron pre-treatment offers neuroprotection to Nigral and retinal dopaminergic cells of MPTP-Treated mice," *Journal of Parkinson's Disease* 3 (2013):77–83.

822. Khazdair, M.R., et al., "The effects of Crocus sativus (saffron) and its constituents on nervous system: A review," *Avicenna Journal of Phytomedicine* 5 (2015):376–391.

823. Akhondzadeh, S., et al., "Saffron in the treatment of patients with mild to moderate Alzheimer's disease: A 16-week, randomized and placebo-controlled trial," *Journal of Clinical Pharmacy Therapeutics* 35 (2010):581–588.

824. Akhondzadeh, S., et al. "Saffron in the treatment of patients with mild to moderate Alzheimer's disease: A 16-week, randomized and placebo–controlled trial," *Journal of Clinical Pharmacy and Therapeutics* 35 (2010):581–88.

825. Farokhnia, M., et al., "Comparing the efficacy and safety of Crocus sativus L. with memantine in patients with moderate to severe Alzheimer's disease: a double-blind randomized clinical trial," *Human Psychopharmacology* 29 (2014):351-9. doi: 10.1002/hup.2412. PMID: 25163440.

826. Wu, A., et al., "Curcumin boosts dha in the brain: Implications for the prevention of anxiety disorders," *BBA Molecular Basis of Disease* 1852 (2015):951–961; Hishikawa, Nozomi, et al., "Effects of turmeric on Alzheimer's disease with behavioral and psychological symptoms of dementia.," *Ayu* 33 (2012):499-504; Dias, Gisele Pereira, et al., "The Role of Dietary Polyphenols on Adult Hippocampal Neurogenesis:

Molecular Mechanisms and Behavioural Effects on Depression and Anxiety," *Oxidative Medicine and Cellular Longevity* (2012). doi.org/10.1155/2012/541971; Sun, C.Y., et al., "Neurobiological and pharmacological validity of curcumin in ameliorating memory performance of senescence-accelerated mice," *Pharmacology Biochemistry and Behavior* 105 (2013): 76–82.

827. Hishikawa, Nozomi, et al., "Effects of turmeric on Alzheimer's disease with behavioral and psychological symptoms of dementia," *AYU* 33 (2012):499–504.

828. Small, Gary, et al., "Memory and Brain Amyloid and Tau Effects of a Bioavailable Form of Curcumin in Non-Demented Adults: A Double-Blind, Placebo-Controlled 18-Month Trial," *American Journal of Geriatric Psychiatry* (2017): https://doi.org/10.1016/j.jagp.2017.10.010

829. Zhang, L., et al., "Curcuminoids enhance amyloid-beta uptake by macrophages of Alzheimer's disease patients," *Journal of Alzheimer's Disease* 10 (2006):1–7.

830. Mishra, Shrikant, et al., "The effect of curcumin (turmeric) on Alzheimer's disease: An overview," *Annals of Indian Academy of Neurology* 11 (2008):13–19.

831. Yang, F., et al., "Curcumin inhibits formation of amyloid beta oligomers and fibrils, binds plaques, and reduces amyloid in vivo," *Journal of Biological Chemistry* 280 (2005):5892–901.

832. Frautshy, S. A., et al., "Phenolic anti-inflammatory antioxidant reversal of b induced cognitive deficits and neuropathology," *Neurobiology & Aging* 22 (2001):993-1005.

833. Chandran, B., et al., "A randomized, pilot study to assess the efficacy and safety of curcumin in patients with active rheumatoid arthritis," *Phytotherapy Research* 26 (2012):1719–25.

834. Chandra, V., et al., "Prevalence of Alzheimer's disease and other dementias in rural India: The Indo-U.S. study," *Neurology* 51 (1998):1000–1008.

835. Reiley, Laura, "Some turmeric, wellness potion of the moment, may owe its yellow color to lead contamination, a study says." *The Washington Post* September 28, 2019.

836. Preedy, Victor R.; Watson, Ronald Ross; Patel, Vinood B., eds (2011) *Nuts and Seeds in Health and Disease Prevention* (1st ed.) Burlington, MA: Academic Press. p. 678

837. Shurtleff, William; Aoyago, Akiko, (2007) *History of Soybeans and Soyfoods: 1100 B.C. to 1980s.* www.soyinfocenter.com

838. Mark P. Mattson, et al., "Effects of Intermittent Fasting on Health, Aging, and Disease," *New England Journal of Medicine* 381 (2019): 2541. DOI: 10.1056/NEJMra1905136

839. Jordan, Stefan, et al., "Dietary intake regulates the circulating inflammatory monocyte pool," *Cell* 178 (2019): P1102-1114.

840. Sutton, E. F., et al., "Early Time-Restricted Feeding Improves Insulin Sensitivity, Blood Pressure, and Oxidative Stress Even without Weight Loss in Men with Prediabetes," *Cell Metabolism* 27 (2018):1212-122.

841. Malinowski, B., et al., "Intermittent Fasting in Cardiovascular Disorders-An Overview," *Nutrients* 11 (2019):673. doi:10.3390/nu11030673; Sutton, E. F., et al., "Early Time-Restricted Feeding Improves Insulin Sensitivity, Blood Pressure, and

Oxidative Stress Even without Weight Loss in Men with Prediabetes," *Cell Metabolism* 27 (2018):1212-122.

842. Popkin, B., et al., "Water, hydration and health," *Nutrition Reviews* 68 (2010):439–58.

843. Pivarnik, J.M., et al., "Nutrition in Exercise and Sport," CRC Press; Boca Raton, FL, USA: 1994. Water and electrolyte balance during rest and exercise; pp. 245–262; Zhang, Jianfen, et al., "The Effects of Hydration Status on Cognitive Performances among Young Adults in Hebei, China: A Randomized Controlled Trial (RCT)," *International Journal of Environmental Research and Public Health* 15 (2018):1477.

844. Watso, J.C., et al., "Hydration Status and Cardiovascular Function," *Nutrients* 11 (2019):1866.doi:10.3390/nu11081866

845. Armstrong, L.E, et al., "Mild dehydration affects mood in healthy young women," *Journal of Nutrition* 142 (2012):382–388; Ganio, M.S, et al., "Mild dehydration impairs cognitive performance and mood of men," *British Journal of Nutrition* 106 (2011):1535–1543.

846. Environmental Protection Agency, "Drinking water contaminant candidate list 5-draft," *Federal Register* July 19, 2021. https://www.federalregister.gov/documents/2021/07/19/2021-15121/drinking-water-contaminant-candidate-list-5-draft

847. Phillips, Anna M., et al., "California finds widespread water contamination of 'forever chemicals'," *Los Angeles Times* October 14, 2019.

848. Evlampidou, Iro, et al., "Trihalomethanes in drinking water and bladder cancer burden in the European union," *Environmental Health* Perspectives 128 (2020). Doi. org/10.1289/EHP4495

849. Grandjeane, Philip, et al., "Neurobehavioural effects of developmental toxicity," *Lancet* 13 (2014):330–38.

850. Bhatnagar M.L., et al., "Neurotoxicity of fluoride: neurodegeneration in hippocampus of female mice," *Indian Journal of Experimental Biology* 40 (2002):546-54; Choi, Anna L., et al., "Developmental Fluoride Neurotoxicity: A Systematic Review and Meta-Analysis," *Environmental Health Perspectives* 120 (2012):1362-68; Bashash, Morteza, et al., "Prenatal Fluoride Exposure and Cognitive Outcomes in Children at 4 and 6–12 Years of Age in Mexico," *Environmental Health Perspectives* (2017): / doi.org/10.1289/EHP655

851. McDonagh, Marianne, et all., "A Systematic Review of Public Water Fluoridation, NHS Centre for Reviews and Dissemination," University of York (2000): https://www.nhs.uk/conditions/fluoride/documents/crdreport18.pdf; Maupome, G., et al., "Patterns of dental caries following the cessation of water fluoridation," *Community Dentistry and Oral Epidemiology* 29 (2001):37-47; Iheozor-Ejiofor, Zipporah, et al., "Water fluoridation for the prevention of dental caries," *Cochrane Database of Systematic Reviews* (2015): /doi.org/10.1002/14651858.CD010856.pub2

852. Cheng, K.K./, et al. "Adding fluoride to water supplies," *BMJ* 335 (2007): 699-702.

853. Benotti, Mark J., et al., "Pharmaceuticals and Endocrine Disrupting Compounds in U.S. Drinking Water," *Environmental Science and Technology* 43 (2009):597-603.

854. Kolpin, Dana W., et al., "Pharmaceuticals, hormones, and other organic wastewater contaminants in U.S. streams, 1999-2000: A national reconnaissance," *Environmental Science and Toxicology* 36 (2002):1202-11; Harvard Health Letter, "Drugs in the water," June 2011, https://www.health.harvard.edu/newsletter_article/drugs-in-the-water

855. Pell, M.B., et al., "The thousands of U.S. locales where lead poisoning is worse than in Flint," *Reuters Investigates* December 19, 2016

856. DeNoon, Daniel J., "Heavy metals found in wine," *WebMD* October 29, 2008; Puzo, Daniel P., "600 Wines Contain Lead, U.S. Tests Find: Health: FDA has not established a risk level for the substance in wine. But the amounts measured far exceed the EPA's standard for drinking water," *Los Angeles Times* August 1, 1991.

857. Juresa, D., et al., "Mercury, arsenic, lead and cadmium in fish and shellfish from the Adriatic Sea," *Food Additives and Contaminants* 20 (2003):241–46; Mallongi, Anwar, et al., "Health Risk Analysis of Lead Exposure from Fish Consumption among Communities along Youtefa Gulf, Jayapura," *Pakistan Journal of Nutrition* 15 (2016): 929-935: Zaza, Silvia, et al., "Human exposure in Italy to lead, cadmium and mercury through fish and seafood product consumption from Eastern Central Atlantic Fishing Area," *Journal of Food Composition and Analysis* 40 (2015):148-53.

858. Bernstein, Lenny, "How much lead is in your chocolate," *Washington Post* February 11, 2015. https://www.washingtonpost.com/news/to-your-health/wp/2015/02/11/lead-and-cadmium-in-chocolate-nooooooooooooo/, accessed online, Feb. 11, 2015.

859. "Health risks of protein drinks. You don't need the extra protein or the heavy metals our tests found," *Consumer Reports* July 2010

860. Schwalfenberg, Gerry, et al., "The Benefits and Risks of Consuming Brewed Tea: Beware of Toxic Element Contamination," *Journal of Toxicology* 2013 (2013): doi.org/10.1155/2013/370460

861. Wong, M. H., et al., "Aluminum and fluoride contents of tea, with emphasis on brick tea and their health implications," *Toxicology Letters* 137 (2003):111–20.

862. "Toxicological profile for aluminum," U.S. Department of Health and Human Services, Sept. 2008; Agency for Toxic Substances and Disease Registry: http://www.atsdr.cdc.gov/toxprofiles/tp22.pdf, accessed online, Apr. 15, 2015.

863. DaSilva, E., et al., "Aluminum and strontium in calcium supplements and antacids: a concern to haemodialysis patients?" *Food Additives and Contaminants: Part A Chemistry, Analysis, Control, Exposure and Risk Assessment* 27 (2010):1405-14.

864. Veríssimo, M.I, et al., "Aluminum migration into beverages: are dented cans safe?," *Science and the Total Environment* 405 (2008):385-8. doi: 10.1016/j.scitotenv.2008.05.045. Epub 2008 Jul 30. PMID: 18672271; Duggan, J.M., et al., "Aluminum beverage cans as a dietary source of aluminum," *Medical Journal of Australia* 156 (1992):604-5. doi: 10.5694/j.1326-5377.1992.tb121455.x. PMID: 1625612.

865. St-Onge, M.P., et al., "Fiber and Saturated Fat Are Associated with Sleep Arousals and Slow Wave Sleep," *Journal of Clinical Sleep and Medicine* 12 (2016):19-24. doi: 10.5664/jcsm.5384. PMID: 26156950; PMCID: PMC4702189.

St Onge, Marie-Pierre, et al., "Effects of diet on sleep quality," *Advances in Nutrition* 7 (2016):938–949;

Zuraikat, Faris M., et al., "Measures of poor sleep quality are associated with higher energy intake and poor diet quality in a diverse sample of women from the Go Red for Women Strategically Focused Research Network," *JAHA* (2020). doi.org/10.1161/JAHA.119.014587

866. West, Kathleen E., et al., "Blue light from light-emitting diodes elicits a dose-dependent suppression of melatonin in humans," *Journal of Applied Physiology* 110 (2011):619-26.

867. Zhang, Jun, et al., "Acute effects of radiofrequency electromagnetic field emitted by mobile phone on brain function," *Bioelectromagnetics* 38 (2017): DOI: 10.1002/bem.22052

868. Aminoff, M.J., et al., "We spend about one-third of our life either sleeping or attempting to do so," *Handbook of Clinical Neurology* 98 (2011).

869. Hsin, Shih, et al., "An Increased Risk of Reversible Dementia May Occur After Zolpidem Derivative Use in the Elderly Population," *Medicine* 94 (2015):1.

870. Wilson, R. S, et al., "Chronic psychological distress and risk of Alzheimer's disease in old age," *Neuroepidemiology* 27 (2006): 143–53.

871. Katz, Mindy J., et al., "Influence of perceived stress on incident amnestic mild cognitive impairment: Results from the Einstein Aging Study," *Alzheimer's Disease & Associated Disorders* 30 (2015):93–98.

872. Peavy, G. M., et al., "The effects of prolonged stress and APOE genotype on memory and cortisol in older adults," *Biological Psychiatry* 62 (2007): 472–78; Heim, C., et al., "Long term neuroendocrine effect of childhood maltreatment," *JAMA* 284 (2000): 2321; Bornstein, A. R., et al., "Early-life risk factors for Alzheimer disease," *Alzheimer Disease and Associated Disorders* 20 (2006): 6372; Wilson, R. S, et al., "Vulnerability to stress, anxiety, and development of dementia in old age," *American Journal of Geriatric Psychiatry* 19 (2011): 327–34.

873. Baum, A., et al., "Control and intrusive memories as possible determinants of chronic stress," *Psychosomatic Medicine* 55 (1993):274–286; McEwen, B.S., "The Brain on Stress: Toward an Integrative Approach to Brain, Body and Behavior," *Perspectives on Psychological Science* 8 (2013):673–675; Keinan, G., "The effect of stress on the suppression of erroneous competing responses," *Anxiety, Stress, and Coping* 12 (1999):455–476.

874. Ricci, S., Fuso, et al., "Stress-induced cytokines and neuronal dysfunction in Alzheimer's disease. *Journal of Alzheimer's Disease* 28 (2012):11–24.

875. Schwabe, Lars, et al., "Learning under stress impairs memory formation," *Neurobiology of Learning and Memory* 93 (2010):183-88; Kim E.J., et al., "Stress effects on the hippocampus: a critical review," *Learning & Memory* 22 (2015):411–416. doi:10.1101/lm.037291.114

876. Bremner, J. Douglas, "Stress and brain atrophy," *CNS Neurological Disorders and Drug Targets* 5 (2006):503–12.

877. McEwen, B., "Protective and damaging effects of stress mediators," *New England Journal of Medicine* 338 (1998): 171–79; Innes, K. E et al., "Meditation as a therapeutic intervention for adults at risk for Alzheimer's disease—potential benefits and underlying mechanisms," *Frontiers in Psychiatry* 5 (2014): 40.

878. Bremmer, J. Douglas, "Traumatic stress: effects on the brain," *Dialogues in Clinical Neuroscience* 8 (2006):445-61.

879. Miller, G. E., et al., "Chronic psychological stress and the regulation of pro-inflammatory cytokines: A glucocorticoid-resistance model," *Health Psychology* 21 (2002):531–41.

880. UCI MIND. "Stress and its influence on Alzheimer's disease," University of California Irvine Alzheimer's Disease Research Center. http://www.mind.uci.edu/stress-and-its-influence-on-alzheimer%E2%80%99s-disease/, accessed online, Oct. 13, 2015.

881. Epel, E. S., et al., "Dynamics of telomerase activity in response to acute psychological stress," *Brain Behavior and Immunity* 24 (2010): 531–39; Lukens, J. N., et al., "Comparisons of telomere length in peripheral blood and cerebellum in Alzheimer's disease," *Alzheimer's & Dementia* 5 (2009): 463–69; Davalos, Albert R., et al., "Senescent cells as a source of inflammatory factors for tumor progression," *Cancer Metastasis Reviews* 29 (2010):273-83.

882. Libby, P., et al., "Leukocytes link local and systemic inflammation in ischemic cardiovascular disease: An expanded cardiovascular continuum," *Journal of the American College of Cardiology* 67 (2016):1091–103.

883. Hunter, MaryCarol R., et al., "Urban Nature Experiences Reduce Stress in the Context of Daily Life Based on Salivary Biomarkers," *Frontiers in Psychology* (2019): doi.org/10.3389/fpsyg.2019.00722

884. Kobayashi, H., et al., "Population-based study on the effect of a forest environment on salivary cortisol concentration," *International Journal of Environmental Research and Public Health* 14 (2017) doi: 10.3390/ijerph14080931; Park, B.J., et al., "Effect of the forest environment on physiological relaxation—The results of field tests at 35 sites throughout Japan," *Forest Medicine*, ed. Q. Li (New York, NY, 2012: Nova Science Publishers), 55–65.

885. Ricci, S., et al., "Stress-induced cytokines and neuronal dysfunction in Alzheimer's disease," *Journal of Alzheimer's Disease* 28 (2012):11–24.

886. Chetelat, Gael, et al., "Reduced age-associated brain changes in expert meditators: a multimodal neuroimaging pilot study," *Scientific Reports—Nature* 7 (2017): :10160. doi: 10.1038/s41598-017-07764-x.

887. Schneirder, Robert H., et al., "Stress reduction in the prevention of cardiovascular disease: Randomized, controlled trial of Transcendental Meditation and health education in blacks," *Circulation: Cardiovascular Quality and Outcomes* 5 (2012):750–58.

888. Rosenthal, Joshua, et al., "Effects of Transcendental Meditation in veterans of Operation Enduring Freedom and Operation Iraqi Freedom with posttraumatic stress disorder: A pilot study," *Military Medicine* 176 (2011):626–30.

889. Brooks, James S., et al., "Transcendental Meditation in the treatment of post-Vietnam adjustment," *Journal of Counseling and Development* 64 (1985):212–15.

890. Nidich, S. I., et al., "A randomized controlled trial on effects of the Transcendental Meditation program on blood pressure, psychological distress, and coping in young adults," *American Journal of Hypertension* 22 (2009):1326–31.

891. Jevning, R., et al., "Adrenocortical activity during meditation," *Hormones and Behavior* 10 (1978):54–60.

892. Travis, F., et al., "Effects of transcendental meditation practice on brain functioning and stress reactivity in college students," *International Journal of Psychophysiology* 71 (2009): 170–76.

893. Epel, E., et al., "Can meditation slow rate of cellular aging? Cognitive stress, mindfulness, and telomeres," *Annals of the New York Academy of Science* 1172 (2009):34–53. doi:10.1111/j.1749-6632.2009.04414.x

894. Duraimani, S., et al., "Effects of Lifestyle Modification on Telomerase Gene Expression in Hypertensive Patients: A Pilot Trial of Stress Reduction and Health Education Programs in African Americans," *PLOS ONE* 10 (2015), published online: http://journals.plos.org/plosone/article?id=10.1371/journal.pone.0142689

895. Newberg, A. N., et al., "Cerebral blood flow differences between long-term meditators and non-meditators," *Consciousness and Cognition* 19 (2010):899–905.

896. Creswell, J. David, et al., "Alterations in Resting-State Functional Connectivity Link Mindfulness Meditation with Reduced Interleukin-6: A Randomized Controlled Trial," *Biological Psychiatry* 80 (2016):53-61.

897. Lazar, S., et al., "Meditation experience is associated with increased cortical thickness," *Neuroreport* 16 (2005):1893–97; Hölzel, B. K., et al., "Investigation of mindfulness meditation practitioners with voxel-based morphometry," *Social Cognitive and Affective Neuroscience* 3 (2008): 55–61.

898. Holzel, B. K., et al., "Mindfulness practice leads to increases in regional brain gray matter density," *Psychiatry Research* 191 (2011):36–43.

899. Wallace, R.K., et al., "The Effects of the Transcendental Meditation and TM-Sidhi program on the Aging Process," *International Journal of Neuroscience* 16 (1982): 53-58.

900. Herron, R., et al., "Can the Transcendental Meditation program reduce the expenditures of older people? A longitudinal cost reduction study in Canada," *Journal of Social Behavior and Personality* 17 (2005):415–42.

901. Eyre, H.A., et al., "Changes in neural connectivity and memory following a yoga intervention for older adults: A pilot study," *Journal of Alzheimer's Disease* 52 (2016):673–84.

902. Afonso, Rui F., et al., "Greater Cortical Thickness in Elderly Female Yoga Practitioners—A Cross-Sectional Study," Frontiers in Aging Neuroscience 9 (2017): 10.3389/fnagi.2017.00201

903. Mortimer, J. A., et al., "Changes in brain volume and cognition in a randomized trial of exercise and social interaction in a community-based sample of non-demented Chinese elders," *Journal of Alzheimer's Disease* 30 (2012):757–66.

904. Lam, L.C.W., et al., "Interim follow-up of a randomized controlled trial comparing Chinese style mind body (Tai Chi) and stretching exercises on cognitive function in subjects at risk of progressive cognitive decline," *International Journal of Geriatric Psychiatry* 26 (2012):733–740.

905. Northey, Joseph Michael, et al., "Exercise interventions for cognitive function in adults older than 50: a systematic review with meta-analysis," *British Journal of Sports Medicine* 54 (2018):154-160.

906. Xue-Qiang Wang, et al., "Traditional Chinese Exercise for Cardiovascular Diseases: Systematic Review and Meta-Analysis of Randomized Controlled Trials," *Journal of the American Heart* Association 5 (2016). doi.org/10.1161/JAHA.115.002562

907. Nyman, Samuel, et al., "Randomised controlled trial of the effect of tai chi on postural balance of people with dementia," *Clinical Interventions in Aging (2019)* doi:10.2147/CIA.S228931.

908. Byeonsang, Oh, et al., "Effect of medical Qigong on cognitive function, quality of life, and a biomarker of inflammation in cancer patients: a randomized controlled trial," *Supportive Care in Cancer* 20 (2012):1235-42.

909. Higuchi et al., "Endocrine and Immune Response during Guolin New Qigong," *Journal of the International Society of Life Information Science* 15 (1997):138; Yuanliang, Liu, et al., "Clinical observation of the treatment of 158 cases of cerebral arteriosclerosis by qigong," 2nd World Conference for Academic Exchange of Medical Qigong, 125.

910. Tao, J., et al., "Tai Chi Chuan and Baduanjin Increase Grey Matter Volume in Older Adults: A Brain Imaging Study," *Journal of Alzheimer's Disease* 60 (2017):389-400. doi:10.3233/JAD-170477

911. Aranda, Julie H., et al., "Proceedings of the 20th International Conference on Human-Computer Interaction with Mobile Devices and Services, Article No. 19," Barcelona, Spain, September3-6, 2018.

912. Cardinal, Bradley J., et al., "If Exercise is Medicine, Where is Exercise in Medicine? Review of U.S. Medical Education Curricula for Physical Activity-Related Content," *Journal of Physical Activity and Health* 12 (2014):1336-43.

913. Hillman CH, "Be smart, exercise your heart: exercise effects on brain and cognition," National Review of Neuroscience 9 (2008):58-65.

914. Gomez-Pinilla, F., "Collaborative effects of diet and exercise on cognitive enhancement," *Nutrition and Health 20* (2011):165–169.

915. Vaynman, S., "Hippocampal BDNF mediates the efficacy of exercise on synaptic plasticity and cognition," *European Journal of Neuroscience* 20 (2004):2580-90.

916. Seals, D.R., et al., "Edward F. Adolph Distinguished Lecture: The remarkable anti-aging effects of aerobic exercise on systemic arteries," *Journal of Applied Physiology* (1985) 117 (2014):425-39. doi: 10.1152/japplphysiol.00362.2014.

917. Gaitán, Julian M., et al., 'Brain Glucose Metabolism, Cognition, and Cardiorespiratory Fitness Following Exercise Training in Adults at Risk for Alzheimer's Disease," *Brain Plasticity* 5 (2019): 83–95.

918. Dimitrov, Stoyan, et al., "Inflammation and exercise: Inhibition of monocytic intracellular TNF production by acute exercise via B_2-adrenergic activation," *Brain, Behavior, and Immunity* 61 (2017):60-68.

919. Won, J., et al., "Semantic Memory Activation After Acute Exercise in Healthy Older Adults," *Journal of the International Neuropsychological Society* 25 (2019):557-568. doi:10.1017/S1355617719000171

920. da Silveira, M.P., et al., "Physical exercise as a tool to help the immune system against COVID-19: an integrative review of the current literature," *Clinical and Experimental Medicine* 21 (2021):15-28. doi:10.1007/s10238-020-00650-3; Sallis, R., et al., "Physical inactivity is associated with a higher risk for severe COVID-19 outcomes: a study in 48 440 adult patients," *British Journal of Sports Medicine* 55 (2021):1099-1105.

921. Alfini, Alfonso, et al., "Hippocampal and cerebral blood flow after exercise cessation in master athletes," *Frontiers in Aging Neuroscience* 2016; doi:10.3389/fnagi.2016.00184

922. Buchman, A. S., et al., "Total daily physical activity and the risk of AD and cognitive decline in older adults," *Neurology* 78 (2012):1323–29.

923. Cassandra, Szoeke, et al., "Predictive factors for verbal memory performance over decades of aging: data from the women's healthy ageing project," *American Journal of Geriatric Society* 24 (2016):857-67.

924. Sofi, F., et al., "Physical activity and risk of cognitive decline: A meta-analysis of prospective studies," *Journal of Internal Medicine* 269 (2011):107–17.

925. Stern, Yaakov, et al., "Effect of aerobic exercise on cognition in younger adults: A randomized clinical trial," *Neurology* (2019): DOI: https://doi.org/10.1212/WNL.0000000000007003

926. inu P. Thomas, et al., "Brain Perfusion Change in Patients with Mild Cognitive Impairment After 12 Months of Aerobic Exercise Training," *Journal of Alzheimer's Disease* 75 (2020):617 DOI: 10.3233/JAD-190977

927. Tari, Atefe, R., et al., "Temporal changes in cardiorespiratory fitness and risk of dementia incidence and mortality: a population-based prospective cohort study," *Lancet* (2019): https://doi.org/10.1016/S2468-2667(19)30183-5

928. Rashid, M.H., et al., "The Neuroprotective Effects of Exercise on Cognitive Decline: A Preventive Approach to Alzheimer Disease," *Cureus* (2020): e6958. DOI:10.7759/cureus.6958

929. Lin, T.W, et al., "Running exercise delays neurodegeneration in amygdala and hippocampus of Alzheimer's disease (APP/PS1) transgenic mice," *Neurobiology Learning and Memory* 118 (2015):189–97; Maesako, M, et al., "Exercise is more effective than diet control in preventing high fat diet induced β-amyloid deposition and memory deficit in amyloid precursor protein transgenic mice," *Journal of Biological Chemistry* 287 (2012):23024–33.

930. Casaletto, Kaitlin, et al., "Late-life physical activity relates to brain tissue synaptic integrity markers in older adults," *Alzheimer's & Dementia* (2022). DOI: 10.1002/alz.12530

931. Huang, L., et al., "Decreased serum levels of the angiogenic factors VEGF and TGF-B1 in Alzheimer's disease and amnestic mild cognitive impairment," *Neuroscience Letters* 550 (2013):60-3.

932. Robinson, C.J, et al., "The splice variants of vascular endothelial growth factor (VEGF) and their receptors," *Journal of Cell Science* 114 (2001):853-865

933. Kim, Oh Yoen, et al., "The Role of Irisin in Alzheimer's Disease," *Journal of Clinical Medicine* 7 (2018): doi:10.3390/jcm7110407

934. Gottmann K., et al., "BDNF signaling in the formation, maturation and plasticity of glutamatergic and gabaergic synapses," *Experimental Brain Research* 199 (2009):203–234.

935. Shen, H., et al. "Physical activity elicits sustained activation of the cyclic AMP response element-binding protein and mitogen-activated protein kinase in the rat hippocampus," *Neuroscience* 107(2001):219–29.

936. Bezprozvanny, Ilya, "Calcium signaling and neurodegenerative diseases," *Trends in Molecular Medicine* 15 (2009):89-100.

937. Bednarski, E., et al., "Lysosomal dysfunction reduces brain-derived neurotrophic factor expression," *Experimental Neurology* 150 (1998):128–35.

938.   Weinstein, G., et al., "Serum brain-derived neurotrophic factor and the risk for dementia: the Framingham Heart Study," *JAMA Neurology* 71 (2014):55–61. doi:10.1001/jamaneurol.2013.4781; Buchman, Aron S., et al., "Higher brain *BDNF* gene expression is associated with slower cognitive decline in older adults," *Neurology* 86 (2016):735-41.

939.   H.Y. Moon et al., "Running-induced systemic cathepsin B secretion is associated with memory function," *Cell Metabolism* doi:10.1016/j.cmet.2016.05.025, 2016.

940.   Dubal, D.B., et al., "Life extension factor Klotho enhances cognition," *Cell Reports* 7 (2014):1065-1076.

941.   Querido, J. S., et al., "Regulation of cerebral blood flow during exercise," *Sports Medicine* 37 (2009):765–82.

942.   Elizabeth Bullitt, M.D., Laurence, Katz, M.D., and Bonita Marks, Ph.D. Presented at the meeting of the Radiological Society of North America (RSNA), December 1, 2008., Fauber, John, "Exercise builds small blood vessels in brain, study says," *Journal Sentinel* December 1, 2008.

943.   Schmitz, Christiana, "MRA explains benefits of exercise for aging adults," *Psychiatric Times* December 1, 2008.

944.   Bailey, D.M., et al., "Elevated aerobic fitness sustained throughout the adult lifespan is associated with improved cerebral hemodynamics," *Stroke* 44 (2013):3235-8. doi: 10.1161/STROKEAHA.113.002589. Epub 2013 Aug 20. PMID: 23963329.

945.   Firth, Joseph, et al., "Effect of aerobic exercise on hippocampal volume in humans: A systematic review and meta-analysis," *NeuroImage* 166 (2018):230-38.

946.   Smith, J., Carson, et al., "Physical activity reduces hippocampal atrophy in elders at genetic risk for Alzheimer's disease," *Frontiers in Aging Neuroscience* 6 (2014):61.

947.   Erickson, Kirk I., e al., "Exercise training increases size of hippocampus and improves memory," *PNAS* 108 (2011):3017–3022

948.   Killgore, W., et al., "Physical Exercise Habits Correlate with Gray Matter Volume of the Hippocampus in Healthy Adult Humans," *Science Reports* 3457 (2013). doi.org/10.1038/srep03457

949.   Colmenares, Andrea Mendez, et al., "White matter plasticity in healthy older adults: The effects of aerobic exercise," *NeuroImage* 239 (2021). doi.org/10.1016/j.neuroimage.2021.118305

950.   Clark, Peter J., et al., "New neurons generated from running are broadly recruited into neuronal activation associated with three different hippocampus-involved tasks," *Hippocampus* 22 (2009):1860–67.

951.   Hotting, K., et al., "Beneficial effects of physical exercise on neuroplasticity and cognition," *Neuroscience and Biobehavioral Reviews* 37 (2013):2243–57.

952.   Amrita Vijay, et al., "The anti-inflammatory effect of bacterial short chain fatty acids is partially mediated by endocannabinoids," *Gut Microbes* 13 (2021). DOI: 10.1080/19490976.2021.1997559

953.   Gleeson, M., "Immune function in sport and exercise," *Journal of Applied Physiology* 103 (2007):693-9.

954. Kaitlin B. et al., "Microglial correlates of late life physical activity: relationship with synaptic and cognitive aging in older adults," *Journal of Neuroscience* (2021). DOI: https://doi.org/10.1523/JNEUROSCI.1483-21.2021

955. Pan, X.R., et al., "Effects of diet and exercise in preventing NIDDM in people with impaired glucose tolerance, The Da Qing IGT and Diabetes Study," *Diabetes Care* 20 (1997):537–544; Handschin, C., et al., "The role of exercise and PGC1alpha in inflammation and chronic disease," *Nature* 454 (2008):463–9.

956. Gaitán, Julian M., et al., 'Brain Glucose Metabolism, Cognition, and Cardiorespiratory Fitness Following Exercise Training in Adults at Risk for Alzheimer's Disease," *Brain Plasticity* 5 (2019): 83–95.

957. Diaz, Keith M., et al., "Physical Activity and the Prevention of Hypertension," *Current Hypertension Reports* 15 (2013):659-668.

958. Laaksonen, D.E., et al., "Physical activity in the prevention of type 2 diabetes: the Finnish diabetes prevention study," *Diabetes* 54 (2005):158–165; Cederholm, J., "The relationship of blood pressure to blood glucose and physical leisure time activity. A study of hypertension in a survey of middle-aged subjects in Uppsala 1981-82," *Acta Medica Scandinavica* 219 (1986):37–46.

959. Naci, H., et al., "How does exercise treatment compare with antihypertensive medications? A network meta-analysis of 391 randomised controlled trials assessing exercise and medication effects on systolic blood pressure," *British Journal of Sports Medicine* 53 (2019):859-869.

960. Muller, Stephan, et al., "Relationship between physical activity, cognition, and Alzheimer pathology in autosomal dominant Alzheimer's disease," *Alzheimer's & Dementia* 14 (2018):1427-37.

961. Ahlskog, J. Eric., et al., Physical exercise as a preventive or disease-modifying treatment of dementia and brain aging," *Mayo Clinic Proceedings* 86 (2011):876–84; Northey, J.M., et al., "Exercise interventions for cognitive function in adults older than 50: a systematic review with meta-analysis," *British Journal of Sports Medicine* 52 (2018):154-160.

962. Baker, Laura D., et al., "Effects of aerobic exercise on mild cognitive impairment: A controlled trial," *Archives of Neurology* 67 (2009):71–79.

963. Lautenschlager, N. T., et al., "Effect of physical activity on cognitive function in older adults at risk for Alzheimer disease: a randomized trial," *JAMA* 300 (2008):1027–1037.

964. Liu-Ambrose, Teresa, et al., "Vascular cognitive impairment and aerobic exercise: A 6-month randomized controlled trial," *Alzheimer's & Dementia* 11 (2015):323-24.

965. Venturelli, M., et al., "Six-Month Walking Program Changes Cognitive and ADL Performance in Patients with Alzheimer," *American Journal of Alzheimer's Disease & Other Dementias* (2011):381-388. doi:10.1177/1533317511418956; Winchester, J., et al., "Walking stabilizes cognitive functioning in Alzheimer's disease (AD) across one year," *Archives of Gerontology and Geriatrics* 56 (2013):96–103

966. Knopf, David, "Memory-care centers develop specialized treatments to slow Alzheimer's disease," *The Kansas City Star* June 20, 2017.

967. Holthoff, V.A., et al., "Effects of physical activity training in patients with Alzheimer's dementia: results of a pilot RCT study," *PLoS One* 10 (2015): e0121478. doi: 10.1371/journal.pone.0121478.eCollection 2015.

968. Roland, Y., et al., "Exercise program for nursing home residents with Alzheimer's disease: A 1-year randomized, controlled trial," *Journal of the American Geriatric Society* 55 (2007):158–65.

969. Sobol, N.A., et al., "Effect of aerobic exercise on physical performance in patients with Alzheimer's disease," *Alzheimer's & Dementia* 12 (2016):1207-15.

970. Baker, Laura D., et al., "Aerobic exercise reduces phosphorylated tau protein in cerebrospinal fluid in older adults with mild cognitive impairment," *Alzheimer's & Dementia* 11 (2015):324S. DOI: https://doi.org/10.1016/j.jalz.2015.07.467

971. Shah, C., et al., "Exercise Therapy for Parkinson's Disease: Pedaling Rate Is Related to Changes in Motor Connectivity," *Brain Connections* 6 (2016):25-36. doi:10.1089/brain.2014.0328

972. Blumenthal, J.A., et al., "Is Exercise a Viable Treatment for Depression?" *ACSMs Health and Fitness Journal* 16 (2012):14–21. doi:10.1249/01.FIT.0000416000.09526. eb; Craft, L.L., et al., "The Benefits of Exercise for the Clinically Depressed," *Primary Care Companion Journal of Clinical Psychiatry* 6 (2004):104–111. doi:10.4088/pcc. v06n0301

973. Alfini, Alfonso, et al., "Hippocampal and cerebral blood flow after exercise cessation in master athletes," *Frontiers in Aging Neuroscience* (2016). doi"10.3389/fnagi.2016.00184

974. Northey, Joseph Michael, et al., "Exercise interventions for cognitive function in adults older than 50: a systematic review with meta-analysis," *British Journal of Sports Medicine* 52 (2018): doi.org/10.1136/bjsports-2016-096587

975. Abe, K., "Total daily physical activity and the risk of AD and cognitive decline in older adults," *Neurology* 79 (2012):1071–1071.

976. Beeri, M. S., et al., "Being physically active may protect the brain from Alzheimer disease," *Neurology* 78 (2012):1290–91; Buchman, A. S., et al., "Total daily physical activity and the risk of AD and cognitive decline in older adults," *Neurology* 10 (2012).

977. Angevaren, M., et al., "Physical activity and enhanced fitness to improve cognitive function in older people without known cognitive impairment," *Cochrane Database Systematic Reviews* 2 (2008):CD005381.

978. Herring, Arne, et al., "Exercise during pregnancy mitigates Alzheimer-like pathology in mouse offspring," *FASEB Journal* 10 (2011).

979. Lee, M., et al., "Associations of light, moderate, and vigorous intensity physical activity with longevity. The Harvard Alumni Health Study," *American Journal of Epidemiology* 151 (2000):293-9; Manini, Todd M., "Energy Expenditure and Aging," *Ageing Research Reviews* 9 (2010):1.

980. Lossi, L., et al., "Synapse-independent and synapse-dependent apoptosis of cerebellar granule cells in postnatal rabbits occur at two subsequent but partly overlapping developmental stages," *Neuroscience* 112 (2002):509–23.

981. Wilson, R. S., et al., "Relation of cognitive activity to risk of developing Alzheimer's disease," *Neurology* 69 (2007):1911–20.

982. Rebok, George, et al., "Ten-Year Effects of the ACTIVE Cognitive Training Trial on Cognition and Everyday Functioning in Older Adults," *Journal of the American Geriatric Society* 62 (2014):16-24.

983. Johnson, Lorie, "Slowing down Alzheimer's one exercise at a time," CBN News August 28, 2015. http://www1.cbn.com/cbnnews/healthscience/2015/August/Slowing-Down-Alzheimers-One-Exercise-at-a-Time. Related video: https://www.youtube.com/watch?v=iTYYAgcqLjE

984. Hoang, Tina, et al., "Effect of early adult patterns of physical activity and television viewing on midlife cognitive function," *JAMA Psychiatry* 73 (2016):73–79.

985. http://www.nielsen.com/us/en/insights/news/2009/americans-watching-more-tv-than-ever.html.

986. Draganski, B., et al., "Neuroplasticity: Changes in grey matter induced by training," *Nature* 427 (2004):311–12.

987. University Of Illinois at Urbana-Champaign, "Brains of Those in Certain Professions Shown to Have More Synapses," *Science Daily* December 3, 1999.

988. Maguire, Eleanor A., et al., "London taxi drivers and bus drivers: A structural MRI and neuropsychological analysis," *Hippocampus* 16 (2006):1091–1101.

989. Wilson, Robert S., et al., "Life-span cognitive activity, neuropathologic burden, and cognitive aging," *Neurology* 81 (2013):314–21.

990. Landau, Susan M., et al., "Association of lifetime cognitive engagement and low B-amyloid deposition," *JAMA Neurology* 69 (2012):623–29.

991. James E. Galvin, MD, MPH, professor of neurology, psychiatry, nursing, nutrition and population health, and director, Pearl Barlow Center for Memory Evaluation and Treatment, Langone School of Medicine, New York University, New York City; Heather M. Snyder, PhD, director, medical and scientific operations, Alzheimer's Association, Chicago; July 15, 2013, presentation, Alzheimer's Association International Conference, Boston.

992. Hulette, C. M., et al., "Neuropathological and neuropsychological changes in 'normal' aging: Evidence for preclinical Alzheimer disease in cognitively normal individuals," *Journal of Neuropathology and Experimental Neurology* 57 (1998):1168–74.

993. Fischer, Corinne, et al., "How does speaking another language reduce the risk of dementia?" *Expert Review of Neurotherapeutics* 14 (2014):469–71; Craik, F. L., et al., "Delaying the onset of Alzheimer disease: Bilingualism as a form of cognitive reserve," *Neurology* 75 (2010):1726–29.

994. Chertkow, H., et al., "Multilingualism (but not always bilingualism) delays the onset of Alzheimer's disease: Evidence from a bilingual community," *Alzheimer's Disease and Associated Disorders* 24 (2010):118–25.

995. Kovelman, Loulia, et al., "Bilingual and monolingual brains compared: A functional magnetic resonance imaging investigation of syntactic processing and a possible "neural signature" of bilingualism," *Journal of Cognitive Neuroscience* 20 (2008):153–69.

996. Gaser, C., et al., "Brain structures differ between musicians and non-musicians," *Journal of Neuroscience* 23 (2003):9240–45.

997. Anguera, J. A., et al., "Video game training enhances cognitive control in older adults," *Nature* 501 (2013):97–101.

998. Edwards, Jerri D., et al., "Speed of processing training results in lower risk of dementia," *Alzheimer's & Dementia: Translational Research & Clinical Interventions* 3 (2017):603-11.

999. Dresler, Martin, et al., "Mnemonic training reshapes brain networks to support superior memory," *Neuron* 93 (2017):1227-235. DOI: 10.1016/j.neuron.2017.02.003

1000. Greenwood, Pamela, et al., "Neuronal and cognitive plasticity: A neurocognitive framework for ameliorating cognitive aging," *Frontiers in Aging Neuroscience* 2 (2010):1–14.

1001. Maguire, Elanor, et al., "Recalling routes around London: Activation of the right hippocampus in taxi drivers," *Journal of Neuroscience* 17 (1997):7103–10.

1002. Clow, Angela, et al., "Normalization of salivary cortisol levels and self-report stress by a brief lunchtime visit to an art gallery by London City workers," *Journal of Holistic Healthcare* 3 (2006):29–32.

1003. Bolwerk, Anne, et al., "How art changes your brain: Differential effects of visual art production and cognitive art evaluation on functional brain connectivity," *PLOS* 9 July 1, 2014. http://journals.plos.org/plosone/article?id=10.1371/journal.pone.0101035.

1004. Gawande, Atul, "Hellhole: The United States holds tens of thousands of inmates in long-term solitary confinement. Is this torture?" *New Yorker* Mar. 30, 2009.

1005. Barnes, L. L., et al., "Social resources and cognitive decline in a population of older African Americans and whites," *Neurology* 63 (2004):2322-26.

1006. Luo, Ye, et al., "Loneliness, health, and mortality in old age: A national longitudinal study," *Social Science and Medicine* 74 (2012):907–14.

1007. "Cigna U.S Loneliness Index. Survey of 20,000 Americans examining behaviors driving loneliness in the United States." May 2018. https://www.cigna.com/assets/docs/newsroom/loneliness-survey-2018-updated-fact-sheet.pdf

1008. Brayne, Carol, "Social relationships and mortality risk: A meta-analytic review," *PLOS Medicine* 7 (2010).

1009. Frankish, Helen, et al. "Prevention and management of dementia: a priority for public health," *The Lancet* 390 (2017): DOI: 10.1016/S0140-6736(17)31756-7

1010. Steyaert, K., et al., Interdem Taskforce on Prevention of Dementia, "Putting primary prevention of dementia on everybody's agenda," *Aging and Mental Health* (2020):1-5.

1011. Reeves, M.J., et al., "Healthy lifestyle characteristics among adults in the United States, 2000," *Archives of Internal Medicine* 165 (2005):854-7.

1012. Steyaert, K., et al., Interdem Taskforce on Prevention of Dementia, "Putting primary prevention of dementia on everybody's agenda," *Aging and Mental Health* (2020):1-5.

1013. Grosse, S. D., et al., "Economic gains resulting from the reduction in children's exposure to lead in the United States," *Environmental Health Perspectives* 110 (2002):563–69.